Non-Viral Gene Therapy

Volume II

Non-Viral Gene Therapy Volume II

Edited by **Harvey Summers**

FOSTER
ACADEMICS

New Jersey

Published by Foster Academics,
61 Van Reypen Street,
Jersey City, NJ 07306, USA
www.fosteracademics.com

Non-Viral Gene Therapy
Volume II
Edited by Harvey Summers

International Standard Book Number: 978-1-63242-292-7 (Hardback)

Contents

Preface

This book deals with current developments in the study of gene delivery structures. With interdisciplinary inputs in gene delivery, the book covers a number of aspects in the gene therapy enhancement, covering nanoparticles for gene therapy, nanomedicine based approaches to cancer diagnosis and therapy. This book will assist experts in comprehending the fundamental knowledge of gene delivery vehicles, DNA molecular biology and DNA management.

All of the data presented henceforth, was collaborated in the wake of recent advancements in the field. The aim of this book is to present the diversified developments from across the globe in a comprehensible manner. The opinions expressed in each chapter belong solely to the contributing authors. Their interpretations of the topics are the integral part of this book, which I have carefully compiled for a better understanding of the readers.

At the end, I would like to thank all those who dedicated their time and efforts for the successful completion of this book. I also wish to convey my gratitude towards my friends and family who supported me at every step.

Editor

1

Medical Polymer-Based Gene Therapy

Hu-Lin Jiang[1], You-Kyoung Kim[2], Chong-Su Cho[2]
and Myung-Haing Cho[1,3,4,5,6]
[1]College of Veterinary Medicine, Seoul National University
[2]Department of Agricultural Biotechnology and Research Institute for Agriculture and Life
Sciences, Seoul National University
[3]Department of Nanofusion Technology
Graduate School of Convergence Science and Technology, Seoul National University
[4]Advanced Institute of Convergence Technology, Seoul National University
[5]Graduate Group of Tumor Biology, Seoul National University
[6]Center for Food Safety and Toxicology, Seoul National University
Korea

1. Introduction

Gene therapy provides great opportunities for treatment of diseases resulting from genetic disorders, infections, and cancer (Park, et al., 2006). Gene therapy has also been regarded as a suitable substitute for conventional protein therapy, since it can overcome inherent problems associated with administration of protein drugs in terms of bioavailability, systemic toxicity, *in vivo* clearance rate, and manufacturing cost (Ledley, 1996). Gene therapy refers to local or systemic administration of a nucleic acid construct capable of prevention, treatment, and even cure of disease through change of expression of genes responsible for the pathological condition (Bhavsar & Amiji, 2007). In theory, gene therapy is a simple concept that holds great promise as a cure for disease. However, in practice, considerable obstacles need to be overcome, including problems associated with safe and efficient gene delivery and stable gene expression. Many problems need to be solved in development of any gene therapy approach, including definition of cells that constitute the target, entry of DNA into those cells, expression of useful levels of gene product over an appropriate time period, and avoidance of the almost inevitable response of the host to the introduced materials, and so on (Grosshans, 2000, Smith, 1995).

Current gene therapy consists of two key factors: a gene that encodes a specific therapeutic protein, and a gene delivery system that controls delivery of gene expression plasmids to specific locations within the body (Mahato, et al., 1999, Park, et al., 2006). Due to several problems, including their instability in body fluids, non-specificity to target cells, degradation by enzymes, and low transfection efficiency, the lack of effective vectors is a major barrier to progress in gene therapy. Therefore, the ideal gene delivery method will be capable of high efficiency transfection of genes to a specific cell type; delivery to the nucleus, where it will become integrated into the host genome in a non mutagenic fashion and be expressed or regulated; efficient transduction of cells, independent of the mitotic potential of the recipient; be non-infectious, non-toxic, and non-immunogenic; and be easy to manufacture and apply clinically (Chaum & Hatton, 2002).

Vehicles for gene delivery can be divided into two major groups: viral and non-viral vectors. Although such viral vectors have been commonly employed in clinical trials due to their high transfection efficiency, compared with non-viral vectors (Quong & Neufeld, 1998), their application to the human body is often frustrated by immunogenicity, potential infectivity, complicated production, and inflammation (Smith, 1995). Non-viral vectors involving use of cationic polymer and cationic lipid based carriers continue to enjoy a high profile due to the advantages offered by these systems, including safety, lower immunogenicity, and the ability to transfer larger DNA molecules, when compared with viruses (Anderson, 1998, Brown, et al., 2001). Previous efforts have focused primarily on cationic liposomes, such as N-[1-(2,3-dioleyloxy)propyl]-N,N,N-trimethyl ammonium chloride (DOTMA) (Felgner, et al., 1987), N-[1-(2,3-dioleoyloxy) propyl]-N,N,N-trimethyl ammonium ethyl sulphate (DOTAP) (Alexander & Akhurst, 1995), dimethylaminoethane-carbamoyl cholesterol (DC-Chol) and/or dioleoyl phosphatidylethanolamine (DOPE) (Farhood, et al., 1995) which incorporate with DNA and are transferred effectively into cell membranes. However, the major limitation of liposomes is their fast elimination from the bloodstream and localization in the reticuloendothelial system, primarily Kupfer cells of liver (Klibanov, et al., 1990). In addition, DNA/liposome complexes have been restricted due to cellular toxicity. Cellular changes, including cell shrinkage, reduced number of mitoses, and vacuolization of the cytoplasm (Friend, et al., 1996, Lappalainen, et al., 1994) and consequently leading to cell death via the apoptosis pathway, caused by lipoplexes, already been reported (Nguyen, et al., 2007). An alternative approach to development of non-viral vectors has been proposed for cationic polymers. In general, cationic polymers are widely accepted because of their ability for efficient condensation of DNA and interaction with cells due to the charge interaction between positively charged polymer/DNA complexes and negatively charged cellular membranes. Polymer/DNA complexes are more stable than those involving cationic lipids. In addition, they protect DNA against nuclease degradation (Jiang, et al., 2007, Jiang, et al., 2009).

Therefore, the objective of this chapter was to summarize the use of medical polymers, such as cyclodextrin, chitosan, polyethylenimine, poly(β-amino ester)s (PAEs), and their derivatives as non-viral vectors in the area of gene therapy.

2. Medical polymer-based gene therapy

2.1 Cyclodextrin

Cyclodextrins (CDs) are naturally occurring cyclic oligosaccharides composed of (1-4)-linked glucose units arising from enzymatic degradation of starch, which have been approved by the FDA for use as food additives (Mellet, et al., 2011). CDs comprised of 6, 7, and 8 glucose units are called α-, β-, and γ-CDs, respectively. Table. 1 shows the chemical structure and properties of α-, β-, and γ-CDs.

They feature a basket-shaped topology in which glucose hydroxyls orient to the outer space flanking the upper and lower rims, while methinic protons (H-5 and H-3), which point to the inner cavity cup-shaped cyclic oligomers of glucose, can form inclusion complexes with small, hydrophobic molecules (Forrest, et al., 2005). Due to their unique capability for formation of inclusion complexes in inner cavities, as well as many other favourable physicochemical and biological properties, natural CDs, and their derivatives have been applied in both drug delivery systems (Loftsson, et al., 2005, Uekama, et al., 1998) and gene delivery systems (Challa, et al., 2005, Dass, 2002, Redenti, et al., 2001).

The capability of CDs and their derivatives to interact with nucleotides is of great importance for exploitation of their properties of increasing resistance to nucleases as well as delivery of genes. CDs can improve cellular uptake of genes and can also delay their degradation by increasing their stability against endonucleases. Zhao et al. reported that CDs can increase the cellular uptake of phosphorothioate ODNs (Zhao, et al., 1995). Cellular uptake of [35]S- and fluorescence-labeled antisense agents has been studied in human T cell leukemia cell lines (H9, CEM, or Molt-3) in the presence of CDs, including α-, β-, γCD, methyl-βCD, trimethyl sulfated βCD, HPγCD, HPβCD, hydroxyethyl βCD (HECD), trimethyl, sulfated βCD, and a mixture of various HPβCDs. Cellular uptake was found to be concentration and time dependent in the presence of CDs, and up to a two- and three-fold increase in cellular uptake was observed within 48 h. Interaction between βCD and cellular cholesterol in living cells was well reviewed by Zidovetzki et al. (Zidovetzki & Levitan, 2007). CDs can solve many of the problems associated with *in vivo* delivery of genetic materials, such as their limited ability to extravasate from the blood stream and traverse cellular membranes, high degree of susceptibility to endonucleases with potential toxicity of their breakdown products, polyanionic nature leading to nonspecific interactions with extracellular and intracellular cationic molecules, and potential immunogenicity (Challa, et al., 2005). For further efficient gene delivery, CDs were conjugated with cationic polymers. The most important feature of the CD-containing cationic polymer gene delivery system is that formation of polyplexes between polymers and DNA can be further modified by formation of inclusion complexes, since there are a large number of CD moieties (Davis & Brewster, 2004, Pack, et al., 2005). The first example of cationic polymers containing β-CD in the polymer backbone for gene delivery was reported by Davis and co-workers (Gonzalez, et al., 1999). β-CD containing cationic polymers efficiently condensed DNA to small particles and showed nontoxic and high gene transfection efficiency. The same group has developed a set of such CD-containing polymers and studied the structural effects of the polymers on gene delivery (Popielarski, et al., 2003, Reineke & Davis, 2003, 2003). In general, the CD-containing cationic polymers showed lower cytotoxicity and efficient gene transfection *in vitro*.

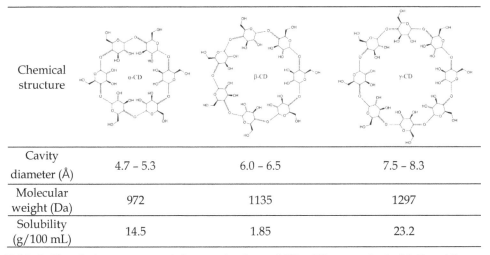

Chemical structure	α-CD	β-CD	γ-CD
Cavity diameter (Å)	4.7 – 5.3	6.0 – 6.5	7.5 – 8.3
Molecular weight (Da)	972	1135	1297
Solubility (g/100 mL)	14.5	1.85	23.2

Table 1. Chemical structures and characterizations of CDs. CDs comprised of 6, 7, and 8 glucose units are called α-, β-, and γ-CDs, respectively.

The Uekama group synthesized dendrimer conjugates with α-, β-, and γ-CDs [Fig. 1], in anticipation of the following synergic effect; i.e., (1) dendrimer has the ability to complex with plasmid DNA (pDNA) and to enhance cellular uptake of pDNA and (2) CDs have a disruptive effect on biological membranes by complexation with membrane constituents, such as phospholipids and cholesterols (Arima, et al., 2001). Dendrimer-conjugated CD (CDE) provided the greatest transfection activity (approximately 100 times higher than those of dendrimer alone and the physical mixture of dendrimer and α-CD) in NIH3T3 fibroblasts and RAW264.7 macrophage cells (Arima, et al., 2001).

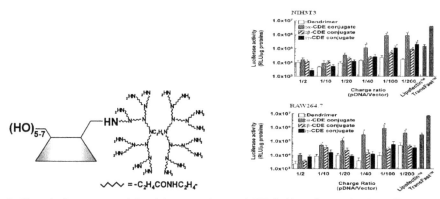

Fig. 1. Chemical structure of dendrimer-conjugated CD (left) and transfection efficiency of the complexes of pDNA/dendrimer or pDNA/CDE conjugates complexes at various charge ratios (right). [Source from Ref. (Arima, et al., 2001)].

They also studied the effect of dendrimer structure on gene transfection efficiency by preparation of CDEs with different dendrimer generations (Kihara, et al., 2002). The generation3 (G3) CDE showed the highest gene expression levels. More recently, the same group developed a lactose moiety-bearing CDE (Lac-α-CDE) for hepatocyte targeting (Arima, et al., 2010). Lac-α-CDE provided higher gene transfer activity than jetPEI™-Hepatocyte to hepatocytes with significantly fewer changes of blood chemistry values 12 h after intravenous administration in mice.

As shown in Fig. 2, Pun et al. synthesized linear and branched poly(ethylenimines) (PEIs) grafted with β-CD (CD-lPEI and CD-bPEI, respectively) by reaction of a mono-tosylated cyclodextrin with PEI amines and evaluated gene delivery ability as non-viral gene delivery agents *in vitro* and *in vivo* (Pun, et al., 2004).

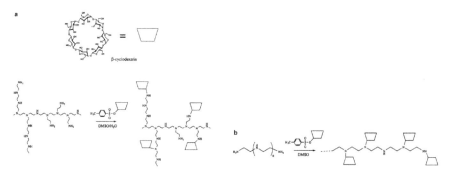

Fig. 2. (a) Synthesis of β-CD-bPEI. (b) Synthesis of β-CD-lPEI. [Source from Ref. (Pun, et al., 2004)].

Transfection efficiency of the polymers was impaired as cyclodextrin grafting increased, and toxicity was affected by cyclodextrin grafting due to the increasing polymer solubility, by capping primary amines, or by reducing polycation binding affinity [Fig. 3].

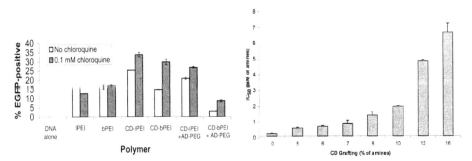

Fig. 3. Comparison of transgene expression from PEI and CD-PEI polymers in the presence or absence of 0.1 mM chloroquine (left) and effect of cyclodextrin grafting on CD-bPEI toxicity to PC3 cells (right). [Source from Ref. (Pun, et al., 2004)].

Recently, Huang et al. also used CDs for crosslinking of low MW branched PEI (MW 600) in order to form high MW cationic polymers (average MW 61K), which displayed lower cytotoxicity and high gene transfection in cultured cells (Huang, et al., 2006). As shown in Fig. 4, a series of new cationic star polymers were also synthesized by conjugation of multiple oligoethylenimine (OEI) arms onto an α-CD core as non-viral gene delivery vectors (Yang, et al., 2007).

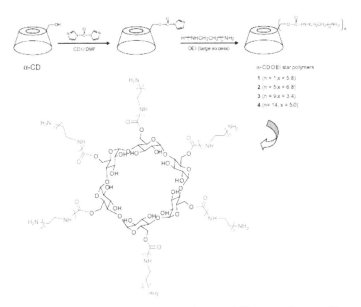

Fig. 4. Synthesis procedures and the structures of α-CD-OEI star polymers. [Source from Ref. (Yang, et al., 2007)].

All of the α-CD-OEI star polymers inhibited migration of pDNA on agarose gel through formation of complexes with pDNA, and the complexes formed nanoparticles with sizes ranging from 100-200 nm at N/P ratios of 8 or higher. Star polymers displayed much lower *in vitro* cytotoxicity than that of branched PEI 25 kD. α-CD-OEI star polymers showed excellent gene transfection efficiency in HEK293 and Cos7 cells. In general, transfection efficiency increased with an increase in OEI arm length. Star polymers with longer and branched OEI arms showed higher transfection efficiency. α-CD-OEI star polymers with different OEI arms have shown promise as new non-viral gene delivery vectors with low cytotoxicity and high gene transfection efficiency for use in future gene therapy applications.

In summary, CD-conjugated polymeric gene carriers showed enhanced transfection efficiency and reduced cytotoxicity, suggesting that CD is a material of potential interest for use in non-viral gene therapy, because these CD-conjugated polymeric gene delivery systems have been evaluated extensively in animal studies as well as clinical trials.

2.2 Chitosan

Chitosan [Fig. 5], a (1→4) 2-amino-2-deoxy-β-D-glucan, is a linear cationic polysaccharide derived by partial alkaline deacetylation of chitin, a polymer abundant in nature. The backbone of chitosan consists of two subunits, D-glucosamine and N-acetyl-D-glucosamine (Muzzarelli, 1997). It is a biocompatible, biodegradable polycationic polymer, which has minimum immunogenicity and low cytotoxicity (Mansouri, et al., 2004). Therefore, chitosan and chitosan derivatives may represent potentially safe cationic carriers for use in gene delivery.

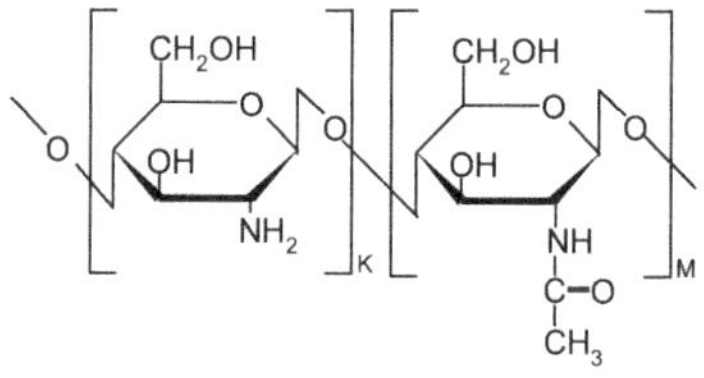

Fig. 5. Chemical structure of chitosan.

Factors including the degree of deacetylation, molecular weight, and charge of chitosan, and the media pH are important in determination of the transfection efficiency of polyplexes containing chitosan and DNA (Huang, et al., 2005, Ishii, et al., 2001, Lavertu, et al., 2006). The increased degree of deacetylation resulted in an increased level of DNA binding ability, and high transgene expression due to higher charge density along the chain (Kiang, et al., 2004, Lavertu, et al., 2006, Saranya, et al., 2011). The effect of the molecular weight of chitosan on complex formulation with DNA can be attributed to the chain entanglement effect (Kiang, et al., 2004). Chain entanglement contributes less to complex formulation as the molecular weight of chitosan decreases. The high molecular weight of chitosan resulted in easier entanglement of free DNA once the initial electrostatic interaction had occurred (Kiang, et al., 2004). Huang et al. reported that low molecular weight chitosan was less efficient at retaining DNA upon dilution, and, consequentially, less capable of protecting condensed DNA from degradation by DNase and serum components, and resulted in low transfection efficiency (Huang, et al., 2005). At acidic pH, below 5.5 or so, the primary amines in chitosan become positively charged due to the pKa value of chitosan around 6.3-6.4 (Li, et al., 1996). At this acidic pH, the primary amine groups are protonated, resulting in a cationic polymer of high charge density, which can form stable complexes with plasmid DNA, protecting DNA from nuclease degradation (Mao, et al., 2001).

N,N,N-trimethyl chitosan chloride (TMC) was synthesized in order to induce an increase of charge density and solubility of chitosan at physiological pH. TMC induced more effective condensation of DNA at physiological pH, compared with chitosan, and the transfection efficiency of TMC/DNA complex showed a 30-fold increase over that of chitosan/DNA (Thanou, et al., 2002). Of particular interest, the presence of fetal calf serum (FCS) did not affect the transfection efficiency of the complexes, whereas the transfection efficiency of DOTAP–DNA complexes was decreased. Cells remained approximately 100% viable in the presence of chitosan oligomers, whereas viability of DOTAP treated cells decreased to about 50% in both cell lines (Thanou, et al., 2002). In addition, folate conjugated TMC (folate-TMC) was recently studied as a target gene delivery carrier (Zheng, et al., 2009). Transfection efficiency of folate-TMC/pDNA complexes in KB cells and SKOV3 cells (folate receptor over-expressing cell lines) increased with increasing N/P ratio and was enhanced up to 1.6-fold and 1.4-fold, compared with that of TMC/pDNA complexes; however, no significant difference was observed between transfection efficiencies of the two complexes in A549 cells and NIH/3T3 cells (folate receptor deficient cell lines), indicating that the increase in transfection efficiencies of folate-TMC/pDNA complexes were attributed to folate receptor mediated endocytosis (Zheng, et al., 2009).

PEGylation of proteins, drugs, and liposomes has been proven to be an effective approach in extending circulation in the blood stream (Patel, 1992). Therefore, in order to reduce the aggregation of complexes and increase circulation time, Jiang et al. synthesized and characterized chitosan-g-PEG [Fig. 6] as a gene carrier (Jiang, et al., 2006).

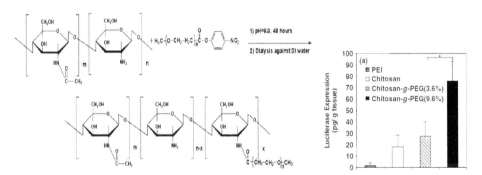

Fig. 6. Sythesis of chitosan-g-PEG polymers (left) and luciferase expression in rat liver after infusion of the complexes from common bile duct (right). [Source from Ref. (Jiang, et al., 2006)].

PEG grafting to chitosan efficiently shields the positive charge on the surface of chitosan/DNA complexes, improving particle stability in bile and serum; therefore, higher transfection efficiency was observed after infusion of the complexes through the bile duct [Fig. 6]. Chitosan-g-PEG mediated 3-fold higher luciferase expression in the liver than unmodified chitosan following intrabiliary infusion. Chitosan-g-PEG also exhibited slightly lower acute toxicity to the liver than chitosan.

Although chitosan showed good properties as a non-viral gene carrier, low transfection efficiency and low cell specificity of chitosan need to be overcome for clinical trials. Many research studies have been conducted for enhancement of transfection efficiency, such as pH-sensitive modification (Jiang, et al., 2007, Jones, et al., 2003, Kim, et al., 2003, Wong, et al., 2006), temperature-sensitive modification (Cho, et al., 2004, Dang, et al., 2006, Sun, et al., 2005), specific target ligand modification (Hashimoto, et al., 2006, Kim, et al., 2004, Kim, et al., 2006, Mansouri, et al., 2006, Wu & Wu, 1998, Zhang, et al., 2006) and so on. Among the chemical modifications of chitosan, PEI grafted chitosan showed some benefit due to high transfection efficiency. Wong et al. prepared PEI-graft-chitosan [Fig. 7] through cationic polymerization of aziridine in the presence of water-soluble oligo-chitosan (Wong, et al., 2006).

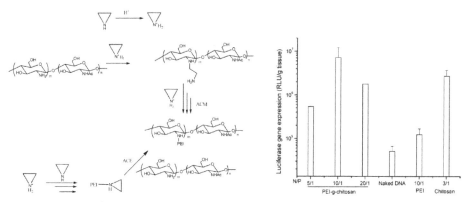

Fig. 7. Preparation of PEI-g-chitosan (left) and in vivo transfection efficiency of the complexes of PEI-g-chitosan/DNA in comparison with that of PEI (25 kDa) and chitosan after administration into common bile duct in rat liver (right). [Source from Ref. (Wong, et al., 2006)].

Results indicated that PEI-g-chitosan had a lower cytotoxicity than PEI 25K and PEI-g-chitosan showed higher transfection efficiency than PEI 25K both *in vitro* and *in vivo*. In addition, improved biocompatibility and long-term safety will be expected for PEI-g-chitosan due to the degradable chitosan main chain and short PEI side chains.

Wong et al. synthesized PEI-graft-chitosan using water-soluble chitosan; however, commercial chitosan is insoluble at neutral and alkaline pH values due to a weak base with a pKa value of the D-glucosamine residue of about 6.2-7.0. Using commercial chitosan, Cho's group synthesized a chitosan-g-PEI copolymer [Fig. 8] by an imine reaction between periodate-oxidized chitosan and an amine group of PEI (Jiang, et al., 2007).

In addition, the same group developed specific ligand-conjugated chitosan-g-PEI, such as galactosylated- (Jiang, et al., 2007), mannosylated- (Jiang, et al., 2009), and folate-conjugated (Jiang, et al., 2009). The specific ligand-conjugated chitosan-g-PEI showed low cytotoxicity and high transfection efficiency with specific cell targeting.

In summary, the transfection efficiency was dependent on the degree of deacetylation, molecular weight of the chitosan, and medium pH. Also, specific ligand-conjugation will increase the transfection efficiency depending on the targeting ability of the ligands. A number of *in vitro* and *in vivo* studies have shown that modified-chitosan is a suitable material for use in efficient non-viral gene therapy.

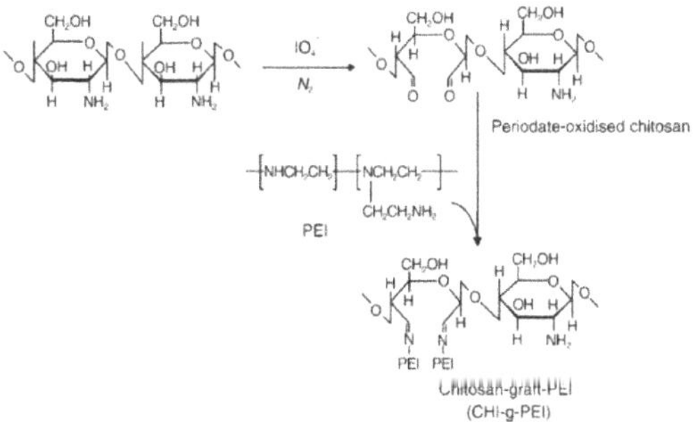

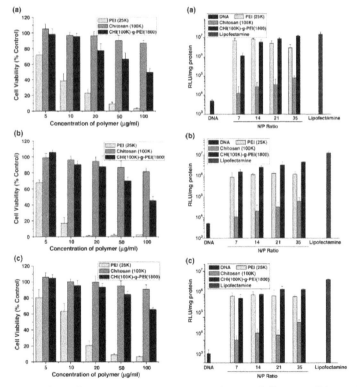

Fig. 8. Proposed reaction scheme for synthesis of CHI-g-PEI. [Source from Ref. (Jiang, et al., 2007)].

Similarly, according to Wong's results, the chitosan-g-PEI copolymer showed higher transfection efficiency and lower cytotoxicity than PEI 25K due to the buffering capacity of low moleculer weight PEI and biocompatible chitosan [Fig. 9].

Fig. 9. Cytotoxicity of copolymer at various concentrations in different cell lines (a) 293T, (b) HeLa and (c) HepG2 (left) and transfection efficiency of copolymer/DNA (pGL3-control) complex at various N/P ratios and in various cell lines. (a) 293T, (b) HeLa and (c) HepG2 (right). [Source from Ref. (Jiang, et al., 2007)].

2.3 Polyethylenimine (PEI)

PEI has received much attention due to its high transfection efficiency. In 1995, Behr's group made the first use of this polymer for delivery of DNA and oligonucleotides (Boussif, et al., 1995). As shown in Fig. 10, PEI exists in two principal forms, branched and linear, with a wide range of molecular weights (Lungwitz, et al., 2005).

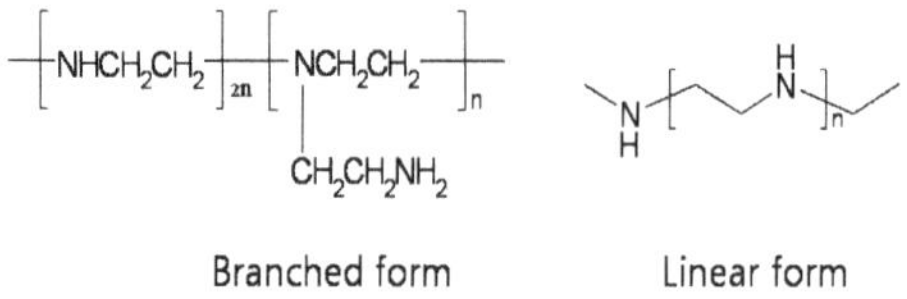

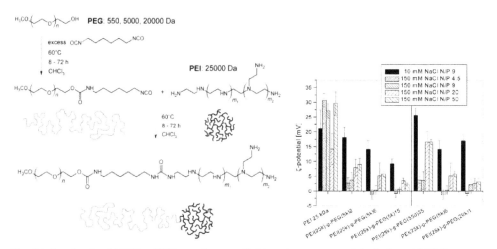

Branched form   Linear form

Fig. 10. Chemical structures of branched and linear PEI.

It is widely accepted that the high transfection ability of PEI is due to its high buffering capacity over a broad pH, which is called "the proton sponge effect" (Akinc, et al., 2005). In addition, the high content of primary amino groups enables chemical coupling of targeting moieties or intracellular active components; high density of positive charges in the molecule allows for a tight compaction of nucleic acids. However, high molecular weight of PEI shows high cytotoxicity, and when further decreasing the molecular weight, both cellular toxicity and transfection efficiency are decreased (Godbey, et al., 2001, Kunath, et al., 2003). One way to reduce toxicity of PEI is to reduce or mask the surface charge by attachment of vesicles with hydrophilic molecules, such as PEG. PEG chains of different length were used for modification of low-molecular weight PEIs (2 kDa), as well as high-molecular weight PEIs, such as the branched PEI (b-PEI) of 25 kDa [Fig. 11] (Petersen, et al., 2002) and the linear PEI (L-PEI) of 22 kDa (Kichler, et al., 2002). One beneficial effect of PEGylation is that PEG-PEI conjugates are less cytotoxic than non-modified polymers.

Fig. 11. Synthesis of bPEI-g-PEG copolymers (left) and zeta-potential of plasmid DNA complexes with PEI 25 kDa and bPEI-g-PEG block copolymers at different ionic strength and at different N/P ratios (right). [Source from Ref. (Petersen, et al., 2002)].

In all of the studies, covalent modification of PEI with PEG reduced the positive surface charge (zeta-potential) of the polyplexes, whereas it only marginally affected their size. However, PEGylation also reduces the DNA-binding capacity of the polymer and sterically hinders interactions of the polyplexes with the target cells. Therefore, in order to increase its usefulness, stealth technology must be combined with the use of ligands that allow specific cell targeting. Different types of ligands, such as sugar residues, peptides, proteins, and antibodies have been used for targeting of PEGylated PEI/DNA complexes [Table 2].

PEGylated PEI	
Ligand	References
Galactose	(Sagara & Kim, 2002)
Folate	(Benns, et al., 2002)
Transferrin	(Kursa, et al., 2003)
Epidermal growth factor	(Blessing, et al., 2001)

Table 2. Specific cell-targeting ligands conjugated with PEG-PEI.

Specific cell-targeting ligand-conjugated PEG-PEI showed low cytotoxicity and high transfection efficiency with specific cell targeting ability.

In summary, PEI is one of the successful and widely used gene delivery polymers, which has become the gold standard of non-viral gene delivery due to its high transfection efficiency. However, concerns over the cytotoxicity of PEI have to be solved for clinical trials. Cytotoxicity of PEI is dependent on its molecular weight; a lower molecular weight PEI has a lower cytotoxicity. Therefore, it is an attractive strategy by combination of lower molecular weight of PEI and biocompatible polymers as gene vectors for reduction of the toxicity of PEI. Also, similar to other cationic gene carriers, specific ligand-conjugation will be a way to increase transfection efficiency with specific cell-targeting.

2.4 Poly(β-amino ester)s (PAEs)

PAEs are one of the biodegradable cationic gene carriers. Biodegradable cationic PAEs are of interest both from the standpoint of mitigating the toxicity of conventional materials as well as a potential means through which to effect the timely release of DNA inside transfected cells (Lim, et al., 2000, Lim, et al., 2002, Luo & Saltzman, 2000). The Langer group has been particularly interested in PAEs as gene carriers, as they are easily synthesized via conjugate addition of either primary or bis(secondary) amine to diacrylate compounds, as shown in Fig. 12.

The Langer group reported a parallel approach suitable for synthesis of hundreds to thousands of structurally unique PAEs and application of these libraries to rapid and high throughput identification of new gene delivery agents and structure-function trends (Lynn, et al., 2001). The advantage of combinatorial chemistry and automated highthroughput synthesis is that it has revolutionized modern drug discovery by rapid synthesis and evaluation with greater precision. As shown in Fig. 13, 140 different PAEs (the set of 7 diacrylate monomers and 20 amine-based monomers) were synthesized as a screening library. Most of the PAEs showed low transfection efficiencies, compared with Lipofectamine 2000, a commercially available lipid-based vector system. However, B14 and G5 yielded higher gene transfection efficiencies. In particular, B14 showed higer transfection efficiency, compared with

Lipofectamine 2000, due to the high endosomal pH buffering capacity, similar to that of other imidazole-substituted polymers (Benns, et al., 2000, Pack, et al., 2000), suggesting that polymer B14 may be the more promising polymer as a gene delivery carrier.

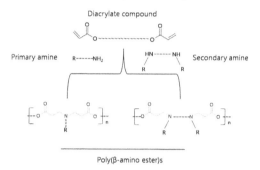

Fig. 12. Synthesis scheme of PAEs.

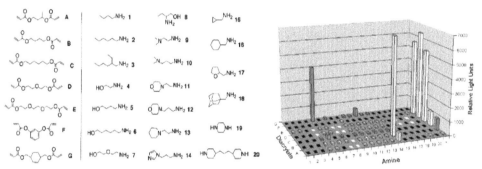

[Source from Ref. (Zugates, et al., 2006)].

Fig. 13. Diacrylate (A-G) and amine (1-20) monomers chosen for the synthesis of an initial screening library (left) and transfection data as a function of structure for an assay employing pCMV-Luc (600 ng/well, DNA/polymer = 1:20, right). [Source from Ref. (Lynn, et al., 2001)].

As shown in Fig. 14, using high throughput methods, over 2,350 PAEs were synthesized (Anderson, et al., 2003). Biodegradable PAEs demonstrated efficient transfection of cells and 26 of these polymers showed higher gene expression, compared with Lipofectamine 2000.

Response to intracellular stimuli, such as pH, is a major advantage of a gene delivery system (Stayton, et al., 2005). Zugates et al synthesized new PAEs using a primary amine monomer, 2-(pyridyldithio)-ethylamine (PDA), speculating that pyridyldithio groups in these side chains display fast and selective reactivity with thiols without alteration of the charge density of the polymer backbone, as shown in Fig. 15 (Zugates, et al., 2006). This property of PDA-based PAEs further led to conjugation of cell-targeting peptides or ligands for targeted and site-specific delivery. As one potential application, they conjugated the mercaptoethylamine (MEA) and the RGDC peptide to PDA PAEs. MEA-based PAE has an advantage that it is sensitive to glutathione. The MEA-based polymer delivery system has demonstrated relative stability in the extracellular space; however, it is responsive to intracellular conditions in which partial unpacking is triggered.

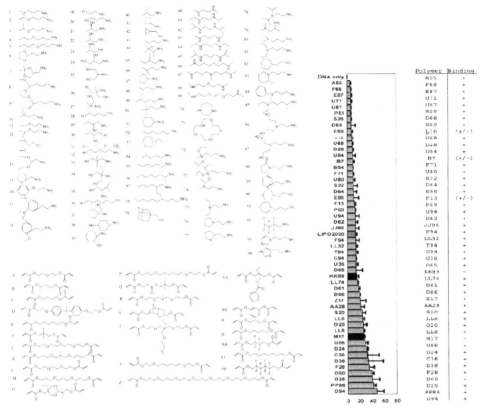

Fig. 14. Amino (numbers) and diacrylate (letters) monomers (left) and optimized transfection efficiency of the top 50 polymers relative to PEI and Lipofectamine 2000. [Source from Ref. (Anderson, et al., 2003)].

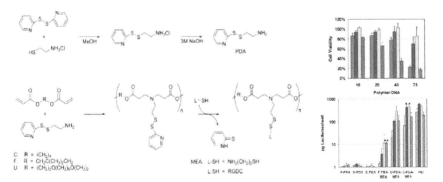

Fig. 15. Synthesis scheme of MEA (left) and cytotoxicity [C-PDA (blue), C-PDA-MEA (Redenti, et al.), 2-mercaptopyridine (2-MP, yellow), and PEI (green)] and transfection studies (right). [Source from Ref. (Zugates, et al., 2006)].

As shown in Fig. 16, Cho's group synthesized novel biodegradable PAEs composed of gamma-aminopropyl-triethoxysilane (APES) and poly (ethylene glycol) diacrylate (PEGDA) for gene delivery (Jere, et al., 2008).

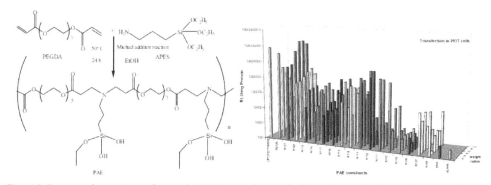

Fig. 16. Proposed reaction scheme for PAE copolymer (left) and transfection efficiency of PAE/DNA complexes in serum free-media at various mass ratios in a 293T cells (right). [Source from Ref. (Jere, et al., 2008)].

They reported that addition of PEGDA over APES resulted in a novel PAE, which shows high safety and transfection efficiency, especially in R121. PAE obtained from R121 showed good DNA binding and condensation with average particle sizes of 133 nm. In addition, PAE-mediated gene expression in the lung and liver was higher than that of the conventional PEI carrier. Of particular interest, non-invasive aerosol delivery induced higher gene expression in all organs, compared with an intravenous method, in an *in vivo* mice study (Park, et al., 2008). The same group developed a new PAE based on hydrophobic polycaprolactone (PCL) and low molecular weight branched PEI following the Michael addition reaction (Arote, et al., 2007). The synthesized PAE showed controlled degradation and was essentially non-toxic in all three cells (293T, HepG2 and HeLa) in contrast with PEI 25K. PAEs revealed much higher transfection efficiencies in three cell lines, compared with PEI 25K, and were also successfully transfected *in vivo*, compared with PEI 25K after aerosol administration. Targeting confers another important criterion in gene delivery. Recently, Arote et al. coupled folic acid moiety for a folate receptor targeting the PAE backbone using PEG (MW: 5000 Da) as a linker (Arote, et al., 2010). At the initial stage, folate-conjugated PAE revealed folate receptor-mediated endocytosis with elevated levels of luciferase expression in folate receptor positive cancer cell lines, suggesting application of specific ligand-modified PAE. They also developed folate-PEG-PAE (FP-PAE) as a gene carrier, which mediated high level folate receptor mediated endocytosis *in vitro* as well as *in vivo* [Fig. 17]. FP-PAE showed marked anti-tumor activity against folate receptor-positive human KB tumors in nude mice with no evidence of toxicity during and after therapy using the TAM67 gene. Anti-tumor activity with PAE without folic acid moiety (PEG-PAE, P-PAE) proved ineffective against a xenograft mice model with KB cells when administered at the same dose as that of FP-PAE, suggesting that FP-PAE is a highly effective gene carrier capable of producing a therapeutic benefit in a xenograft mice model without any signs of toxicity.

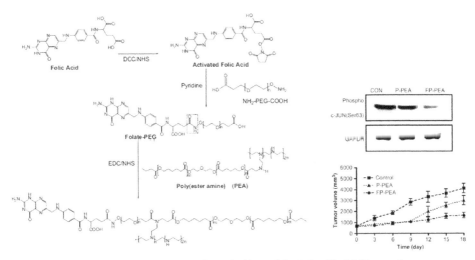

Fig. 17. Synthesis scheme of FP-PEA (left) and effect of FP-PEA/TAM67 complexes on tumor growth (right). Expression level of phospho-c-Jun and suppression of tumor growth by FP-PEA/TAM67 complexes. [Source from Ref. (Arote, et al., 2010)].

In summary, PAEs have excellent characteristics as gene carriers. PAEs comprise a class of degradable cationic polymers with many desirable properties in the context of gene delivery, including condensation of DNA into nanoscale-size particles, which facilitates cellular uptake of DNA and protects DNA from endogenous nucleases as well as efficient delivery of DNA with low toxicity. Tissue targeting, endosome disruption, and nuclear transport should be combined for development of an effective PAE for use in gene therapy. Also, extensive *in vitro* and *in vivo* evaluation and optimization of PAEs will provide valuable information for safe and efficient gene therapy applications.

3. Conclusion

Gene therapy shows tremendous promise for a broad spectrum of clinical applications. Development of a safe and efficient gene delivery system is one of the main challenges to be solved before this strategy can be adopted for routine use in clinical trails. In this chapter, medical polymers, including CD, chitosan, PEI, PAEs, and their derivatives as non-viral vectors in the area of gene therapy have been described. Although more development of structure-function relationships and fundamental research into cellular processes *in vitro* and *in vivo* should be performed for future direction of medical polymer based gene carriers, combination of these polymers will be a way to reduce toxicity and enhance tranfection efficiency. Also, selective tissue or cell targeting ligand conjugation will provide cell-specificity or improve transfection efficiency. Nowadays, multiple targeting gene therapy with multiple-functionalized genes and delivery system are possible. Suitable formulations of these polyplexes with low toxicity and high transfection efficiency must be chosen for *in vivo* use, which will allow for multiple applications of therapeutic genes; however, for this idea to be realized, much work lies ahead.

4. Acknowledgements

This work was partly supported by the R&D Program of MKE/KEIT (10035333, Development of anti-cancer therapeutic agent based on regulating cell cycle or cell death) as well as by the National Research Foundation (NRF-2011-0000380), Ministry of Education, Science and Technology (MEST) in Korea.

5. References

Akinc, A.; Thomas, M.; Klibanov, A. M. & Langer, R. (2005). Exploring polyethylenimine-mediated DNA transfection and the proton sponge hypothesis. *Journal of Gene Medicine*, Vol. 7, No. 5, (May 2005), pp. 657-663, ISSN 1099-498X

Alexander, M. Y. & Akhurst, R. J. (1995). Liposome-medicated gene transfer and expression via the skin. *Human Molecular Genetics*, Vol. 4, No. 12, (Dec 1995), pp. 2279-2285, ISSN 0964-6906

Anderson, D. G.; Lynn, D. M. & Langer, R. (2003). Semi-automated synthesis and screening of a large library of degradable cationic polymers for gene delivery. *Angewandte Chemie. International Ed. In English*, Vol. 42, No. 27, (Jul 14 2003), pp. 3153-3158, ISSN 1433-7851

Anderson, W. F. (1998). Human gene therapy. *Nature*, Vol. 392, No. 6679 Suppl, (Apr 30 1998), pp. 25-30, ISSN 0028-0836

Arima, H.; Kihara, F.; Hirayama, F. & Uekama, K. (2001). Enhancement of gene expression by polyamidoamine dendrimer conjugates with alpha-, beta-, and gamma-cyclodextrins. *Bioconjugate Chemistry*, Vol. 12, No. 4, (Jul-Aug 2001), pp. 476-484, ISSN 1043-1802

Arima, H.; Yamashita, S.; Mori, Y.; Hayashi, Y.; Motoyama, K.; Hattori, K.; Takeuchi, T.; Jono, H.; Ando, Y.; Hirayama, F. & Uekama, K. (2010). In vitro and in vivo gene delivery mediated by Lactosylated dendrimer/alpha-cyclodextrin conjugates (G2) into hepatocytes. *Journal of Controlled Release*, Vol. 146, No. 1, (Aug 17 2010), pp. 106-117, ISSN 1873-4995

Arote, R.; Kim, T. H.; Kim, Y. K.; Hwang, S. K.; Jiang, H. L.; Song, H. H.; Nah, J. W.; Cho, M. H. & Cho, C. S. (2007). A biodegradable poly(ester amine) based on polycaprolactone and polyethylenimine as a gene carrier. *Biomaterials*, Vol. 28, No. 4, (Feb 2007), pp. 735-744, ISSN 0142-9612

Arote, R. B.; Yoon, M. K.; Kim, T. H.; Jere, D.; Jiang, H. L.; Kim, Y. K.; Park, I. K. & Cho, C. S. (2010). Folate conjugated poly(ester amine) for lung cancer therapy. *Journal of Nanoscience and Nanotechnology*, Vol. 10, No. 5, (May 2010), pp. 3294-3298, ISSN 1533-4880

Benns, J. M.; Choi, J. S.; Mahato, R. I.; Park, J. S. & Kim, S. W. (2000). pH-sensitive cationic polymer gene delivery vehicle: N-Ac-poly(L-histidine)-graft-poly(L-lysine) comb shaped polymer. *Bioconjugate Chemistry*, Vol. 11, No. 5, (Sep-Oct 2000), pp. 637-645, ISSN 1043-1802

Benns, J. M.; Mahato, R. I. & Kim, S. W. (2002). Optimization of factors influencing the transfection efficiency of folate-PEG-folate-graft-polyethylenimine. *Journal of Controlled Release*, Vol. 79, No. 1-3, (Feb 19 2002), pp. 255-269, ISSN 0168-3659

Bhavsar, M. D. & Amiji, M. M. (2007). Polymeric nano- and microparticle technologies for oral gene delivery. *Expert Opin Drug Deliv,* Vol. 4, No. 3, (May 2007), pp. 197-213, ISSN 1742-5247

Blessing, T.; Kursa, M.; Holzhauser, R.; Kircheis, R. & Wagner, E. (2001). Different strategies for formation of pegylated EGF-conjugated PEI/DNA complexes for targeted gene delivery. *Bioconjugate Chemistry,* Vol. 12, No. 4, (Jul-Aug 2001), pp. 529-537, ISSN 1043-1802

Boussif, O.; Lezoualc'h, F.; Zanta, M. A.; Mergny, M. D.; Scherman, D.; Demeneix, B. & Behr, J. P. (1995). A versatile vector for gene and oligonucleotide transfer into cells in culture and in vivo: polyethylenimine. *Proceedings of the National Academy of Sciences of the United States of America,* Vol. 92, No. 16, (Aug 1 1995), pp. 7297-7301, ISSN 0027-8424

Brown, M. D.; Schatzlein, A. G. & Uchegbu, I. F. (2001). Gene delivery with synthetic (non viral) carriers. *International Journal of Pharmaceutics,* Vol. 229, No. 1-2, (Oct 23 2001), pp. 1-21, ISSN 0378-5173

Challa, R.; Ahuja, A.; Ali, J. & Khar, R. K. (2005). Cyclodextrins in drug delivery: an updated review. *AAPS PharmSciTech,* Vol. 6, No. 2, 2005), pp. E329-357, ISSN 1530-9932

Chaum, E. & Hatton, M. P. (2002). Gene therapy for genetic and acquired retinal diseases. *Survey of Ophthalmology,* Vol. 47, No. 5, (Sep-Oct 2002), pp. 449-469, ISSN 0039-6257

Cho, J. H.; Kim, S. H.; Park, K. D.; Jung, M. C.; Yang, W. I.; Han, S. W.; Noh, J. Y. & Lee, J. W. (2004). Chondrogenic differentiation of human mesenchymal stem cells using a thermosensitive poly(N-isopropylacrylamide) and water-soluble chitosan copolymer. *Biomaterials,* Vol. 25, No. 26, (Nov 2004), pp. 5743-5751, ISSN 0142-9612

Dang, J. M.; Sun, D. D.; Shin-Ya, Y.; Sieber, A. N.; Kostuik, J. P. & Leong, K. W. (2006). Temperature-responsive hydroxybutyl chitosan for the culture of mesenchymal stem cells and intervertebral disk cells. *Biomaterials,* Vol. 27, No. 3, (Jan 2006), pp. 406-418, ISSN 0142-9612

Dass, C. R. (2002). Vehicles for oligonucleotide delivery to tumours. *Journal of Pharmacy and Pharmacology,* Vol. 54, No. 1, (Jan 2002), pp. 3-27, ISSN 0022-3573

Davis, M. E. & Brewster, M. E. (2004). Cyclodextrin-based pharmaceutics: past, present and future. *Nature Reviews Drug Discovery,* Vol. 3, No. 12, (Dec 2004), pp. 1023-1035, ISSN 1474-1776

Farhood, H.; Serbina, N. & Huang, L. (1995). The role of dioleoyl phosphatidylethanolamine in cationic liposome mediated gene transfer. *Biochimica et Biophysica Acta,* Vol. 1235, No. 2, (May 4 1995), pp. 289-295, ISSN 0006-3002

Felgner, P. L.; Gadek, T. R.; Holm, M.; Roman, R.; Chan, H. W.; Wenz, M.; Northrop, J. P.; Ringold, G. M. & Danielsen, M. (1987). Lipofection: a highly efficient, lipid-mediated DNA-transfection procedure. *Proceedings of the National Academy of Sciences of the United States of America,* Vol. 84, No. 21, (Nov 1987), pp. 7413-7417, ISSN 0027-8424

Forrest, M. L.; Gabrielson, N. & Pack, D. W. (2005). Cyclodextrin-polyethylenimine conjugates for targeted in vitro gene delivery. *Biotechnology and Bioengineering,* Vol. 89, No. 4, (Feb 20 2005), pp. 416-423, ISSN 0006-3592

Friend, D. S.; Papahadjopoulos, D. & Debs, R. J. (1996). Endocytosis and intracellular processing accompanying transfection mediated by cationic liposomes. *Biochimica et Biophysica Acta,* Vol. 1278, No. 1, (Jan 12 1996), pp. 41-50, ISSN 0006-3002

Godbey, W. T.; Wu, K. K. & Mikos, A. G. (2001). Poly(ethylenimine)-mediated gene delivery affects endothelial cell function and viability. *Biomaterials*, Vol. 22, No. 5, (Mar 2001), pp. 471-480, ISSN 0142-9612

Gonzalez, H.; Hwang, S. J. & Davis, M. E. (1999). New class of polymers for the delivery of macromolecular therapeutics. *Bioconjugate Chemistry*, Vol. 10, No. 6, (Nov-Dec 1999), pp. 1068-1074, ISSN 1043-1802

Grosshans, H. (2000). Gene therapy--when a simple concept meets a complex reality. Review on gene therapy. *Funct Integr Genomics*, Vol. 1, No. 2, (Sep 2000), pp. 142-145, ISSN 1438-793X

Hashimoto, M.; Morimoto, M.; Saimoto, H.; Shigemasa, Y. & Sato, T. (2006). Lactosylated chitosan for DNA delivery into hepatocytes: the effect of lactosylation on the physicochemical properties and intracellular trafficking of pDNA/chitosan complexes. *Bioconjugate Chemistry*, Vol. 17, No. 2, (Mar-Apr 2006), pp. 309-316, ISSN 1043-1802

Huang, H.; Tang, G.; Wang, Q.; Li, D.; Shen, F.; Zhou, J. & Yu, H. (2006). Two novel non-viral gene delivery vectors: low molecular weight polyethylenimine cross-linked by (2-hydroxypropyl)-beta-cyclodextrin or (2-hydroxypropyl)-gamma-cyclodextrin. *Chemical Communications (Camb)*, No. 22, (Jun 14 2006), pp. 2382-2384, ISSN 1359-7345

Huang, M.; Fong, C. W.; Khor, E. & Lim, L. Y. (2005). Transfection efficiency of chitosan vectors: effect of polymer molecular weight and degree of deacetylation. *Journal of Controlled Release*, Vol. 106, No. 3, (Sep 2 2005), pp. 391-406, ISSN 0168-3659

Ishii, T.; Okahata, Y. & Sato, T. (2001). Mechanism of cell transfection with plasmid/chitosan complexes. *Biochimica et Biophysica Acta*, Vol. 1514, No. 1, (Sep 3 2001), pp. 51-64, ISSN 0006-3002

Jere, D.; Yoo, M. K.; Arote, R.; Kim, T. H.; Cho, M. H.; Nah, J. W.; Choi, Y. J. & Cho, C. S. (2008). Poly (amino ester) composed of poly (ethylene glycol) and aminosilane prepared by combinatorial chemistry as a gene carrier. *Pharmaceutical Research*, Vol. 25, No. 4, (Apr 2008), pp. 875-885, ISSN 0724-8741

Jiang, H. L.; Kim, Y. K.; Arote, R.; Nah, J. W.; Cho, M. H.; Choi, Y. J.; Akaike, T. & Cho, C. S. (2007). Chitosan-graft-polyethylenimine as a gene carrier. *J Control Release*, Vol. 117, No. 2, (Feb 12 2007), pp. 273-280, ISSN 0168-3659

Jiang, H. L.; Kwon, J. T.; Kim, Y. K.; Kim, E. M.; Arote, R.; Jeong, H. J.; Nah, J. W.; Choi, Y. J.; Akaike, T.; Cho, M. H. & Cho, C. S. (2007). Galactosylated chitosan-graft-polyethylenimine as a gene carrier for hepatocyte targeting. *Gene Therapy*, Vol. 14, No. 19, (Oct 2007), pp. 1389-1398, ISSN 0969-7128

Jiang, H. L.; Kim, Y. K.; Arote, R.; Jere, D.; Quan, J. S.; Yu, J. H.; Choi, Y. J.; Nah, J. W.; Cho, M. H. & Cho, C. S. (2009). Mannosylated chitosan-graft-polyethylenimine as a gene carrier for Raw 264.7 cell targeting. *International Journal of Pharmaceutics*, Vol. 375, No. 1-2, (Jun 22 2009), pp. 133-139, ISSN 1873-3476

Jiang, H. L.; Xu, C. X.; Kim, Y. K.; Arote, R.; Jere, D.; Lim, H. T.; Cho, M. H.& Cho, C. S. (2009). The suppression of lung tumorigenesis by aerosol-delivered folate-chitosan-graft-polyethylenimine/Akt1 shRNA complexes through the Akt signaling pathway. *Biomaterials*, Vol. 30, No. 29, (Oct 2009), pp. 5844-5852, ISSN 1878-5905

Jiang, X.; Dai, H.; Leong, K. W.; Goh, S. H.; Mao, H. Q. & Yang, Y. Y. (2006). Chitosan-g-PEG/DNA complexes deliver gene to the rat liver via intrabiliary and intraportal infusions. *Journal of Gene Medicine,* Vol. 8, No. 4, (Apr 2006), pp. 477-487, ISSN 1099-498X

Jones, R. A.; Cheung, C. Y.; Black, F. E.; Zia, J. K.; Stayton, P. S.; Hoffman, A. S. & Wilson, M. R. (2003). Poly(2-alkylacrylic acid) polymers deliver molecules to the cytosol by pH-sensitive disruption of endosomal vesicles. *Biochemical Journal,* Vol. 372, No. Pt 1, (May 15 2003), pp. 65-75, ISSN 0264-6021

Kiang, T.; Wen, J.; Lim, H. W. & Leong, K. W. (2004). The effect of the degree of chitosan deacetylation on the efficiency of gene transfection. *Biomaterials,* Vol. 25, No. 22, (Oct 2004), pp. 5293-5301, ISSN 0142-9612

Kichler, A.; Chillon, M.; Leborgne, C.; Danos, O. & Frisch, B. (2002). Intranasal gene delivery with a polyethylenimine-PEG conjugate. *Journal of Controlled Release,* Vol. 81, No. 3, (Jun 17 2002), pp. 379-388, ISSN 0168-3659

Kihara, F.; Arima, H.; Tsutsumi, T.; Hirayama, F. & Uekama, K. (2002). Effects of structure of polyamidoamine dendrimer on gene transfer efficiency of the dendrimer conjugate with alpha-cyclodextrin. *Bioconjugate Chemistry,* Vol. 13, No. 6, (Nov-Dec 2002), pp. 1211-1219, ISSN 1043-1802

Kim, T. H.; Ihm, J. E.; Choi, Y. J.; Nah, J. W. & Cho, C. S. (2003). Efficient gene delivery by urocanic acid-modified chitosan. *Journal of Controlled Release,* Vol. 93, No. 3, (Dec 12 2003), pp. 389-402, ISSN 0168-3659

Kim, T. H.; Park, I. K.; Nah, J. W.; Choi, Y. J. & Cho, C. S. (2004). Galactosylated chitosan/DNA nanoparticles prepared using water-soluble chitosan as a gene carrier. *Biomaterials,* Vol. 25, No. 17, (Aug 2004), pp. 3783-3792, ISSN 0142-9612

Kim, T. H.; Nah, J. W.; Cho, M. H.; Park, T. G. & Cho, C. S. (2006). Receptor-mediated gene delivery into antigen presenting cells using mannosylated chitosan/DNA nanoparticles. *Journal of Nanoscience and Nanotechnology,* Vol. 6, No. 9-10, (Sep-Oct 2006), pp. 2796-2803, ISSN 1533-4880

Klibanov, A. L.; Maruyama, K.; Torchilin, V. P. & Huang, L. (1990). Amphipathic polyethyleneglycols effectively prolong the circulation time of liposomes. *FEBS Letters,* Vol. 268, No. 1, (Jul 30 1990), pp. 235-237, ISSN 0014-5793

Kunath, K.; von Harpe, A.; Fischer, D.; Petersen, H.; Bickel, U.; Voigt, K. & Kissel, T. (2003). Low-molecular-weight polyethylenimine as a non-viral vector for DNA delivery: comparison of physicochemical properties, transfection efficiency and in vivo distribution with high-molecular-weight polyethylenimine. *Journal of Controlled Release,* Vol. 89, No. 1, (Apr 14 2003), pp. 113-125, ISSN 0168-3659

Kursa, M.; Walker, G. F.; Roessler, V.; Ogris, M.; Roedl, W.; Kircheis, R. & Wagner, E. (2003). Novel shielded transferrin-polyethylene glycol-polyethylenimine/DNA complexes for systemic tumor-targeted gene transfer. *Bioconjugate Chemistry,* Vol. 14, No. 1, (Jan-Feb 2003), pp. 222-231, ISSN 1043-1802

Lappalainen, K.; Urtti, A.; Soderling, E.; Jaaskelainen, I.; Syrjanen, K. & Syrjanen, S. (1994). Cationic liposomes improve stability and intracellular delivery of antisense oligonucleotides into CaSki cells. *Biochimica et Biophysica Acta,* Vol. 1196, No. 2, (Dec 30 1994), pp. 201-208, ISSN 0006-3002

Lavertu, M.; Methot, S.; Tran-Khanh, N. & Buschmann, M. D. (2006). High efficiency gene transfer using chitosan/DNA nanoparticles with specific combinations of molecular weight and degree of deacetylation. *Biomaterials,* Vol. 27, No. 27, (Sep 2006), pp. 4815-4824, ISSN 0142-9612

Ledley, F. D. (1996). Pharmaceutical approach to somatic gene therapy. *Pharmaceutical Research*, Vol. 13, No. 11, (Nov 1996), pp. 1595-1614, ISSN 0724-8741

Li, J.; Revol, J. F. & Marchessault, R. H. (1996). Rheological Properties of Aqueous Suspensions of Chitin Crystallites. *Journal of Colloid and Interface Science*, Vol. 183, No. 2, (Nov 10 1996), pp. 365-373, ISSN 1095-7103

Lim, Y. B.; Han, S. O.; Kong, H. U.; Lee, Y.; Park, J. S.; Jeong, B. & Kim, S. W. (2000). Biodegradable polyester, poly[alpha-(4-aminobutyl)-L-glycolic acid], as a non-toxic gene carrier. *Pharmaceutical Research*, Vol. 17, No. 7, (Jul 2000), pp. 811-816, ISSN 0724-8741

Lim, Y. B.; Kim, S. M.; Suh, H. & Park, J. S. (2002). Biodegradable, endosome disruptive, and cationic network-type polymer as a highly efficient and nontoxic gene delivery carrier. *Bioconjugate Chemistry*, Vol. 13, No. 5, (Sep-Oct 2002), pp. 952-957, ISSN 1043-1802

Loftsson, T.; Jarho, P.; Masson, M. & Jarvinen, T. (2005). Cyclodextrins in drug delivery. *Expert Opininon on Drug Delivery*, Vol. 2, No. 2, (Mar 2005), pp. 335-351, ISSN 1742-5247

Lungwitz, U.; Breunig, M.; Blunk, T. & Gopferich, A. (2005). Polyethylenimine-based non-viral gene delivery systems. *European Journal of Pharmaceutics and Biopharmaceutics*, Vol. 60, No. 2, (Jul 2005), pp. 247-266, ISSN 0939-6411

Luo, D. & Saltzman, W. M. (2000). Synthetic DNA delivery systems. *Nature Biotechnology*, Vol. 18, No. 1, (Jan 2000), pp. 33-37, ISSN 1087-0156

Lynn, D. M.; Anderson, D. G.; Putnam, D. & Langer, R. (2001). Accelerated discovery of synthetic transfection vectors: parallel synthesis and screening of a degradable polymer library. *Journal of the American Chemical Society*, Vol. 123, No. 33, (Aug 22 2001), pp. 8155-8156, ISSN 0002-7863

Mahato, R. I.; Smith, L. C. & Rolland, A. (1999). Pharmaceutical perspectives of nonviral gene therapy. *Advances in Genetics*, Vol. 41, 1999), pp. 95-156, ISSN 0065-2660

Mansouri, S.; Lavigne, P.; Corsi, K.; Benderdour, M.; Beaumont, E. & Fernandes, J. C. (2004). Chitosan-DNA nanoparticles as non-viral vectors in gene therapy: strategies to improve transfection efficacy. *European Journal of Pharmaceutics and Biopharmaceutics*, Vol. 57, No. 1, (Jan 2004), pp. 1-8, ISSN 0939-6411

Mansouri, S.; Cuie, Y.; Winnik, F.; Shi, Q.; Lavigne, P.; Benderdour, M.; Beaumont, E. & Fernandes, J. C. (2006). Characterization of folate-chitosan-DNA nanoparticles for gene therapy. *Biomaterials*, Vol. 27, No. 9, (Mar 2006), pp. 2060-2065, ISSN 0142-9612

Mao, H. Q.; Roy, K.; Troung-Le, V. L.; Janes, K. A.; Lin, K. Y.; Wang, Y.; August, J. T. & Leong, K. W. (2001). Chitosan-DNA nanoparticles as gene carriers: synthesis, characterization and transfection efficiency. *Journal of Controlled Release*, Vol. 70, No. 3, (Feb 23 2001), pp. 399-421, ISSN 0168-3659

Mellet, C. O.; Fernandez, J. M. & Benito, J. M. (2011). Cyclodextrin-based gene delivery systems. *Chemical Society Reviews*, Vol. 40, No. 3, (Mar 22 2011), pp. 1586-1608, ISSN 1460-4744

Muzzarelli, R. A. (1997). Human enzymatic activities related to the therapeutic administration of chitin derivatives. *Cellular and Molecular Life Sciences*, Vol. 53, No. 2, (Feb 1997), pp. 131-140, ISSN 1420-682X

Nguyen, L. T.; Atobe, K.; Barichello, J. M.; Ishida, T. & Kiwada, H. (2007). Complex formation with plasmid DNA increases the cytotoxicity of cationic liposomes.

Biological and Pharmaceutical Bulletin, Vol. 30, No. 4, (Apr 2007), pp. 751-757, ISSN 0918-6158

Pack, D. W.; Putnam, D. & Langer, R. (2000). Design of imidazole-containing endosomolytic biopolymers for gene delivery. *Biotechnology and Bioengineering*, Vol. 67, No. 2, (Jan 20 2000), pp. 217-223, ISSN 0006-3592

Pack, D. W.; Hoffman, A. S.; Pun, S. & Stayton, P. S. (2005). Design and development of polymers for gene delivery. *Nature Reviews Drug Discovery*, Vol. 4, No. 7, (Jul 2005), pp. 581-593, ISSN 1474-1776

Park, M. R.; Kim, H. W.; Hwang, C. S.; Han, K. O.; Choi, Y. J.; Song, S. C.; Cho, M. H. & Cho, C. S. (2008). Highly efficient gene transfer with degradable poly(ester amine) based on poly(ethylene glycol) diacrylate and polyethylenimine in vitro and in vivo. *Journal of Gene Medicine*, Vol. 10, No. 2, (Feb 2008), pp. 198-207, ISSN 1099-498X

Park, T. G.; Jeong, J. H. & Kim, S. W. (2006). Current status of polymeric gene delivery systems. *Advanced Drug Delivery Reviews*, Vol. 58, No. 4, (Jul 7 2006), pp. 467-486, ISSN 0169-409X

Patel, H. M. (1992). Serum opsonins and liposomes: their interaction and opsonophagocytosis. *Critical Reviews in Therapeutic Drug Carrier Systems*, Vol. 9, No. 1, 1992), pp. 39-90, ISSN 0743-4863

Petersen, H.; Fechner, P. M.; Martin, A. L.; Kunath, K.; Stolnik, S.; Roberts, C. J.; Fischer, D.; Davies, M. C. & Kissel, T. (2002). Polyethylenimine-graft-poly(ethylene glycol) copolymers: influence of copolymer block structure on DNA complexation and biological activities as gene delivery system. *Bioconjugate Chemistry*, Vol. 13, No. 4, (Jul-Aug 2002), pp. 845-854, ISSN 1043-1802

Popielarski, S. R.; Mishra, S. & Davis, M. E. (2003). Structural effects of carbohydrate-containing polycations on gene delivery. 3. Cyclodextrin type and functionalization. *Bioconjugate Chemistry*, Vol. 14, No. 3, (May-Jun 2003), pp. 672-678, ISSN 1043-1802

Pun, S. H.; Bellocq, N. C.; Liu, A.; Jensen, G.; Machemer, T.; Quijano, E.; Schluep, T.; Wen, S.; Engler, H.; Heidel, J. & Davis, M. E. (2004). Cyclodextrin-modified polyethylenimine polymers for gene delivery. *Bioconjugate Chemistry*, Vol. 15, No. 4, (Jul-Aug 2004), pp. 831-840, ISSN 1043-1802

Quong, D. & Neufeld, R. J. (1998). DNA protection from extracapsular nucleases, within chitosan- or poly-L-lysine-coated alginate beads. *Biotechnology and Bioengineering*, Vol. 60, No. 1, (Oct 5 1998), pp. 124-134, ISSN 0006-3592

Redenti, E.; Pietra, C.; Gerloczy, A. & Szente, L. (2001). Cyclodextrins in oligonucleotide delivery. *Advanced Drug Delivery Reviews*, Vol. 53, No. 2, (Dec 17 2001), pp. 235-244, ISSN 0169-409X

Reineke, T. M. & Davis, M. E. (2003). Structural effects of carbohydrate-containing polycations on gene delivery. 2. Charge center type. *Bioconjugate Chemistry*, Vol. 14, No. 1, (Jan-Feb 2003), pp. 255-261, ISSN 1043-1802

Reineke, T. M. & Davis, M. E. (2003). Structural effects of carbohydrate-containing polycations on gene delivery. 1. Carbohydrate size and its distance from charge centers. *Bioconjugate Chemistry*, Vol. 14, No. 1, (Jan-Feb 2003), pp. 247-254, ISSN 1043-1802

Sagara, K. & Kim, S. W. (2002). A new synthesis of galactose-poly(ethylene glycol)-polyethylenimine for gene delivery to hepatocytes. *Journal of Controlled Release*, Vol. 79, No. 1-3, (Feb 19 2002), pp. 271-281, ISSN 0168-3659

Saranya, N.; Moorthi, A.; Saravanan, S.; Devi, M. P. & Selvamurugan, N. (2011). Chitosan and its derivatives for gene delivery. *International Journal of Biological Macromolecules*, Vol. 48, No. 2, (Mar 1 2011), pp. 234-238, ISSN 1879-0003

Smith, A. E. (1995). Viral vectors in gene therapy. *Annual Review of Microbiology*, Vol. 49, 1995), pp. 807-838, ISSN 0066-4227

Stayton, P. S.; El-Sayed, M. E.; Murthy, N.; Bulmus, V.; Lackey, C.; Cheung, C. & Hoffman, A. S. (2005). 'Smart' delivery systems for biomolecular therapeutics. *Orthodontics & Craniofacial Research*, Vol. 8, No. 3, (Aug 2005), pp. 219-225, ISSN 1601-6335

Sun, S.; Liu, W.; Cheng, N.; Zhang, B.; Cao, Z.; Yao, K.; Liang, D.; Zuo, A.; Guo, G. & Zhang, J. (2005). A thermoresponsive chitosan-NIPAAm/vinyl laurate copolymer vector for gene transfection. *Bioconjugate Chemistry*, Vol. 16, No. 4, (Jul-Aug 2005), pp. 972-980, ISSN 1043-1802

Thanou, M.; Florea, B. I.; Geldof, M.; Junginger, H. E. & Borchard, G. (2002). Quaternized chitosan oligomers as novel gene delivery vectors in epithelial cell lines. *Biomaterials*, Vol. 23, No. 1, (Jan 2002), pp. 153-159, ISSN 0142-9612

Uekama, K.; Hirayama, F. & Irie, T. (1998). Cyclodextrin Drug Carrier Systems. *Chemical Reviews*, Vol. 98, No. 5, (Jul 30 1998), pp. 2045-2076, ISSN 1520-6890

Wong, K.; Sun, G.; Zhang, X.; Dai, H.; Liu, Y.; He, C. & Leong, K. W. (2006). PEI-g-chitosan, a novel gene delivery system with transfection efficiency comparable to polyethylenimine in vitro and after liver administration in vivo. *Bioconjugate Chemistry*, Vol. 17, No. 1, (Jan-Feb 2006), pp. 152-158, ISSN 1043-1802

Wu, C. H. & Wu, G. Y. (1998). Receptor-mediated delivery of foreign genes to hepatocytes. *Advanced Drug Delivery Reviews*, Vol. 29, No. 3, (Feb 2 1998), pp. 243-248, ISSN 1872-8294

Yang, C.; Li, H.; Goh, S. H. & Li, J. (2007). Cationic star polymers consisting of alpha-cyclodextrin core and oligoethylenimine arms as nonviral gene delivery vectors. *Biomaterials*, Vol. 28, No. 21, (Jul 2007), pp. 3245-3254, ISSN 0142-9612

Zhang, H.; Mardyani, S.; Chan, W. C. & Kumacheva, E. (2006). Design of biocompatible chitosan microgels for targeted pH-mediated intracellular release of cancer therapeutics. *Biomacromolecules*, Vol. 7, No. 5, (May 2006), pp. 1568-1572, ISSN 1525-7797

Zhao, Q.; Temsamani, J. & Agrawal, S. (1995). Use of cyclodextrin and its derivatives as carriers for oligonucleotide delivery. *Antisense Research and Development*, Vol. 5, No. 3, (Fall 1995), pp. 185-192, ISSN 1050-5261

Zheng, Y.; Cai, Z.; Song, X.; Yu, B.; Bi, Y.; Chen, Q.; Zhao, D.; Xu, J. & Hou, S. (2009). Receptor mediated gene delivery by folate conjugated N-trimethyl chitosan in vitro. *International Journal of Pharmaceutics*, Vol. 382, No. 1-2, (Dec 1 2009), pp. 262-269, ISSN 1873-3476

Zidovetzki, R. & Levitan, I. (2007). Use of cyclodextrins to manipulate plasma membrane cholesterol content: evidence, misconceptions and control strategies. *Biochimica et Biophysica Acta*, Vol. 1768, No. 6, (Jun 2007), pp. 1311-1324, ISSN 0006-3002

Zugates, G. T.; Anderson, D. G.; Little, S. R.; Lawhorn, I. E. & Langer, R. (2006). Synthesis of poly(beta-amino ester)s with thiol-reactive side chains for DNA delivery. *Journal of the American Chemical Society*, Vol. 128, No. 39, (Oct 4 2006), pp. 12726-12734, ISSN 0002-7863

Chitosan-DNA/siRNA Nanoparticles for Gene Therapy

Qin Shi[1], Marcio J. Tiera[2], Xiaoling Zhang[3], Kerong Dai[3],
Mohamed Benderdour[1] and Julio C. Fernandes[1]
*[1]Orthopedic Research Laboratory, Hôpital du Sacré-Cœur de Montréal
Université de Montréal
[2]Departamento de Quimica e Ciencias Ambientais, UNESP-Universidade Estadual
Paulista- Brazil
[3]The key laboratory of Stem Cell Biology, Institute of Health Sciences
Shanghai Jiao Tong University School of Medicine (SJTUSM) & Shanghai
Institutes for Biological Sciences (SIBS), Chinese Academy of Sciences (CAS)
[1]Canada
[2]Brazil
[3]China*

1. Introduction

Human diseases can be treated by the transfer of therapeutic genes (transgene) into specific cells or tissues of patients to correct or supplement defective, causative genes. Gene therapy offers a solution to controlled and specific delivery of genetic materials (DNA and RNA) to targeted cells. The success of gene therapy depends on the ability to deliver these therapeutic materials to targeted site. Viral vectors (e.g. adenovirus) are very effective in term of transfection efficiency, but they have limitations *in vivo*, particularly by their safety concern and non tissue-specific transfection. Non-viral gene transfer systems are limited by their lower gene transfer efficiency, low tissue specificity and transient gene expression.

Chitosan is a polysaccharide usually obtained from deacetylation of chitin, which may be extracted from various sources, particularly from exoskeletons of arthropods such as crustaceans. The goal of this chapter is to introduce the readers to chitosan as a DNA/small interfering RNA (siRNA) delivery vector, as well as different variable strategies to improve cellular transfection and its potential clinical application. the first section is to present of chapter (section 1). The second section presents the discussion about barriers to DNA/siRNA delivery *in vitro* and *in vivo*. It is important to have a clear overview of obstacles to the *in vivo* treatment with DNA/siRNAs. Different *in vivo* administration routes will encounter different physiological barriers, and complications may be furthered by different cells in organs and tissues (section 2). The third section provides the readers with an understanding of the key steps of cellular internalization of DNA/siRNA non viral vectors. Internalization of non viral vector-based DNA/siRNA delivery system into cells typically occurs through endocytosis (section 3). the fourth section describes chitosan as a vector for gene therapy (section 4) followed by chitosan structure and physicochemical behaviour (section 5), general strategies for chitosan modification (section 6), chitosan-DNA delivery system (section 7), chitosan-siRNA delivery system (section 8), and potential applications of chitosan–DNA/siRNA nanoparticles (section 9). Our current research will be summarized in the section of conclusion.

2. Barriers to gene delivery using non-viral vectors

2.1 Viral gene vectors

Gene transfer can occur through 2 delivery systems: viral or non-viral vectors. Viral gene therapy consists of using viral vectors which, given their structure and mechanisms of action, are good candidates or models to carry therapeutic genes efficiently, leading to long-term expression. Viruses are obvious first choices as gene transport. They have the natural ability to enter cells and express their own proteins. Nowadays, most viral vectors used are retroviruses, herpes virus, adenoviruses and lentiviruses. Unfortunately, certain viral vectors (for example, adenoviruses) can elicit a robust cellular immune response against viral and some transgenic proteins, so their use has been limited to studies in immune-compromised animals (Seiler et al., 2007). Adeno-associated viruses (AAV), which have been considered safe, appear to be immunogenic in several experimental settings (Vandenberghe & Wilson, 2007) and in a clinical trial (Mingozzi & High, 2007). Some serious adverse events have occurred with viral gene therapy. One patient died of fatal systemic inflammatory response syndrome after adenoviral gene transfer in 1999 (Raper et al., 2003). Two children developed leukemia-like clonal lymphocyte proliferation after recombinant retroviral gene transfer in 2000 (Hacein-Bey-Abina et al., 2003), and 1 of them died after unsuccessful chemotherapy late in 2004. Attention focused recently on the tragic death of a young female patient in a gene therapy study (intra-articular injection of AAV vectors) of severe RA in 2007 (Kaiser, 2007).

2.2 Non-viral gene vectors

Non-viral gene transfer systems offer several potential advantages over virus vectors. They are non-infectious, relatively non-immunogenic, have low acute toxicity, can accommodate large DNA plasmids or RNA, and may be produced on a large scale (Castanotto & Rossi, 2009; Gary et al., 2007). Non-viral gene therapy has been explored by physical approaches (transfer by gene gun, electroporation, ultrasound-facilitated and hydrodynamic delivery) as well as chemical approaches (cationic lipid-mediated gene delivery and cationic polymer-mediated gene transfer). Numerous chemical non-viral gene transfer systems have been proposed, including naked DNA, cationic liposomes, histones, and polymers (Gao et al., 2007; Ulrich-Vinther, 2007). The main drawback of non-viral vectors as gene carriers is their typically low transfection efficiency (Gao et al., 2007; Giannoudis et al., 2006). Furthermore, the *in vivo* delivery of non-viral liposome/plasmid DNA complex triggers an immune response (Sakurai et al., 2008). Non-viral gene therapy with cationic liposomes has already been tested in clinical trials that dealt with the treatment of inherited genetic disorders (for example, cystic fibrosis) (Hyde et al., 2000) and cancer (Ramesh et al., 2001). Synthetic and natural cationic polymers (positively-charged) have been widely used to carry DNA or siRNA (both negatively-charged) and condense it into small particles, facilitating cellular internalization via endocytosis through charge-charge interactions with anionic sites on cell surfaces. Although existing non-viral vectors have been found to enable DNA expression after *in vivo* delivery, the efficiency and duration of ensuing gene expression have proven to be unsatisfactory. Research efforts to improve the *in vivo* DNA-delivery efficacy of non-viral vectors are ongoing.

2.3 Barriers to DNA delivery

Systemic gene delivery involves a systemic approach in which exogenous genes are delivered to cells in a certain tissues, and secreted gene products are released into the circulatory system where they could modulate disease processes throughout the body. Systemic non-viral gene delivery has become an attractive alternative to viral vectors because of their safety, versatility and ease of preparation (Li & Huang, 2006). Genes can be delivered systemically (intramuscularly, intravenously, subcutaneously or, in animals, intraperitoneally). Otherwise, hydrodynamic-based gene delivery through systemic DNA injection offers a convenient, efficient and powerful means for high-level gene expression in animals (Liu & Knapp, 2001; Suda & Liu, 2007). This method is expected to be evaluated in patients soon (Romero et al., 2004). The limitations of the systemic approach to gene therapy are essentially the advantages of local delivery: exposure of non-target tissues to the therapeutic agent may have toxic effects or may compromise the immune system of the patient. Certain proteins will likely require very high levels of synthesis to achieve therapeutic function.

Ideally, gene therapy must protect DNA against degradation by nucleases in intercellular matrices so that the availability of macromolecules is not affected. Transgenes should be brought across the plasma membrane and into the nucleus of targeted cells but should have no detrimental effects. Hence, interaction with blood components, vascular endothelial cells and uptake by the reticuloendothelial system must be avoided. For DNA-based gene therapy to succeed, small-sized systems must internalize into cells and pass to the nucleus. Also, flexible tropisms allow applicability to a range of disease targets. Last but not least, such systems should be able to escape endosome-lysosome processing for endocytosis.

2.4 Barriers to siRNA delivery

The discovery of small interfering RNAs (siRNAs) has given renewed vision to the treatment of incurable diseases and genetically-associated disorders. Short double stranded (ds) RNA of 21-23 bp was cleaved by the RNAse III-like protein Dicer and incorporated into RNA-induced silencing complexes (RISC) (Hammond et al., 2000). Chemically-synthesized siRNAs and short hairpin RNA (shRNA) expression plasmids, which are sequence-specific for mRNA targeting, are methods commonly employed to mimic Dicer cleavage (Chen et al., 2007). However, siRNAs are susceptible to nuclease destruction and cannot penetrate the cell membrane because of their highly-charged backbone. An effective delivery system would enclose siRNA in carriers for protection and transport to the cytoplasm of targeted cells but should have no detrimental effects such as specific and non-specific off-targeted effects. Off-target effects can be divided into two categories: specific and non-specific off-targeted effects. Off-targeted effects may cause inflammation including interferon response, cell toxicity, and unintended gene knockdown.

Turning siRNA into drugs is a 3-step process. The design and *in vitro* screening of target siRNAs are followed by incorporating stabilizing chemical modifications in lead siRNAs, as required, and end in the selection as well as *in vivo* evaluation of delivery technologies that are appropriate for the target cell type/organ and disease setting (Vaishnaw et al., 2010). After nearly 10 years of study and development, many problems have been resolved, such as improving the stability of siRNAs, and avoiding 2 types of off-target effects. A recent anti-influenza study showed that the anti-viral activity of siRNA as found to be due to active siRNA. However, a different non-targeting control siRNA also had significant anti-viral activity (Mook et al., 2007). siRNA targeting vascular endothelial growth factor for patients with age-related macular degeneration (AMD) are currently in clinical trial. But further study showed that the inhibition is a siRNA classic effect, which is sequence- and target-independent (Jackson & Linsley, 2010). The off-target effect can be minimized by optimizing the rules and algorithms for siRNA design (Vaishnaw et al., 2010). However, several other factors limit the utility of siRNAs as therapeutic agents, such as competition with endogenous RNA, induction of immune responses, degradation in lysosomes after endocytosis (Dominska & Dykxhoorn, 2010; Wang et al., 2010). Unprotected, naked siRNAs are relatively unstable in blood and serum and have short half-lives *in vivo* (Gao et al., 2009). Naked siRNAs do not freely cross cellular membranes because of their large molecular weight (~13 kDa) and strong anionic charge. They are rapidly degraded by nuclease. Physiological barriers hinder siRNAs from reaching their targets, thereby reducing their therapeutic efficacy. Moreover, siRNA molecules have unfavorable physicochemical properties (negative charge, large molecular weight and instability). Therefore, they need delivery systems to overcome physiological obstacles and prolong vascular circulation by reducing renal clearance, protecting them from serum nucleases, improving their effective bio-distribution as well as targeted cellular uptake with endosomal escape and, finally, promoting trafficking to the cytoplasm and loading onto RISC. Therefore, delivery systems are required to facilitate siRNA access to intracellular sites of action.Barriers to siRNA delivery depend on the targeted organ and routes of administration. For example, intravenous (IV) administration is the most commonly used technique. The endothelial wall in the vasculature presents the primary delivery barrier to siRNAs. The endothelial barrier is often altered by inflammatory processes (e.g., RA, infection) (Moghimi et al., 2005). siRNAs leave a blood vessel to enter tissue. After reaching target cells, they undergo internalization via endocytosis, escape from endosomes, and release into the cytosol and, finally, load onto RISC. At the same time, siRNAs undergo elimination. The mononuclear phagocyte system is responsible for removing circulating foreign particles from the bloodstream by the phagocytosis of resident macrophages (Moghimi et al., 2005).

3. Cellular internalization of non-viral vector delivery system

There are seven steps should be overcome before the expression of exogenous DNA. They are (1) complexation, (2) *in vivo* administration, (3) endocytosis, (4) escape from endolysosome, (5) release of DNA, (6) trafficking through cytoplasm and (7) finally import of DNA into nucleus. (If siRNA is used as exogenous nucleotide, the last two steps can be ignored; but if vector-expressed siRNA is used, the process remains the same.) During each step, many factors may come into play, inducing toxicity, immunogenicity or affecting transfection efficiency. (1) During complexation, the non-viral vectors-DNA interaction is driven mainly by the electrostatic interaction between the polycation and the charged phosphate groups leading to reversible linear to globule transition of DNA. The ability of the non-viral vectors to condense DNA into nanoparticles is often critical for transfection efficiency since DNA must be protected from DNase degradation. (2) Different *in vivo* administration routes will meet different physiological barriers. Therefore, it is suggested that the corresponding primary cells and similar physiological barriers should be tested *in vitro* as far as possible, before *in vivo* administration is attempted. (3) The following step is to reach its target, the cell by endocytosis. In this respect it is well accepted that the polyelectrolyte complex polycation-DNA exhibiting a net positive charge binds to negatively charged cell membrane. (4) After the internalization the following crucial step in gene delivery with cationic polymers is the escape of the polymer/DNA complexes from the endosome. (5) The inefficient release of the DNA/polymer complex from endocytic vesicles into the cytoplasm is indicated as one of the primary causes of poor gene delivery. (6) and (7) the following step, the nuclear envelope is the ultimate obstacle to the nuclear entry of plasmid DNA. This obstacle is also considered crucial and two main mechanisms were proposed to explain how plasmid DNA enters into the nucleus: (i) a passive DNA entry into the nucleus during cell division when the nuclear membrane is temporarily disintegrated or (ii) an active transport of the DNA through the nuclear pores.

4. Chitosan as a vector for gene therapy

Cationic polymers, such as chitosan, are promising candidates for DNA transport in non-viral delivery systems (Kean & Thanou, 2010; Tong et al., 2009). Chitosan, a linear polysaccharide composed of randomly distributed β-(1-4)-linked D-glucosamine (deacetylated unit) and N-acetyl-D-glucosamine (acetylated unit), and has once been considered as an attractive gene transfer candidate for its superior biocompatibility, superior biodegradability and low cell toxicity. In recent years, with more researching methods involved, a more accurate and subtle view on the process of the entry of chitosan/DNA complexes into the cell nucleus has been developed. The enabling characteristics of Chitosan-DNA nanoparticles include biocompatibility, multiple ligand affinity, and a capacity of taking up large DNA fragments, while remaining small in size (Techaarpornkul et al., 2010). Chitosan and its derivatives, as favorable non-viral vectors involved in plasmid DNA delivery, have attracted attention in the field of siRNA delivery *in vitro* and *in* vivo (Andersen et al., 2009; Howard et al., 2009). Chitosan was once believed to be less effective than most other non-viral vectors because of its low stability and buffering capacity. However, recent technological advances in the chemical modification of chitosan have instituted improvements of its transfection efficiency without disturbing its biocompatibility and biodegradability. It has been demonstrated that transfection level is closely related to the molecular weight of polymers (Godbey et al., 1999). Chitosan (10-150 kDa), with a specific degree of deacetylation, allows maximum transgenic expression *in vitro* (Lavertu et al., 2006). Another strategy for improving transfection is to take advantage of the mechanism of ligand-mediated uptake by cells to promote targeting and internalization, enhancing transfection efficiency. Ligand-mediated transfection has been shown to facilitate DNA internalization into cells via membrane receptors both *in vitro* and *in vivo*. Cell-specific ligand modification such as galactose, transferrin, folate and mannose can also effectively enhance the specificity of transfection through receptor-mediated endocytosis. Galactose ligand modification has been used to target HepG2 cells through the interaction with asialoglycoprotein receptors (ASGP-R) (Gao et al., 2003). A transferrin receptor is found on many mammalian cells, therefore it can be used as a universal ligand (Dautry-Varsat, 1986). Folate is not only over-expressed on macrophage surfaces, but is also over-expressed on many human cancer cell surfaces (Lee et al., 2006). Antigen presenting cells (APCs), the ideal targets of DNA vaccine, such as macrophages and immature dendritic cells are the target cells of mannose ligand (Kim et al., 2006). The specificity of these modifications can be demonstrated through ligand competitive inhibition experiments.

The low stability, low buffering capacity and low cell-specificity have also hindered its clinical applications. However, as a nature resource-based polysaccharide, chitosan has more functional groups that can be chemically modified than other cationic polymers, thus has many more potential chemical derivatives to overcome the deficiencies. Chitosan has been experimentally modified using hydrophilic, hydrophobic, pH-sensitive, thermosensitive and cell-specific ligand groups for enhancement of transfection efficiency (Ishii et al., 2001). The degree of deacetylation (DDA) and the molecular weight (MW) of chitosan or its derivatives, can affect the ultimate transfection efficiency. Most chitosan/DNA complexes are highly deacetylated (above 80%), because chitosan with a high degree of deacetylation exhibits an increased DNA binding efficacy (Kiang et al., 2004). Through chain entanglement, chitosan with a higher MW (longer chain length) can become more readily enmeshed with free DNA, once the initial electrostatic interaction has occurred. But it will also delay the disassociation of chitosan and DNA (Huang et al., 2005). Consequently, low MW chitosan requires a higher charge ratio to stably condense DNA for the same DDA, and a lower DDA requires a higher charge ratio to stably condense DNA at equal MW (Lavertu et al., 2006). The charge ratio for minimum complexation can be determined by agarose gel electrophoresis.

5. Chitosan structure and physicochemical behaviour

The structure of chitin and chitosan correspond to those of poly [$\beta(1{\rightarrow}4)$-2-acetamido-2-deoxy-d-glucopyranose] and poly[$\beta(1{\rightarrow}4)$-2-amino-2-deoxy-d-glucopyranose], respectively (Figure 1). Chitosan is mainly manufactured from crustaceans (crab, krill and crayfish) primarily because a large amount of the crustacean exoskeleton is available as a byproduct of food processing. However, depending on the organism considered chitin can adopt polymorphic structures denominated alpha (α), beta (β) and gamma (γ) chitin (Jang et al., 2004).The polymorphism of chitin is due to different arrangements of chitin chains in the lamellas that constitute the crystalline portions. Alpha (α) chitin found in arthropods corresponds to an antiparallel chain packing at which intramolecular and intermolecular hydrogen bonding is favored. β-Chitin, typically extracted from squid pens, is less widely used although it can have higher reactivity than that of α-chitin. The parallel arrangement of the lamellas is responsible for a loose-packing fashion with weak intermolecular interactions. In the gamma (γ) chitin structure arrangements, beta and alpha occur, i.e., two lamellas in a parallel arrangement is intercalated by a lamella arranged in antiparallel packing (Roberts, 1992). The source from which chitosan is prepared is considered very important since chitosan derived from β-chitin exhibits higher reactivity than that derived from α-chitin (Kuritia et al., 1994; Shimojohay 1998).

In general the isolation of chitin from crustacean shell waste consists of three basic steps: demineralization (DM-calcium carbonate and calcium phosphate separation), deproteinization (DP-protein separation), and decolorization (DC-removal of pigments). These three steps are the standard procedure for chitin production (No et al., 1989). Chitosan is obtained after hydrolysis of the acetamide groups of chitin. However in the commercialized samples both units are commonly found, since chitosans having high deacetylation degrees (DA> 99%) are obtained only through of successive hydrolysis with strong bases as KOH and NaOH, and the degree of deacetylation is strongly dependent of the alkali concentration and temperature (Figure.1). The source of chitin and the deacetylation process can change dramatically the properties of the final product and the deacetylation in alkaline medium leads to the depolimerization (Domard & Rinaudo, 1983; Tolaimate et al., 2000). However it has been reported that chitin extracted from squid pens can be hydrolyzed under conditions that it allows obtaining chitosans of high molecular weight (Tolaimate et al., 2003).

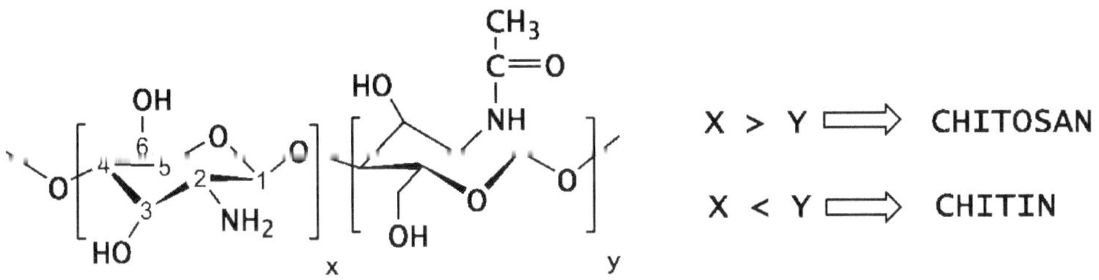

$$X > Y \implies \text{CHITOSAN}$$

$$X < Y \implies \text{CHITIN}$$

Fig. 1. Chemical structure of chitin and chitosan. In the 2-amino-2-deoxy-d-glucopyranose ring is shown the commonly used numbering for the carbon atoms.

The homopolymer is a weak base with a pKa value of the D-glucosamine residue of about 6.3 and is therefore insoluble at neutral and alkaline pH values. In acidic mediums, the amine groups will be positively charged, conferring to the polysaccharide a high charge density. As in all polyelectrolytes, the dissociation constant of chitosan is not constant, but depends on the degree of dissociation at which it is determined. The pka value can be calculated using the Katchalsky's equation (Roberts, 1992).

$$Pk_a = pH + \log [(1-\alpha)/\alpha] = pK_0 - \varepsilon \Delta\psi(\alpha)/kT$$

Where $\Delta\psi$ is the difference in electrostatic potential between the surface of the polyion and the reference, α is the degree of dissociation, k is Boltzman's constant, T is the temperature and ε is the electron charge. Extrapolation of the pK_a values to $\alpha = 1$, where the polymer is uncharged and hence the electrostatic potential becomes zero, makes possible the value of the intrinsic dissociation constant of the ionizable groups, pK_0, to be determined. The value obtained does not depend of the degree of N-acetylation, whereas the pKa value is dependent on this parameter, since the electrostatic potential will be varied depending of amount of the free amino groups. The pK_0 value is called the intrinsic pK_a of the chitosan. However chitosans of low molecular weight having degrees of deacetylation higher than 0.4 are also easily soluble in weakly acidic solvents such as acetic acid and formic acid (Lee et al., 1995).

The physicochemical behavior in aqueous solution is highly dependent of pH and degree of acetylation and has received more attention only recently. Bertha et al. working on chitosans from 95 to 175kDa have recently determined the radius of gyration of chitosan (R_G) (Bertha et al., 1998a; 2002b). The R_G is an alternative measure of the size of the polymer chain and it can be measured by light scattering measurements. R_G express the square mean radius of each one of the elements of the chain measured from its center of gravity. The study established the relationship between the molecular weight and radius of gyration (R_G) of chitosan in aqueous solution, and the author indicated that chitosan behaved more like a Gaussian coil instead of the worm-like chain model found in common polyelectrolytes. At the same time the presence of N- acetyl groups on the chitosan backbone imparts hydrophobic properties. Schatz et al. (Schatz et al., 2003) have studied homogeneous series of chitosans with different degrees of acetylation and almost the same degree of polymerization in ammonium acetate buffer. Their results indicate that the aqueous solution behavior depends only on the degree of acetylation (DA). Three distinct domains of DA were defined and correlated to the different behaviors of chitosans: (i) a polyeletrolyte domain for DA below 20%; (ii) a transition domain between DA = 20% and 50% where chitosan loses its hydrophilicity; (iii) a hydrophobic domain for DAs over 50% where polymer associations can arise. Conformations of chitosan chains varying from 160 to 270kDa were studied by the calculations of the persistence lengths (L(p)). The average value was found to be close to 5 nm, in agreement with the wormlike chain model, but no significant variation of L(p) with the degree of acetylation was noticed. Pa et al. (Pa & Yu, 2001) have also reported that that the particle sizes of chitosan molecules in dilute acetic acid/water solutions increased with decreasing pH value. SLS data also demonstrated that the second virial coefficient (A_2) increased with decreasing pH value, suggesting that solubility of chitosan in water increased with increasing acetic acid concentration. Signini et al. (Signini et al., 2000) have also shown that acid-free aqueous solutions of chitosan hydrochloride of variable ionic strengths (0:06 M $\leq$ µ$\leq$ 0.3 M) are free of aggregation as evaluated by the values of the Huggins constants (0.31 $\leq k \leq$ 0.63).

As other polysaccharides the biodegradation and biocompatibility are important properties of chitosan making it an attractive polymer for a variety of biomedical and pharmaceutical applications. Besides the degradation by chitinases (Hung et al., 2002), chitosanases (Kuroiwa et al., 2003), papain (Kumar et al., 2004; Lin et al., 2002; Muzzarelli et al., 2002; Terbojevich et al., 1996) and other proteases (Kumar et al., 2004), partially acetylated chitosan may be also degraded by lyzosymes of the human serum (Varurn et al., 1997), by oxidative-reductive depolymerization (Mao et al., 2004) and by acid hydrolysis reactions (Lee et al., 1999). In the acid hydrolysis the protonation of the glycosidic oxygen is recognized as the first step of the mechanism, which leads to formation of a cyclic carbonium –oxonium ion, yielding after the addition of water the reducing sugar end group (Sinnott et al., 1990; Yip & Withers, 2004). Besides enzymatic and acid hydrolysis the alkaline treatment with ultrasonication can be used to obtain either chitosan of decreasing molecular weight (Tang et al., 2003) or oligomers having a few glucosamine units (Tsaih et al., 2003).

6. General strategies for chitosan modification

In the chitosan structure two groups are particularly susceptible to react through nucleophilics attacks, i.e., the free amine and/or acetamide groups, and the hydroxyl groups linked to the glucopyranose ring. The hydroxyl groups can be modified by substitution of the hydrogen atoms but their reactivities are smaller than that of the amino group. Various procedures targeting the hydroxyl groups employ a sequence of protection/deprotection reactions aiming to obtain derivatives with a well defined structure (Kuitra, 2001). On the other hand under appropriated conditions a variety of other reactions can be easily conducted to selectively modify the free amine groups. The literature presents a wide range of procedures to target the amine group aiming to improve the properties of chitosan for a particular purpose. The modifications include those aiming the separation technologies of chiral molecules (Franco et al., 2001), recovery of metals (Guibal, 2004; Varma et al., 2004), antimicrobial activity (Rabea et al., 2003), anti tumoral carriers (Kato et al., 2004), biomedical applications (Berge et al., 2004a; 2004b) and vectors for gene therapy (Janes et al., 2001; Sinha et al., 2004; Liu et al., 2002; Borchard et al., 2001). Kumar et al (Kumar et al., 2004) and Kurita (Kurta, 2001) reviewed the procedures for the modification of chitosan.

Many strategies have been deployed to improve transfection efficiency, taking into account the biological steps involved in gene delivery. Modifications of chitosan structure to impart properties to NPs, such as to increase endosomal escape (Jiang et al., 2010; Yu et al., 2010), attaching of ligands to mediate cell internalization or to promote the nuclear entry of DNA, are among the most common ways. Figure 2 shows representative structures from these chitosan derivatives tested as carriers for gene therapy. A variety of nucleophilic reactions targeting the groups linked to the glucopyranose ring have been employed to improve the properties of chitosan.

Poly (ethylene glycol) (PEG) has been widely used for attaching to chitosan due to its hydrophilicity and biocompatibility. In general, the terminal hydroxyl group of methoxy poly(ethylene glycol) is modified to generate PEG derivatives able to promote nucleophilic displacements targeting the amino groups of chitosan (Harris et al., 1984; Aiba et al, 1993; Saito et al., 1997; Ouchi et al., 1998). Chitosan nanospheres modified by introducing PEG$_{5000}$ chains to amine groups were more stable during lyophilization (Leong et al., 1998). These chitosan-DNA nanospheres were effective in tranfecting 293 cells but not HeLa cells, and tranfection efficiency was not affected by PEG derivatization.

Polymers can also be attached to the chitosan main chain using different routes. Poly(vinyl pyrrolidone) (PVP) was also grafted on galactosylated chitosan (GCPVP) and displayed improved physicochemical properties over unmodified chitosan (Park et al., 2003). PVP with a single terminus carboxylic group was coupled to galactosylated chitosan via formation of an amide bond between the amino *complex* group of GC and the terminal carboxyl group of the PVP. The terminal carboxyl group of PVP was activated by the N-hydroxysuccinimide (NHS)/EDC. The binding strength of GCPVP 10k/DNA was superior to that of GCPVP 50k/DNA, which was attributed to its higher flexibility because of its smaller size. However, DNase I protection of GCPVP 10k/DNA complex was inferior to that of GCPVP 50k/DNA. The DNA-binding property was shown to be dependent on the MW of chitosan and the composition of PVP (Park et al., 2003). The reaction of chitosan with methoxy poly(ethylene glycol) iodide (mPEG, Mn 2 kDa) in an alkalinized suspension was recently used by Yu *et al.* to attach PEG (Yu et al., 2010). This derivative was subsequently modified by attaching poly(ethylenimine) to the amino groups (Figure 2). Other approaches successfully employed to attach PEI to chitosan were an imine reaction between periodate-oxidized chitosan and amine groups of low MW PEI (Jiang et al., 2007) and the cationic polymerization of aziridine in the presence of water-soluble oligo-chitosan (Wong et al., 2006).

A series of new degradable cationic polymers composed of biocompatible chitosan backbones and poly((2-dimethyl amino) ethylmethacrylate) (P(DMAEMA)) side chains were recently synthesized via atom transfer radical polymerization (ATR) (Ping et al., 2010). This synthesis was carried out by introducing alkyl halide initiators onto chitosan, followed by the reaction with DMAEMA. Bromoisobutyryl-terminated chitosan (CS-Br initiators) was prepared via the reaction of primary amines of chitosan with carboxyl group of 2-bromo-2-methylpropionic acid (BMPA), which was previously converted into reactive esters (succinimidyl intermediates) in the presence of EDAC and NHS. The reactive esters underwent nucleophilic substitution reactions with the amine groups of chitosan to form a stable amide linkage and produce the resultant CS-Br initiators for DMAE polymerization (Ping et al., 2010).

The activation of carboxylic groups is one of the most commonly used procedures to attach different ligands and peptides to chitosan chain. Arginine-modified trimethylated chitosans labeled with folic acid have been prepared by activation of the acid group of arginine using EDC/NHS (Morris et al., 2010). The same procedure was utilized by Gao et al and it has proven to increase the transfection efficiency (Gao et al., 2008) and chitosan properties (Liu et al., 2004). A similar procedure was utilized to attach a short peptide (SP) (Sun et al., 2010) to chitosan. The peptide was further combined with GFP/luciferase reporter gene pDNA to form SP-CS/DNA complex. The NPs were able to transfect multiple cell lines, and the results revealed that, compared with CS, SP-CS could intensively augment transfection efficiency nearly to the level of Lipofectamine 2000 (Sun et al., 2010). Reactions targeting the hydroxyl groups are uncommon, however Sato et al. have prepared 6-Amino-6-deoxychitosan from 6-deoxy-6-halo-N-phthaloylchitosan via 6-azidation. The product had high stereoregularity because of the effective and regioselective reactions (Saito et al., 2004; Satoh et al., 2007).

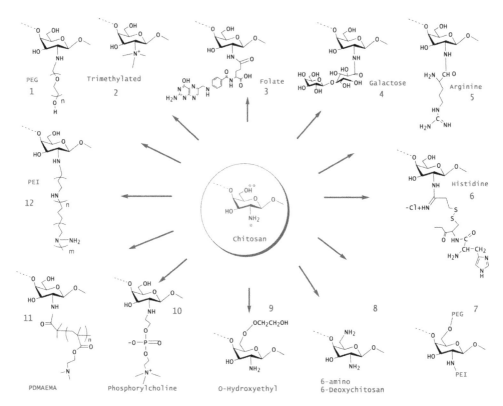

Fig. 2. Chemical structures of chitosan and its derivatives; **1.** PEG (Harris et al., 1984); **2.** trimethylated (Zeng et al., 2007); **3.** folic acid (Mansouri et al., 2006; Fernandes et al., 2008); **4.**galactosylated (Park et al., 2001); **5.** Arginine (Morris et al., 2010); **6.** histidine; **7.** PEI and PEG grafts (Yu et al., 2010); **8.** 6-amino 6-deoxychitosan (Saito et al., 2004; Satoh et al., 2007); **9.** O-hydroethyl (Kwon et al., 2003); **10.** Phosphorylcholine (Case et al., 2009; Tiera et al., 2006); **11.** grafted PDMAEMA (Ping et al., 2010); **12.** PEI (Jiang et al., 2007; Wong et al., 2006).

7. Chitosan-DNA delivery system

Chitosan-DNA gene delivery methods must achieve sufficient efficiency in the transportation of therapeutic genes across various extracellular and intracellular barriers. These barriers include interactions with blood components, vascular endothelial cells and uptake by the reticuloendothelial system. Furthermore, the degradation of therapeutic DNA by serum nucleases is a potential obstacle for functional delivery to target cells. DNA should escape from endosomes and traffic to enter the nucleus. Many factors, including the degree of deacetylation (DDA) and the molecular weight (MW) of the chitosan, the pH of the serum, the charge ratio (in some conditions, it equals the ratio of N/P, 'N': the content of Nitrogen atom in cationic polymer; 'P': the content of Phosohorus atom in DNA or RNA) of chitosan to DNA or RNA and the cell type can all affect the transfection efficiency of chitosan during each step of the process. The pKa value of chitosan is around 6.3-6.4, below which the protonated amines in the chitosan structure facilitate their binding to negatively charged DNA. Sato et al. showed the highest transfection efficiency can be obtained at pH 6.8 to 7.0. When pH of the transfection medium increases to 7.4, the transfection efficiency dramatically decreases due to the dissociation of the free plasmid from the complex (Sato et al., 2001).

Even if chitosan/DNA complexes display high transfection efficiency *in vitro*, their transfection efficiency *in vivo* may be low. Chitosan and its derivatives have become of great interest in the field of controlled release due to their favorable biocompatibility and biodegradability. Thiolated chitosan, which can be oxidized to form inter- and intra-molecular disulfide bonds, allowing the crosslinking of chitosan, shows a significant enhancement of transfection over that of lipofectin (Lee et al., 2007). Chitosan microspheres for micro-encapsulation of adenoviral vectors has been achieved by ionotropic coacervation of chitosan, using bile salts as counter-anions (Lameiro et al., 2006). A 3-D scaffold composed of chitosan-gelatin complexes with entrapped DNA has been proposed as a promoter of cartilage regeneration (Xia et al., 2004).

Although hydrophobic modification is not cell-specific, it can also enhance the attachment of complexes on cell surfaces and the subsequent cell uptake. Amphiphobic deoxycholic acid-modified chitosan oligosaccharide (DACO) nanoparticles showed superior gene condensation and high gene transfection efficiency, even in the presence of serum (Chae et al., 2005). After endocytosis, the endosome containing the complexes has to fuse with a lysosome to form an endolysosome. At this point, the complexes will meet a harsh acidic and multienzymatic environment. Nanocomplexes that are successfully protected against dissociation and degradation will finally escape from the endolysosome and enter the cytoplasm. PEI, a classic synthetic polymer with many amino groups to absorb protons (called a proton sponge mechanism), was found to have a better endolysosome buffering ability and caused a quicker release from the endolysosome in its intact form than did chitosan (Kim et al., 2005). The chemical modifications, such as urocanic acid (UA) (Kim et al., 2003), PEI-graft-chitosan (Wong et al., 2006), chitosan-graft-PEI (Jiang et al., 2007), poly(propyl acrylic acid) (PPAA) (Jones et al., 2003), trimethyl chitosan (Germershaus et al., 2008), have similar effects to PEI. Such modifications can be called pH-sensitive modifications that will not only enhance the escape of chitosan/DNA complexes from endolysosome but also enhance the stability of complexes in different pH situations.

The dissociation of chitosan/DNA complexes and subsequent release of DNA is also a very important step for its rate-limiting effect (Schaffer et al., 2000). Hydrophobic modification, such as deoxycholic acid modification (Lee et al., 1998), or 5β-cholanic acid modification (Yoo et al., 2005), can attenuate the electrostatic attractions between cationic polymers and anionic DNA. It is actually a contradiction between the stability and dissociation ability of complexes. A temperature-sensitive modification of poly(N-isopropylacrylamide) (PNIPAAm) can control the dissociation of PNVLCS (N-isopropylacrylamide/vinyl laurate copolymer with chitosan) complexes with DNA by a temporary reduction in the culture temperature to 20℃ (Sun et al., 2005)

The cytoplasm, a mesh-like network of microfilaments and microtubules, will limit the diffusion of complexes or DNA about 500-1000-fold. Adenovirus particles naturally bind to dynein and are actively transported towards the nuclear pore complexes once they are inside the cytoplasm. Prior to entry into the nucleus, the viruses dissociate into smaller structures and use their attached transport factors such as importins or karyopherins which have nuclear localization signals (NLS) to recognize the nuclear pore complex (NPC) (Whittaker & Helenius, 1998). Justin Hanes et al. used a new method called multiple particles tracking (MPT) to quantify the intracellular transport of non-viral DNA nanocarriers. They found that PEI/DNA complexes can accumulate in the perinuclear area through a subdiffusive transport, which is a combination of diffusive transport and active transport. This discovery is a dispute to the common belief that non-viral vectors go through the cell cytoplasm in a slow random way. Further investigation showed that actively transported complexes of PEI/DNA are in endosomes undergoing motor protein-driven movement guided by microtubules or physically associated with the motor proteins themselves (Suh et al., 2003). As to chitosan and its derivatives, however, few studies have examined how they pass through the highly structured cytoplasm and eventually enter into the nucleus.

8. Chitosan-siRNA delivery system

siRNA silencing technology is exploited in a wide range of biological studies, but has also become one of the most challenging therapeutic strategies. However, because of its poor delivery and susceptibility to nuclease degradation, siRNA-based approaches need a protective delivery system. A variety of polymer formulations have been proposed in the literature as potential carriers (De Fougerolles 2008; Gary et al., 2007; Zhang et al., 2007). Polymer molecular weight, change density, N/P ratio (ratio of protonatable polymer amine groups to nucleic acid phosphate groups) and ionic strength of the medium can affect electrostatic binding between siRNA and cationic polymers. Research over the years has revealed that chitosan is one of the desirable polymeric carriers of siRNA because of its natural biocompatibility, biodegradability, nontoxicity, and high nuclease resistance. The effects of different chitosan (114-kDa or more)-siRNA complexes on transfection activity have been observed previously (Katas et al., 2008; Katas & Alpar, 2006; Liu et al., 2007; Rojanarata et al., 2008). Higher MW and DDA are desirable characteristics for the formation of chitosan nanoparticles, as higher MW chitosan molecules are long and flexible while higher DDA enhances its electrostatic interaction with siRNAs, thus synergically reducing the size of complexes and increasing their stability (Liu et al., 2007). A high charge ratio also enhances the stability of complexes because the loosely bound excess chitosan on the outer surface of nanoparticles can promote binding and uptake across anionic cell surfaces and also provide subsequent protection against siRNA degradation within endosome compartments (Liu et al., 2007). The method of complexation also affects the gene-silencing activity of chitosan/siRNA complexes. Haliza Katas et al. studied the difference between simple complexation, ionic gelation (siRNA entrapment) and adsorption of siRNA onto the surface of preformed chitosan nanoparticles. Ionic gelation gave the strongest stability and the most efficient gene-silencing activity among the three methods tested. For the involvement of tripolyphosphate (TPP) ions during the complexation of ionic gelation, pH became one of the factors that mostly affected the gene-silencing activity. The decrease of pH resulted in a reduction in the charge number of TPP, which subsequently led to the need for more TPP ions for cross-linking of the chitosan by electrostatic forces (Katas & Alpar, 2006). Rojanarata et al. reported that chitosan-thiamine pyrophosphate (TPP)-mediated siRNA enhanced green fluorescent protein (EGFP) gene silencing efficiency depended on the molecular weight and weight ratio of chitosan and siRNA. The chitosan-TPP-siRNA complex with the lowest molecular weight of chitosan (20 kDa) at a weight ratio of 80 showed the strongest inhibition of gene expression (Rojanarata et al., 2008). A novel study of chitosan/siRNA nanoparticles with fluorescent quantum dots was taken to silence HER2/neu and achieved desirable silencing effects (Tahara et al., 2008; Tan et al., 2007). In the field of controlled release, chitosan coating PLGA nanospheres with a high loading efficiency of siRNAs were found to reduce the initial burst of nucleic acid release and to prolong release at later stages, without changing the release pattern (Tahara et al., 2008). Kenneth A. Howard found that the chitosan-based system had the ability for endosome escape through the proton sponge mechanism, because the endosomolytic agent chloroquine did not increase the effect of RNA interference (Howard et al., 2006). In terms of *in vivo* administration of chitosan/siRNAs complexes, only a few studies are available. Nasal administration to silence EGFP expression of the endothelial cells distributed in the bronchioles of transgenic EGFP mouse model has been successfully achieved without showing any adverse effects (Howard et al., 2006). Cross-linking of hyaluronan and chitosan has proven to have a higher efficiency of transfection in ocular tissue over unmodified chitosan (de la Fuente et al., 2008).

9. Potential application of chitosan-DNA/siRNA nanoparticles

Gene therapy offers new possibilities for the clinical management of different disease conditions that are difficult to treat by traditional surgical or medical means. In the last decade, extensive improvements have been made to optimize gene therapy and have been tested on several disease conditions. The success of chitosan-DNA nanoparticles for delivery plasmid DNA to mucosal surfaces such as the oral and nasal mucosa has already shown (Bivas-Benita et al., 2003; Chen et al., 2004; Khatri et al., 2008). Oral delivery is most attractive due to easy administration. The oral delivery of peptide, protein, vaccine and nucleic acid-based biotechnology products is the greatest challenge facing the drug delivery industry. Mice were fed with plasmid pCMVβ (containing LacZ gene), whether it was wrapped by chitosan or no. The study demonstrated that oral chitosan-DNA nanoparticles can efficiently deliver genes to enterocytes, and may be used as a useful tool for gene transfer (Chen et al., 2004). Hepatitis B virus infection is a major global health concern and is the most common cause of chronic liver disease, new generation of HBV vaccines are urgently needed in order to overcome problems encountered with the immunization of immunocompromised people and more importantly with the potential of using active immunotherapy in treating chronic patients. DNA vaccines have the potential to eliminate many of the limitations of current vaccine technologies. Chitosan nanoparticles loaded with plasmid DNA encoding surface protein of Hepatitis B virus. Nasal administration of such nanoparticles resulted in serum anti-HBsAg titre that was less compared to that elicited by naked DNA and alum adsorbed HBsAg, but the mice were seroprotective within 2 weeks and the immunoglobulin level was above the clinically protective level (Khatri et al., 2008). Particulate mucosal delivery systems that encapsulate protein or plasmid DNA encoding antigens have been widely explored for their ability to induce an immune response. Oral delivery of vaccines using chitosan as a carrier material appears to be beneficial for inducing an immune response against *Toxoplasma gondii*. Chitosan microparticles as carriers for GRA-1 protein vaccine were prepared. It was shown that priming with secreted dense granule protein 1 (GRA1) protein vaccine loaded chitosan particles and boosting with GRA1 pDNA vaccine resulted in high anti-GRA1 antibodies, characterized by a mixed IgG2a/IgG1 ratio (Bivas-Benita et al., 2003). The application of chitosan-based delivery system as ocular gene carriers, there is evidence of their ability to transfect the ocular cells in vitro. This capacity of chitosan nanoparticles to transfect the cells, was found to be highly dependent on the molecular weight of chitosan. Only chitosan of low molecular weight (10-12 kDa) was able to transfect plasmid DNA in both cell lines derived from the human cornea and the conjunctives (De la Fuente et al., 2008). In Utero delivery of chitosan-DNA results in postnatal gene expression, and shows promise for non-viral gene transfer in animal models of fetal gene therapy (Yang et al., 2010). The intravenous and intratracheal solutions and the intratracheal powder of pCMV-Muβ encoding murine interferon-β were administered the day after the inoculation of mice with CT26 cells. Lung weight and the number of pulmonary nodules at day 21 were significantly suppressed by the three formulations at a dose of 10 μg (N/P = 5). Reducing the dose to 1 μg resulted in a loss of effect by the intravenous solution (Okamoto et al., 2010). These findings showed that therapeutic gene powders are promising for gene therapy to treat lung cancer or metastasis.

siRNA gene therapy research has focused on several types of viral vectors: adeno-associated viruses (AAV), adenoviruses, retroviruses, lentiviruses, and herpes simplex viruses. siRNA therapeutics have been assessed in numerous diseases, including genetic and viral diseases, cancer, as well as non-lethal disorders, such as arthritis and osteoporosis. Among these viral vectors, lentiviruses have progressed to clinical trials on metastatic melanoma and HIV infection (Baker, 2010a; 2010b). siRNA-based gene therapy has already been tested in clinical trials dealing with the treatment of age-related macular degeneration, viral infection, skin disorders and cancer. Cancer treatment is by the most important proposed application of gene therapy and many clinical trials using gene therapy are under investigation. Non-viral vectors including chitosan derivatives have been used in animal model, but clinical trials are lagging due to low transfection efficiency. Anderson et al. (Andersen et al., 2008) demonstrated that silencing of pro-inflammatory TNFα in the RAW 246.7 murine macrophage cell line was achieved by using lyophilized chitosan/siRNA. Compared to research in vitro with chitosan-based systems, in vivo research is still in the developmental stage. Only a few studies are avaible which *in vivo* demonstration of chitosan/siRNA nanocomplexes in silencing gene expression in animals. Howard et al. (Howard et al., 2009) demonstrated that chitosan nanopaticles contains an anti-TNFα siRNA knock downed efficiently of TNFα expression in primary peritoneal macrophages in vitro. Downregulation of TNFα-induced inflammatory responses arrested systemic and local inflammation in collagen-induced arthritic mice after intraperitoneal injection of chitosan/anti-TNFα siRNA nanoparticles, thereby presenting a novel strategy for arthritis treatment.

10. Conclusion

Clinical trials on gene therapy are limited to naked DNA or plasmid DNAs/siRNA delivered by viral vectors. Among non-viral vectors for DNA and siRNA delivery, chitosan and its derivatives are promising alternatives to viral vectors for targeting DNA and siRNA to specific cells. Chitosan has once been considered as an attractive gene transfer candidate for its superior biocompatibility, superior biodegradability and low cell toxicity, but the low stability, low buffering capacity and low cell-specificity have also hindered its clinical applications. To date, however, no clinical trials of chitosan-DNA or siRNA therapy have been performed. Chitosan based gene therapy remains in the experimental stage due to low transfection efficacy. Many key challenges were involved in DNA and siRNA delivery to targeted cells using chitosan-based carriers. As a nature resource-based polysaccharide, chitosan has more functional groups that can be chemically modified than do the other cationic polymers, thus has many more potential chemical derivatives to make up these deficiencies. Parameters are critical to achieve favourable transfection efficiency and include degree of deacetylation, molecular weight, pH and N/P ratio. For example, a low molecular weight, high degree of deacetylation, small particle size and a moderate, positive, surface zeta potential along with a high N/P ration are advantageous to achieve high siRNA transfection efficiency. Recent technological advances in the chemical modification of chitosan have instituted improvements of its transfection efficiency without disturbing its biocompatibility and biodegradability.

Our work on gene coding for IL-1Ra in dogs (Pelletier et al., 1997) and rabbits (Fernandes et al., 1999) was our previous study with the protein itself. We have improved a non-viral intraarticular transfection technique using lipofection and have tested it in osteoarhtritis animal models. These were the very first published articles in the literature that demonstrated the efficacy of gene therapy in osteoarthritis models *in vivo*. Our recent work on polymeric nanoparticles has led us to develop a much safer and effective system for in vitro transfection of embryonic kidney cells, as well as adult mesenchymal stem cells (Corsi et al., 2003). This new system has been successfully tested in muscle and skin tissues *in vivo* in mice and holds great promise for future application on the field of gene therapy and tissue engineering. We developed a second-generation nanovector by successfully coupling folic acid to the polymer (Mansouri et al., 2006). One strategy for improving transfection is to take advantage of the mechanism of folate-mediated uptake by cells to promote targeting and internalization, hence improving transfection efficiency. Folate-mediated transfection has been shown to facilitate DNA internalization into cells via membrane receptors both *in vitro* and *in vivo* (Sudimack & Lee, 2000). Expression of folate receptor (FR)-β in synovial mononuclear cells and CD14+ cells from patients with RA was described by 1999 (Nakashima-Matsushita et al., 1999). Articular macrophages isolated from rats with adjuvant-induced arthritis overexpress FRs and exhibit significantly higher binding capacity for folate conjugates than macrophages obtained from healthy rats (Turk et al., 2002). The wide distribution of FRs at the surface of activated macrophages in rheumatoid arthritis allows the use of folate as potential ligand for folate-targeted chitosan gene therapy. Our laboratory demonstrated that folate-chitosan DNA nanoparticle containing IL-1Ra has been shown to play a role to prevent abnormal osteoblast metabolism and bone damage in this adjuvant-induced arthritis model (Fernandes et al., 2008). It also allows a significant decrease of the inflammation in the rats' paw compared to untreated rats, proving indirectly the efficacy of the IL-1Ra protein treatment. Various inflammation markers (IL-1β and PGE$_2$)

showed a significant decrease in muscle and serum after the injection of the IL-1Ra protein demonstrating by direct evidence the efficacy of the administration technique to deliver efficient nanoparticles. Therefore, we have already shown it is possible to do gene therapy with IL-1Ra to decrease arthritis and have a positive effect on inflammation.

11. Acknowledgments

This work was supported by the grants from National Natural Science Foundation of China (No. 30811120440 and 30911120261), The Ministry of Science and Technology of China (No. S2011GR0323), Shanghai International Collaboration Foundation (No. 08410701800) and Canadian Institutes of Health Research (CCI-92212, CCL-99636 and CCM 104888). Dr Fernandes and Dr Benderdour are research scholars of *Fonds de la Recherche en santé du Québec* (FRSQ). Dr Tiera holds a post-PH D scholarship from UNESP - Brazil.

12. References

Alexander, B.L.; Ali, R.R.; Alton, E.W.; Bainbridge, J.W.; Braun, S.; Cheng, S.H.; Flotte, T.R.; Gaspar, H.B.; Grez, M.; Griesenbach, U.; Kaplit,t M.G.; Ott, M.G.; Seger, R.; Simons, M.; Thrasher, A.J.; Thrasher, A.Z. & Ylä-Herttuala, S. (2007). Progress and prospects: gene therapy clinical trials (part 1). *Gene Ther.*, 14, 1439-1447, ISSN 0969-7128

Aiba, S. (1993). Reactivity of partially N-acetylated chitosan in aqueous media, *Makromolekulare Chemie.*, 194(1), 65–75, ISSN 0025-116X

Andersen, M.O.; Howard, K.A. & Kjems, J. (2009). RNAi using a chitosan/siRNA nanoparticle system: in vitro and in vivo applications. *Methods Mol. Biol.*, 555, 77-86, ISSN 1064-3745

Andersen, M.O.; Howard, K.A.; Paludan, S.R.; Besenbacher, F. & Kjems,J. (2008). Delivery of siRNA from lyophilized polymeric surfaces. *Biomaterials*, 29, 506-512, ISSN 1043-1802

Baker, M. (2010a). RNA interference: From tools to therapies. *Nature*, 464, 1225, ISSN 0028-0836

Baker, M. (2010b). RNA interference: Homing in on delivery. *Nature*, 464, 1225-1228. ISSN 0028-0836

Berger, J.; Reist, M.; Mayer, J.M.; Felt, O. & Gurny, R. (2004). Structure and interactions in chitosan hydrogels formed by complexation or aggregation for biomedical applications. *Eur. J. Pharm. Biopharm.*, 57, 35-52, ISSN 0928-0987

Berger, J.; Reist, M.; Mayer, J.M.; Felt, O.; Peppas, N.A. & Gurny, R. (2004). Structure and interactions in covalently and ionically crosslinked chitosan hydrogels for biomedical applications. *Eur. J. Pharm. Biopharm.*, 57, 19-34, ISSN 0928-0987

Bertha, G.; Dautzenberg, H. & Peter, M.G. (1998). Physico-chemical characterization of chitosans varying in degree of acetylation. *Carbohydr. Polym.*, 36, 205-216, ISSN 0144-8617

Bertha, G. & Dautzenberg, H. (2002). The degree of acetylation of chitosans and its effect on the chain conformation in aqueous solution. *Carbohydr. Polym.*, 47, 39-51, ISSN 1043-1802

Bivas-Benita, M.; Laloup, M.; Versteyhe, S.; Dewit, J.; De, B.J.; Jongert, E. & Borchard, G. (2003). Generation of Toxoplasma gondii GRA1 protein and DNA vaccine loaded chitosan particles: preparation, characterization, and preliminary in vivo studies. *Int. J. Pharm.*, 266, 17-27, ISSN 0378-5173.

Borchard, G. (2001). Chitosans for gene delivery. *Adv. Drug Deliv. Rev.*, 52, 145-150, ISSN 0169-409X

Casé, A.H.; Picola, I.P.D.; Zaniquelli, M.E.D.Z.; Fernandes, J.C.; Sebastião Taboga, R.; Winnik, F.M. & Tiera, M.J. (2009). Physicochemical characterization of nanoparticles formed between DNA and phosphorylcholine substituted chitosans, *J. Colloid. Interface. Sci.*, 336, 125–133, ISSN 0021-9797

Castanotto, D. & Rossi, J.J. (2009). The promises and pitfalls of RNA-interference-based therapeutics. *Nature*, 457, 426-433, ISSN 0028-0836

Chae, S.Y.; Son, S.; Lee, M.; Jang, M.K. & Nah, J.W. (2005). Deoxycholic acid-conjugated chitosan oligosaccharide nanoparticles for efficient gene carrier. *J. Control Release*, 109, 330-344. ISSN 0168-3659

Chen, J.; Yang, W.L.; Li, G.; Qian, J.; Xue, J.L.; Fu, S.K. & Lu, D.R. (2004). Transfection of mEpo gene to intestinal epithelium in vivo mediated by oral delivery of chitosan-DNA nanoparticles. *World J. Gastroenterol.*, 10, 112-116, ISSN 1007-9327

Chen, M.; Granger, A.J.; Vanbrocklin, M.W.; Payne, W.S.; Hunt, H.; Zhang, H.; Dodgson, J.B. & Holmen, S.L. (2007). Inhibition of avian leukosis virus replication by vector-based RNA interference. *Virology*, 365, 464-472, ISSN 0042-6822

Corsi. K.; Chellat, F.; Yahia, L. & Fernandes, J.C. (2003). Mesenchymal stem cells, MG63 and HEK293 transfection using chitosan-DNA nanoparticles. *Biomaterials*, 24:1255-64, ISSN 0142-09612

Dautry-Varsat, A. (1986). Receptor-mediated endocytosis: the intracellular journey of transferrin and its receptor. *Biochimie*, 68, 375-381, ISSN 0300-9084

De Fougerolles, A.R. (2008). Delivery vehicles for small interfering RNA in vivo. *Hum. Gene Ther.*, 19, 125-132, ISSN 1043-0342

De la Fuente, M.; Seijo, B. & Alonso, M.J. (2008). Bioadhesive hyaluronan-chitosan nanoparticles can transport genes across the ocular mucosa and transfect ocular tissue. *Gene Ther.*, 15, 668-676, ISSN 0969-7128

Domard, A. & Rinaudo, M. (1983). Preparation and characterization of fully deacetylated chitosan. *Int. J. Biol. Macromol.*, 5, 49–53, ISSN 0141-8130

Dominska, M. & Dykxhoorn, D.M. (2010). Breaking down the barriers: siRNA delivery and endosome escape. *J. Cell Sci.*, 123, 1183-1189, ISSN 1477-9137

Fernandes, J.; Tardif, G.; Martel-Pelletier, J., Lascau-Coman, V., Dupuis, M., Moldovan, F., Sheppard, M., Krishnan, B.R. & J.P. (1999). In vivo transfer of interleukin-1 receptor antagonist gene in osteoarthritic rabbit knee joints: prevention of osteoarthritis progression. *Am. J. Pathol.*, 154, 1159-69, ISSN 1525-2191

Fernandes, J.C.; Wang, H.; Jreyssaty, C.; Benderdour, M.; Lavigne, P.; Qiu, X.; Winnik, F.M.; Zhang, X.; Dai, K. & Shi, Q. (2008). Bone-protective effects of nonviral gene therapy with folate-chitosan DNA nanoparticle containing interleukin-1 receptor antagonist gene in rats with adjuvant-induced arthritis. *Mol. Ther.*, 16, 1243-1251, ISSN 1525-0016

Franco, P.; Senso, A.; Oliveros, L. & Minguillon, C. (2001). Covalently bonded polysaccharide derivatives as chiral stationary phases in high-performance liquid chromatography. *J. Chromatogr. A*, 906, 155-170, ISSN 0021-9673

Gao, S.; Chen, J.; Xu, X.; Ding, Z.; Yang, Y.H.; Hua, Z. & Zhang, J. (2003). Galactosylated low molecular weight chitosan as DNA carrier for hepatocyte-targeting. *Int. J. Pharm.*, 255, 57-68, ISSN 0378-5173

Gao, S.; Dagnaes-Hansen, F.; Nielsen, E.J.; Wengel, J.; Besenbacher, F.; Howard, K.A. & Kjems, J. (2009). The effect of chemical modification and nanoparticle formulation on stability and biodistribution of siRNA in mice. *Mol. Ther.*, 17, 1225-1233, ISSN 1525-0016

Gao, X.; Kim, K.S. & Liu, D. (2007). Nonviral gene delivery: what we know and what is next. *AAPS. J.*, 9, E92-104, ISSN 1550-7416

Gao, Y.; Xu, Z.H.; Chen, S.W.; Gu, W.W.; Chen, L.L. & Li, Y.P. (2008). Arginine-chitosan/DNA self-assemble nanoparticles for gene delivery: In vitro characteristics and transfection efficiency. *Int. J. Pharm.*, 359, 241-246, ISSN 0378-5173

Gary, D.J.; Puri, N. & Won, Y.Y. (2007). Polymer-based siRNA delivery: perspectives on the fundamental and phenomenological distinctions from polymer-based DNA delivery. *J. Control Release*, 121, 64-73, ISSN 0168-3659

Germershaus, O.; Mao, S.; Sitterberg, J.; Bakowsky, U. & Kissel, T. (2008). Gene delivery using chitosan, trimethyl chitosan or polyethylenglycol-graft-trimethyl chitosan block copolymers: establishment of structure-activity relationships in vitro. *J. Control Release*, 125, 145-154, ISSN 0168-3659

Giannoudis, P.V.; Tzioupis, C.C. & Tsiridis, E. (2006). Gene therapy in orthopaedics. *Injury*, 37 Suppl 1, S30-S40, ISSN 0020-1383

Godbey, W.T.; Wu, K.K. & Mikos, A.G. (1999). Size matters: molecular weight affects the efficiency of poly(ethylenimine) as a gene delivery vehicle. *J. Biomed. Mater. Res.*, 45, 268-275, ISSN 1549-3296

Guibal, E. (2004). Interactions of metal ions with chitosan-based sorbents: a review. *Separ. Purific. Techn.*, 38, 43-74, ISSN 1383-5866

Guo, T.; Zhao, J.; Chang, J.; Ding, Z.; Hong, H.; Chen, J. & Zhang, J. (2006). Porous chitosan-gelatin scaffold containing plasmid DNA encoding transforming growth factor-beta1 for chondrocytes proliferation. *Biomaterials*, 27, 1095-1103, ISSN 0142-9612

Hacein-Bey-Abina, S.; von, K.C.; Schmidt, M.; Le, D.F.; Wulffraat, N.; McIntyre, E.; Radford, I.; Villeval, J.L.; Fraser, C.C.; Cavazzana-Calvo, M. & Fischer, A. (2003). A serious adverse event after successful gene therapy for X-linked severe combined immunodeficiency. *N. Engl. J Med*, 348, 255-256, ISSN 0028-4793

Hammond, S.M.; Bernstein, E.; Beach, D. & Hannon, G.J. (2000). An RNA-directed nuclease mediates post-transcriptional gene silencing in Drosophila cells. *Nature*, 404, 293-296, ISSN 0028-0836

Harris, J.M., Struk, E.C., Case, M.G., Paley, M.S., Yalpani, M., Van Alstin, J.M. & Brooks, D.E. (1984). Synthesis and Characterization of Poly(ethylene Glycol) Derivatives. J. Polym. Sci. Polym. Chem. Ed. 22, 341–352, ISSN 0360-6376

Hillaireau, H. & Couvreur, P. (2009). Nanocarriers' entry into the cell: relevance to drug delivery. *Cell Mol. Life Sci.*, 66, 2873-2896, ISSN 1420-682X

Howard, K.A., Paludan, S.R., Behlke, M.A., Besenbacher, F., Deleuran, B. & Kjems, J. (2009). Chitosan/siRNA nanoparticle-mediated TNF-alpha knockdown in peritoneal macrophages for anti-inflammatory treatment in a murine arthritis model. *Mol. Ther.*, 17, 162-168, ISSN 1525-0016

Howard, K.A., Rahbek, U.L., Liu, X., Damgaard, C.K., Glud, S.Z., Andersen, M.O., Hovgaard, M.B., Schmitz, A., Nyengaard, J.R., Besenbacher, F. & Kjems, J. (2006). RNA interference in vitro and in vivo using a novel chitosan/siRNA nanoparticle system. *Mol. Ther.*, 14, 476-484, ISSN 1525-0016

Huang, M., Fong, C.W., Khor, E. & Lim, L.Y. (2005). Transfection efficiency of chitosan vectors: effect of polymer molecular weight and degree of deacetylation. *J. Control Release*, 106, 391-406, ISSN 0168-3659

Hung, T.H.; Chang, Y.M.; Sung, H.Y. & Chang, C.T. (2002). Purification and characterization of hydrolase with chitinase and chitosanase activity from commercial stem bromelain, *J. Agric. Food Chem.*, 50, 4666-4673, ISSN 0021-8561

Hyde, S.C., Southern, K.W., Gileadi, U., Fitzjohn, E.M., Mofford, K.A., Waddell, B.E., Gooi, H.C., Goddard, C.A., Hannavy, K., Smyth, S.E., Egan, J.J., Sorgi, F.L., Huang, L., Cuthbert, A.W., Evans, M.J., Colledge, W.H., Higgins, C.F., Webb, A.K. & Gill, D.R. (2000). Repeat administration of DNA/liposomes to the nasal epithelium of patients with cystic fibrosis. *Gene Ther.*, 7, 1156-1165, ISSN 0969-7128

Ishii, T., Okahata, Y. & Sato, T. (2001). Mechanism of cell transfection with plasmid/chitosan complexes. *Biochim. Biophys. Acta*, 1514, 51-64, ISSN 0006-3002

Jackson, A.L. & Linsley, P.S. (2010). Recognizing and avoiding siRNA off-target effects for target identification and therapeutic application. *Nat. Rev. Drug. Discov.*, 9, 57-67, ISSN 1474-1776

Janes, K.A.; Calvo, P. & Alonso, M.J. (2001). Polysaccharide colloidal particles as delivery systems for macromolecules. *Adv. Drug Deliv. Rev.*, 47, 83–97, ISSN 0169-409X

Jang, M.K.; Kong, B.G; Jeong, Y.I.; Lee, C.H. & Nah, J.W. (2004). Physicochemical Characterization of α-Chitin, β-Chitin, and γ-Chitin Separated from Natural Resources. *J. Polym. Sci. Pol. Chem.*, 42, 3423–3432, ISSN 1099-0518.

Jiang, H.L., Kim, Y.K., Arote, R., Nah, J.W., Cho, M.H., Choi, Y.J., Akaike, T. & Cho, C.S. (2007). Chitosan-graft-polyethylenimine as a gene carrier. *J. Control Release*, 117, 273-280, ISSN 0168-3659

Jiang, H.L.; Kim, Y.K.; Lee, S.M.; Park, M.R.; Kim, E.M.; Jin, Y.M.; Arote, R.; Jeong, H.J.; Song, S.C.; Cho, M.H. & Cho, C.S. (2010). Galactosylated chitosan-g-PEI/DNA complexes-loaded poly(organophosphazene) hydrogel as a hepatocyte targeting gene delivery system. *Arch. Pharm. Res.*, 33, 551, ISSN 0253-6269

Jones, R.A., Cheung, C.Y., Black, F.E., Zia, J.K., Stayton, P.S., Hoffman, A.S. & Wilson, M.R. (2003). Poly(2-alkylacrylic acid) polymers deliver molecules to the cytosol by pH-sensitive disruption of endosomal vesicles. *Biochem. J.*, 372, 65-75, ISSN 0264-6021

Kaiser, J. (2007). Clinical research. Death prompts a review of gene therapy vector. *Science*, 317, 580. ISSN 0036-8075

Katas, H. & Alpar, H.O. (2006). Development and characterisation of chitosan nanoparticles for siRNA delivery. *J. Control Release*, 115, 216-225, ISSN 0168-3659

Katas, H., Chen, S., Osamuyimen, A.A., Cevher, E. & Oya, A.H. (2008). Effect of preparative variables on small interfering RNA loaded Poly(D,L-lactide-co-glycolide)-chitosan submicron particles prepared by emulsification diffusion method. *J. Microencapsul.*, 25, 541-548, ISSN 0265-2048

Kato, Y.; Onishi, H. & Machida, Y. (2004). N-succinyl-chitosan as a drug carrier: water-insoluble and water-soluble conjugates. *Biomaterials*, 25, 907-915, ISSN 0142-9612

Kean, T. & Thanou, M. (2010). Biodegradation, biodistribution and toxicity of chitosan. *Adv. Drug Deliv. Rev.*, 62, 3-11. ISSN 0169-409X

Khatri, K., Goyal, A.K., Gupta, P.N., Mishra, N. & Vyas, S.P. (2008). Plasmid DNA loaded chitosan nanoparticles for nasal mucosal immunization against hepatitis B. *Int. J. Pharm.*, 354, 235-241, ISSN 0378-5173

Kiang, T., Wen, J., Lim, H.W. & Leong, K.W. (2004). The effect of the degree of chitosan deacetylation on the efficiency of gene transfection. *Biomaterials*, 25, 5293-5301, ISSN 1043-1802

Kim, T.H., Ihm, J.E., Choi, Y.J., Nah, J.W. & Cho, C.S. (2003). Efficient gene delivery by urocanic acid-modified chitosan. *J. Control Release*, 93, 389-402, ISSN 0168-3659

Kim, T.H., Kim, S.I., Akaike, T. & Cho, C.S. (2005). Synergistic effect of poly(ethylenimine) on the transfection efficiency of galactosylated chitosan/DNA complexes. *J. Control Release*, 105, 354-366, ISSN 0168-3659

Kim, T.H., Nah, J.W., Cho, M.H., Park, T.G. & Cho, C.S. (2006). Receptor-mediated gene delivery into antigen presenting cells using mannosylated chitosan/DNA nanoparticles. *J. Nanosci. Nanotechnol.*, 6, 2796-2803, ISSN 1533-4880

Kumar, M.N.V.R.; Muzzarelli, R.A.A.; Muzzarelli, C.; Sashiwa, H. & Domb, A.J. (2004). Chitosan chemistry and pharmaceutical perspectives. *Chem. Rev.*, 104, 6017-6084, ISSN 0009-2665

Kumar, A.B.V. & Tharanathan, R.N. (2004). A comparative study on depolymerization of chitosan by proteolytic enzymes, *Carbohydr. Polym.* 58, 275-283, ISSN 0144-8617

Kumar, A.B.V.; Varadaraj, M. C.; Lalitha, R.G. & Tharanathan, R.N. (2004). Low molecular weight chitosans: preparation with the aid of papain and characterization, *Biochim. Biophys. Acta-Gen. Sub.* 1670, 137-146, ISSN 0304-4165

Kurita. K. (2001). Controlled functionalization of polysaccharide chitin. *Prog. Polym. Sci.*, 26, 1921-1971, ISSN 0340-255X

Kurita, K.; Ishii, S.; Tomita, K.; Nishimura, S.I. & Shlmoda, K. (1994) Reactivity characteristics of squid beta-chitin as compared with those of shrimp chitin: High potentials of squid chitin as a starting material for facile chemical modifications. *J. Polym. Sci. Pol. Chem.*, 32, 1027-1032, ISSN 1099-0518

Kuroiwa, T.; Ichikawa, S.; Sato, S. & Mukataka, S. (2003). Improvement of the yield of physiologically active oligosaccharides in continuous hydrolysis of chitosan using immobilized chitosanases. *Biotechn. Bioeng.*, 84 , 121-127, ISSN 0006-3592.

Kwon, S.; Park, J.H.; Chung, H.; Kwon, I.C. & Jeong, S.Y. (2003). Physicochemical Characteristics of Self-Assembled Nanoparticles Based on Glycol Chitosan Bearing 5β-Cholanic Acid. *Langmuir*, 19, 10188-10193, ISSN 0743-7463

Lameiro, M.H., Malpique, R., Silva, A.C., Alves, P.M. & Melo, E. (2006). Encapsulation of adenoviral vectors into chitosan-bile salt microparticles for mucosal vaccination. *J. Biotechnol.*, 126, 152-162, ISSN 0168-1656

Lavertu, M., Methot, S., Tran-Khanh, N. & Buschmann, M.D. (2006). High efficiency gene transfer using chitosan/DNA nanoparticles with specific combinations of molecular weight and degree of deacetylation. *Biomaterials*, 27, 4815-4824, ISSN 1043-1802

Lee, K.Y.; Ha, W.S. & Park, W.H. (1995) Blood compatibility and biodegradability of partially N-acylated chitosan derivatives. *Biomaterials*, 16, 1211-1216, ISSN 1043-1802

Lee, K.Y., Kwon, I.C., Kim, Y.H., Jo, W.H. & Jeong, S.Y. (1998). Preparation of chitosan self-aggregates as a gene delivery system. *J. Control Release*, 51, 213-220, ISSN 0168-3659

Lee, D., Lockey, R. & Mohapatra, S. (2006). Folate receptor-mediated cancer cell specific gene delivery using folic acid-conjugated oligochitosans. *J. Nanosci. Nanotechnol.*, 6, 2860-2866, ISSN 1533-4880

Lee, D., Zhang, W., Shirley, S.A., Kong, X., Hellermann, G.R., Lockey, R.F. & Mohapatra, S.S. (2007). Thiolated chitosan/DNA nanocomplexes exhibit enhanced and sustained gene delivery. *Pharm. Res.*, 24, 157-167, ISSN 0724-8741

Lee, M.Y.; Var, F.; Shin-ya, Y.; Kajiuchi, T. & Yang, J.W. (1999). Optimum conditions for the precipitation of chitosan oligomers with DP 5-7 in concentrated hydrochloric acid at low temperature. *Proc. Biochem*, 34, 493–500, ISSN 1359-5113

Leong, K.W.; Mao, H.Q.; Truong-Le, V.L.; Roy, K.; Walsh, S.M. & August, J.T. (1998). DNA-polycation nanospheres as non-viral gene delivery vehicles. *J. Control Release.*, 53, 183–193, ISSN 0168-3659

Li, S.D. & Huang, L. (2006). Gene therapy progress and prospects: non-viral gene therapy by systemic delivery. *Gene Ther.*, 13, 1313-1319, ISSN 0969-7128

Lin, H.; Wang, H. Y.; Xue, C.H. M. Y, (2002). Preparation of chitosan oligomers by immobilized papain. *Enzyme Microbial Technology*, 31,588-592, ISSN 0141- 0229

Liu, D. & Knapp, J.E. (2001). Hydrodynamics-based gene delivery. *Curr. Opin. Mol. Ther.*, 3, 192-197, ISSN 1093-4715

Liu, X., Howard, K.A., Dong, M., Andersen, M.O., Rahbek, U.L., Johnsen, M.G., Hansen, O.C., Besenbacher, F. & Kjems, J. (2007). The influence of polymeric properties on chitosan/siRNA nanoparticle formulation and gene silencing. *Biomaterials*, 28, 1280-1288, ISSN 1043-1802

Liu, W.G.; Zhang, J.R.; Cao, Z.Q.; Xu, F.Y. & Yao, K.D. (2004). A chitosan-arginine conjugate as a novel anticoagulation biomaterial. *J. Mater. Sci. Mater. Med.*, 15, 1199–1203, ISSN 0957-4530.

Liu, W.G. & Yao, K.D. (2002). Chitosan and its derivatives—a promising non-viral vector for gene transfection. *J. Control Release*, 83, 1-11, ISSN 0168-3659

Mansouri, S.; Cui, Y.; Winnik, F.; Shi, Q.; Benderdour, M.; Lavigne, P.; Beaumont, E. & Fernandes, J.C. (2006). Characterization of Folate-Chitosan-DNA nanoparticles for gene therapy. *Biomaterials*, 27, 2060-2065, ISSN 0142-9612

Mao, S.; Shuai, X.; Unger, F. Simona, M., Kissel, D., & Bi, T. (2004). The depolymerization of chitosan: effects on physicochemical and biological properties. *Int. J. Pharm.*, 281, 45–54, ISSN 0378-5173

Mingozzi, F. & High, K.A. (2007). Immune Responses to AAV in Clinical Trials. *Curr. Gene Ther.*, 7, 316-324, ISSN 1566-5232

Moghimi, S.M., Hunter, A.C. & Murray, J.C. (2005). Nanomedicine: current status and future prospects. *FASEB J.*, 19, 311-330, ISSN 0892 6638

Mook, O.R., Baas, F., de Wissel, M.B. & Fluiter, K. (2007). Evaluation of locked nucleic acid-modified small interfering RNA in vitro and in vivo. *Mol. Cancer Ther.*, 6, 833-843, ISSN 1535-7163

Morris, V.B. & Sharma C.P. (2010). Folate mediated in vitro targeting of depolymerised trimethylated chitosan having arginine functionality. *J. Coll. Interf. Sci.*, 348, 360-368, ISSN 0021-9797

Muzzarelli, R.A.A.; Terbojevich, M.; Muzzarelli, C. & Francescangeli, O. (2002). Chitosans depolymerized with the aid of papain and stabilized as glycosylamines. *Carbohydr. Polym.*, 50, 69-78, ISSN 0144-8617

Nakashima-Matsushita, N., Homma, T., Yu, S., Matsuda, T., Sunahara, N., Nakamura, T., Tsukano, M., Ratnam, M. & Matsuyama, T. (1999). Selective expression of folate receptor beta and its possible role in methotrexate transport in synovial macrophages from patients with rheumatoid arthritis. *Arthritis Rheum.*, 42, 1609-1616, ISSN 1529-0131

No, H.K. & Meyers, S.P. (1989). Crawfish chitosan as a coagulant in recovery of organic compounds from seafood processing streams. *J. Agric. Food Chem.* 37, 580-583, ISSN 0021-8561

Okamoto, H., Shiraki, K., Yasuda, R., Danjo, K. & Watanabe, Y. (2010). Chitosan-interferon-beta gene complex powder for inhalation treatment of lung metastasis in mice. *J. Control Release.* 2010 Dec 23. [Epub ahead of print, ISSN 0168-3659

Ouchi, T.; Nishizawa, H. & Ohya, Y. (1998). Aggregation phenomenon of PEG-grafted chitosan in aqueous solution. *Polymer*, 39, 5171-5175, ISSN 0032-3861

Pa, J.H. & Yu T.L. (2001). Light scattering study of chitosan in acetic acid aqueous solutions. *Macromol. Chem. Phys.*, 202, 985-991, ISSN 1022-1352

Park, I.K.; Ihm, J.E.; Park, Y.H.; Choi Y.J.; Kim, S.I.; Kim W.J.; Akaike, T. & Cho, C.S. (2003). Galactosylated chitosan (GC)-graft-poly(vinyl pyrrolidone) (PVP) as hepatocyte-targeting DNA carrier Preparation and physicochemical characterization of GC-graft-PVP/DNA complex. *J. Control Release*, 86: 349-359, ISSN 0168-3659.

Park, I.K., Park, Y.H., Shin, B.A., Choi, E.S., Kim, Y.R., Akaike, T. & Cho, C.S. (2000). Galactosylated chitosan-graft-dextran as hepatocyte-targeting DNA carrier. *J. Control Release*, 69, 97-108, ISSN 0168-3659

Pelletier, J.P., Caron, J.P., Evans, C., Robbins, P.D., Georgescu, H.I., Jovanovic, D., Fernandes, J.C. & Martel-Pelletier, J. (1997). In vivo suppression of early experimental osteoarthritis by interleukin-1 receptor antagonist using gene therapy. Arthritis Rheum., 40, 1012-9, ISSN 1529-0131

Ping, Y.A.; Liu, C.D.; Tang, G.P.; Li, J.S.; Li, J.; Yang, W.T. & Xu, F.J. (2010). Functionalization of chitosan via atom transfer radical polymerization for gene delivery. *Adv. Funct. Mater.*, 20, 3106-3116, ISSN 1616-3028

Rabea, E.I.; Badawy, M.E.T.; Stevens, C.V.; Smagghe, G. & Steurbaut, W. (2003). Chitosan as Antimicrobial Agent: applications and mode of action. *Biomacromolecules*, 4, 1457-1465, ISSN 1525-7797

Ramesh, R., Saeki, T., Templeton, N.S., Ji, L., Stephens, L.C., Ito, I., Wilson, D.R., Wu, Z., Branch, C.D., Minna, J.D. & Roth, J.A. (2001). Successful treatment of primary and disseminated human lung cancers by systemic delivery of tumor suppressor genes using an improved liposome vector. *Mol. Ther.*, 3, 337-350, ISSN 1525-0016

Raper, S.E., Chirmule, N., Lee, F.S., Wivel, N.A., Bagg, A., Gao, G.P., Wilson, J.M. & Batshaw, M.L. (2003). Fatal systemic inflammatory response syndrome in a ornithine transcarbamylase deficient patient following adenoviral gene transfer. *Mol. Genet. Metab,* 80, 148-158, ISSN 1096-7192

Richardson, S.C., Kolbe, H.V. & Duncan, R. (1999). Potential of low molecular mass chitosan as a DNA delivery system: biocompatibility, body distribution and ability to complex and protect DNA. *Int. J. Pharm.,* 178, 231-243, ISSN 0378-5173

Roberts, G.A.F. (1992). *Chitin Chemistry,* Mc Millan Press Ltd, London, ISBN 0333524179

Rojanarata, T., Opanasopit, P., Techaarpornkul, S., Ngawhirunpat, T. & Ruktanonchai, U. (2008). Chitosan-thiamine pyrophosphate as a novel carrier for siRNA delivery. *Pharm. Res.,* 25, 2807-2814. ISSN 0724-8741

Romero, N.B., Braun, S., Benveniste, O., Leturcq, F., Hogrel, J.Y., Morris, G.E., Barois, A., Eymard, B., Payan, C., Ortega, V., Boch, A.L., Lejean, L., Thioudellet, C., Mourot, B., Escot, C., Choquel, A., Recan, D., Kaplan, J.C., Dickson, G., Klatzmann, D., Molinier-Frenckel, V., Guillet, J.G., Squiban, P., Herson, S. & Fardeau, M. (2004). Phase I study of dystrophin plasmid-based gene therapy in Duchenne/Becker muscular dystrophy. *Hum. Gene Ther.,* 15, 1065-1076. ISSN 1043-0342

Sakurai, H., Kawabata, K., Sakurai, F., Nakagawa, S. & Mizuguchi, H. (2008). Innate immune response induced by gene delivery vectors. *Int. J Pharm.,* 354, 9-15, ISSN 0378-5173

Saito, H.; Wu, Sato, T.; Nagasaki, T.; Sakairi, N. & Shinkai, S. (2004). 6-Amino-6-deoxychitosan (2004) Preparation and application as plasmid vector in COS-1 cells. *Chem. Lett.,* 33: 340-341, ISSN 0366-7022

Saito, H.; Wu, X.; Harris, J.M. & Hoffman, A.S. (1997). Graft copolymers of poly(ethylene glycol) (PEG) and chitosan. *Macromol. Rapid Commun.,* 18, 547-550, ISSN 1022-1336

Sato, T., Ishii, T. & Okahata,Y. (2001). In vitro gene delivery mediated by chitosan. effect of pH, serum, and molecular mass of chitosan on the transfection efficiency. *Biomaterials,* 22, 2075-2080, ISSN 0142-9612

Satoh, T.; Kakimoto, S.; Kano, H.; Nakatani, M.; Shinkai, S. & Nagasaki, T. (2007). In vitro gene delivery to HepG2 cells using galactosylated 6-amino-6-deoxychitosan as a DNA carrier. *Carbohydr. Res.,* 342, 1427–1433, ISSN 0008-6215

Schaffer, D.V., Fidelman, N.A., Dan, N. & Lauffenburger, D.A. (2000). Vector unpacking as a potential barrier for receptor-mediated polyplex gene delivery. *Biotechnol. Bioeng.,* 67, 598-606, ISSN 0006 3592

Schatz, C.; Viton, C.; Delair, T.; Pichot, C. & Domard, A. (2003). Typical physicochemical behaviors of chitosan in aqueous solution. *Biomacromolecules,* 4, 641-648, ISSN 1525-7797

Seiler, M.P., Cerullo, V. & Lee, B. (2007). Immune response to helper dependent adenoviral mediated liver gene therapy: challenges and prospects. *Curr. Gene Ther.,* 7, 297-305, ISSN 1566-5232

Shimojohay, M.; Fukushimab, K. & Kurita. K. (1998). Low-molecular-weight chitosans derived from P-chitin: preparation, molecular characteristics and aggregation activity. *Carbohydr. Polym.,* 35, 223-231, ISSN 0144-8617

Signini, R.; Desbrieres, J. & Campana Filho, S.P. (2000). On the stiffness of chitosan hydrochloride in acid-free aqueous solutions. *Carbohydr. Polym.* 43, 351–357. ISSN 1043-1802

Sinha, V.R.; Singla, A.K.; Wadhawan, S.; Kaushik, R.; Kumria, R.; Bansal, K. & Dhawan, S. (2004). Chitosan microspheres as a potential carrier for drugs. *Int. J. Pharm. 274*, 1-33, ISSN 0378-5173

Sinnott, M.L. (1990). Catalytic mechanism of enzymic glycosyl transfer. *Chem. Rev.*, 90, 1171–1202, ISSN 0009-2665

Suda, T. & Liu, D. (2007). Hydrodynamic gene delivery: its principles and applications. *Mol. Ther.*, 15, 2063-2069, ISSN 1525-0016

Sudimack, J. & Lee, R.J. (2000). Targeted drug delivery via the folate receptor. *Adv. Drug Deliv. Rev.*, 41, 147-162, ISSN 0169-409X

Suh, J., Wirtz, D. & Hanes, J. (2003). Efficient active transport of gene nanocarriers to the cell nucleus. *Proc. Natl. Acad. Sci. U. S. A*, 100, 3878-3882. ISSN 2227 8424

Sun, S., Liu, W., Cheng, N., Zhang, B., Cao, Z., Yao, K., Liang, D., Zuo, A., Guo, G. & Zhang, J. (2005). A thermoresponsive chitosan-NIPAAm/vinyl laurate copolymer vector for gene transfection. *Bioconjug. Chem.*, 16, 972-980, ISSN 1043-1802

Sun, B.; Zhao, R.L.; Kong, F.Q.; Ren, Y.P.; Zuo, A.J.; Liang, D.C.; Zhang, J.Y. (2010). Phosphorylatable short peptide conjugation for facilitating transfection efficacy of CS/DNA complex. *Int. J. Pharm.*, 397: 206-210, ISSN 0378-5173

Tahara, K., Sakai, T., Yamamoto, H., Takeuchi, H. & Kawashima, Y. (2008). Establishing chitosan coated PLGA nanosphere platform loaded with wide variety of nucleic acid by complexation with cationic compound for gene delivery. *Int. J. Pharm.*, 354, 210-216, ISSN 0378-5173

Tan, W.B., Jiang, S. & Zhang,Y. (2007). Quantum-dot based nanoparticles for targeted silencing of HER2/neu gene via RNA interference. *Biomaterials*, 28, 1565-1571, ISSN 1043-1802

Tang, E.S.K.; Huang, M. & Lim, L.Y. (2003). Ultrasonication of chitosan and chitosan nanoparticles. *Int. J. Pharm.*, 265,103–114, ISSN 0378-5173

Techaarpornkul, S., Wongkupasert, S., Opanasopit, P., Apirakaramwong, A., Nunthanid, J. & Ruktanonchai, U. (2010). Chitosan-mediated siRNA delivery in vitro: effect of polymer molecular weight, concentration and salt forms. *AAPS. PharmSciTech.*, 11, 64-72, ISSN 1530-9932

Terbojevich, M.; Cosani, A. & Muzzarelli, R.A.A. (1996). Molecular parameters of chitosans depolymerized with the aid of papain, *Carbohydr. Polym.*, 29, 63-68, ISSN 0144-8617

Tiera, M.J.; Qiu, X.P.; Bechaouch, S.; Shi, Q.; Fernandes, J.C. & Winnik, F.M. (2006). Synthesis and Characterization of Phosphorylcholine-Substituted Chitosans Soluble in Physiological pH Conditions. *Biomacromolecules*, 7, 3151-3156, ISSN 1525-7797

Tolaimate, A.; Desbrieres, J.; Rhazi, M.; Alagui, A.; Vincendon, M. & Vottero, P. (2000). On the influence of deacetylation process on the physicochemical characteristics of chitosan from squid chitin. *Polymer*, 41, 2463–2469, ISSN 0032-3861

Tolaimate, A.; Desbrieres, J.; Rhazia, M. & Alagui, A. (2003). Contribution to the preparation of chitins and chitosans with controlled physico-chemical properties, *Polymer*, 44, 7939–7952. ISSN 0032-3861

Tong, H., Qin, S., Fernandes, J.C., Li, L., Dai, K. & Zhang, X. (2009). Progress and prospects of chitosan and its derivatives as non-viral gene vectors in gene therapy. *Curr. Gene Ther.*, 9, 495-502, ISSN 1566-5232

Tsaih, M.L. & Chen, R.H. (2003). Effect of degree of deacetylation of chitosan on the kinetics of ultrasonic degradation of chitosan. *J. Appl. Polym. Sci.* 90, 3526-3531, ISSN 0021-8995

Turk, M.J., Breur, G.J., Widmer, W.R., Paulos, C.M., Xu, L.C., Grote, L.A. & Low, P.S. (2002). Folate-targeted imaging of activated macrophages in rats with adjuvant-induced arthritis. *Arthritis Rheum.*, 46, 1947-1955, ISSN 1529-0131

Ulrich-Vinther, M. (2007). Gene therapy methods in bone and joint disorders. Evaluation of the adeno-associated virus vector in experimental models of articular cartilage disorders, periprosthetic osteolysis and bone healing. *Acta Orthop Suppl*, 78, 1-64, ISSN 1745-3674

Vaishnaw, A.K., Gollob, J., Gamba-Vitalo, C., Hutabarat, R., Sah, D., Meyers, R., de, F.T. & Maraganore, J. (2010). A status report on RNAi therapeutics. *Silence.*, 1, 14, ISSN 1758-907X

Vandenberghe, L.H. & Wilson, J.M. (2007). AAV as An Immunogen. *Curr. Gene Ther.*, 7, 325-333, ISSN 1566-5232

Wang, J., Lu, Z., Wientjes, M.G. & Au, J.L. (2010). Delivery of siRNA Therapeutics: Barriers and Carriers. *AAPS. J.*, 12(4):492-503, ISSN 1550-7416

Whittaker, G.R. & Helenius, A. (1998). Nuclear import and export of viruses and virus genomes. *Virology*, 246, 1-23, ISSN 0042-6822

Wong, K., Sun, G., Zhang, X., Dai, H., Liu, Y., He, C. & Leong, K.W. (2006). PEI-g-chitosan, a novel gene delivery system with transfection efficiency comparable to polyethylenimine in vitro and after liver administration in vivo. *Bioconjug. Chem.*, 17, 152-158, ISSN 1043-1802

Varma, A.J.; Deshpande, S.V. & Kennedy, J.F. (2004). Metal complexation by chitosan and its derivatives: a review. *Carbohydr. Polym.*, 55, 77-93, ISSN 0144-8617

Varurn, K.M.; Myhr, M.M.; Hjerde, R.J.N. & Smidsrod, O. (1997). In vitro degradation rates of partially N-acetylated chitosans in human serum, *Carbohydr. Res.*, 299, 99- 101, ISSN 0144-8617

Xia, W., Liu, W., Cui, L., Liu, Y., Zhong, W., Liu, D., Wu, J., Chua, K. & Cao, Y. (2004). Tissue engineering of cartilage with the use of chitosan-gelatin complex scaffolds. *J Biomed Mater Res B Appl Biomater.*, 15:71(2), 373-80, ISSN 1552-4973

Yang, P.T., Hoang, L., Jia, W.W. & Skarsgard, E.D. (2010). In Utero Gene Delivery Using Chitosan-DNA Nanoparticles in Mice. *J. Surg. Res.*, 2010 Jun 12. [Epub ahead of print], ISSN 0022-4804

Yip, V.L.Y. & Withers, S.G. (2004). Nature's many mechanisms for the degradation of oligosaccharides. *Org. Biol. Chem.*, 2, 2707–2713.

Yoo, H.S., Lee, J.E., Chung, H., Kwon, I.C.& Jeong, S.Y. (2005). Self-assembled nanoparticles containing hydrophobically modified glycol chitosan for gene delivery. *J. Control Release*, 103, 235-243, ISSN 0168-3659

Yu, B., Zhao, X., Lee, L.J. & Lee, R.J. (2009). Targeted delivery systems for oligonucleotide therapeutics. *AAPS. J.*, 11, 195-203, ISSN 1550-7416

Yu, Y.Y.; Wang, Z.; Cai, L.; Wang, G.; Yang, X.; Wan, X.P.; Xu, X.H.; Li, Y. & Gao R. (2010). Synthesis and characterization of methoxy poly(ethylene glycol)-O-chitosan-polyethylenimine for gene delivery. *Carbohydr. Polym.* 81. 269-274, ISSN 0144-8617

Zeng, J.M.; Wang, X. & Wang, S. (2007). Self-assembled ternary complexes of plasmid DNA, low molecular weight polyethylenimine and targeting peptide for nonviral gene delivery into neurons. *Biomaterials*, 28: 1443-1451, ISSN 0142-9612

Zelphati, O., Uyechi, L.S., Barron, L.G. & Szoka, F.C., Jr. (1998). Effect of serum components on the physico-chemical properties of cationic lipid/oligonucleotide complexes and on their interactions with cells. *Biochim. Biophys. Acta*, 1390, 119-133.

Zhang, S., Zhao, B., Jiang, H., Wang, B. & Ma, B. (2007). Cationic lipids and polymers mediated vectors for delivery of siRNA. *J. Control Release*, 123, 1-10, , ISSN 0168-3659

Zhang, Y., Chen, J., Zhang, Y., Pan, Y., Zhao, J., Ren, L., Liao, M., Hu, Z., Kong, L. & Wang, J. (2007). A novel PEGylation of chitosan nanoparticles for gene delivery. *Biotechnol. Appl. Biochem.*, 46, 197-204, ISSN 0885-4513

3

PAMAM Dendrimer as Potential Delivery System for Combined Chemotherapeutic and MicroRNA-21 Gene Therapy

Xuan Zhou, Yu Ren, Xubo Yuan, Peiyu Pu and Chunsheng Kang
Department of Neurosurgery, Laboratory of Neuro-Oncology, Tianjin Medical University
Tianjin research center of basic medical science, Tianjin medical university
First Department of Head and Neck Cancer
Tianjin Medical University Cancer Institute & Hospital
School of Materials Science & Engineering, Tianjin University
China

1. Introduction

Chemotherapeutic drugs are fundamental in cancer management and are responsible for most cases of adjuvant treatment in patients after surgical procedures. However, the median overall survival does not increase in patients treated by concurrent chemo-radiotherapy. Consequently, further studies that could enhance the therapeutic effect should be encouraged [1].

Although the biological functions of microRNAs (miRNA) are not completely revealed, there is growing evidence that miRNA pathways are a new mechanism of gene regulation in both normal and diseased conditions [2]. Recent evidence has shown that miRNA mutations or aberrant expression patterns correlate with various diseases, such as cancer, viral infections, cardiovascular and indicates that miRNAs can function as tumor suppressors and oncogenes and oretically become a target to enhance the chemotherapeutic effect in cancer therapy.

However, although much work has been accomplished, the development of an efficient delivery system still remain a major challenge for the wide application of miRNA. In the following sections -- after a brief introduction of the miRNA strategies -- the potential and contributions of dendrimers in the development of effective non-viral delivery systems for combined the microRNA therapy with drug delivery will be discussed.

2. MicroRNA strategy

MicroRNAs (miRNAs) are a class of naturally occurring small non-coding RNAs, approximately 22 nucleotides in length, that target protein-coding mRNAs at the post-transcriptional level [4]. Generally, mature miRNAs are integrated into a protein RNA complex called a microRNA RNPs (similar to the RISCs (RNA-induced silencing complexes) for siRNA). miRNAs bind through partial sequence homology to the 3_-untranslated regions (3'-UTRs) of target genes. Because of this unique feature, a single miRNA has multiple targets. It is thought that more than 30% of human genes are posttranscriptionally regulated by miRNAs [5]. miRNAs have diverse functions in biological processes, including the regulation of cellular proliferation, differentiation, and cell death. As dysregulation of these biological processes frequently occur in human cancer, miRNAs may, therefore, play a critical role in the process of tumorigenesis.

This regulatory mechanism was first shown in the developmental processes in worms, flies, and plants [6]. Subsequently, miRNAs have been shown to have important roles in many physiological processes of mammalian systems by influencing cell apoptosis, development, and metabolism through regulation of critical signaling molecules including cytokines, growth factors, transcription factors, and pro-apoptotic and anti-apoptotic proteins. Increasing number of miRNAs have been identified in the human genome and they are collectively called the miRNome [7]. Accumulating evidence shows the potential involvement of altered regulation of miRNAs in initiation and progression in a wide range of human cancers. Altered expression profiles of miRNAs are associated with genetic and epigenetic alterations including deletion, amplification, point mutation, and aberrant DNA methylation.

2.1 miR-21 general aspects

MiR-21 has been identified as the best hit in a number of miRNA profiling studies designed for the detection of miRNAs dysregulated in human cancer [8]. MiR-21 could suppress several tumor suppressor proteins translation, including PTEN, PDCD4, TMP1 and p53, to mediated cancer cell malignant phenotype alternation [9-10]. MiR-21 was emerging as key regulators of multiple pathways involved in tumorgenesis and may become the next targeted therapies in human cancers [11]. Previously we identified miR-21's aberrant expression in glioblastoma(GBM), and we focused on in what way miR-21 regulated GBM development and progression. Thus, in the current chapter, we manage to elucidate the view point that miR-21 was an effective molecule with great potential of human cancer gene therapy; of course, we will take miR-21's biological role to GBM as an example.

Recent reports suggested that miR-21 functions as an oncogene in human cancers. Ciafre` et alprofiled the expression of 245 miRNAs in 10 glioblastoma (GBM) cell lines and nine freshly resected GBM samples and observed that miR-21 was overexpressed in human brain tumors [12]. It was shown that when miR-21 was suppressed, cell growth inhibition and caspase-dependent apoptosis were observed in A172, U87, LN229, and LN308 cells. It has been shown that miR-21 modulates breast cancer cell anchorage-independent growth through suppressing TMP1 expression. In human colorectal, breast cancer, and renal cell carcinoma, miR-21 contributes to invasion and metastasis cell by inhibiting Pdcd4 mRNA at the post-transcription level. A recent study showed that miR-21 targets PTEN gene through a binding site on the 3'-UTR in hepatocellular carcinoma [13]. PTEN has been shown to be a critical tumor suppressor gene that is commonly inactivated in GBM by deletion, mutation, or attenuated expression. Thus, increased expression of miR-21 may contribute to the attenuated expression of PTEN in GBM.

2.2 miR-21 was up regulated in GBM cell lines and tissue samples

Microarray assay was used to screen the miRNA expression status in GBM cell lines. Data showed miR-21 exhibited a 7.0-fold increase relative to normal brain tissue [14]. In addition, in-situ hybridization (ISH) of surgery resected glioma samples proved that miR-21 displayed varying degrees of intensity in glioma with different grades and the positive rate increased with the ascending order of the glioma WHO grade. In hence, it was important to note that miR-21 ISH was conducted at both the tissue level and the cellular level to indicate that miR-21 disregulation could be a marker to predict the outcome of glioma patients.

To identify miR-21 that was abnormal upregulated in high-grade gliomas, we used ISH to test miR-21 insitu expression in human non-neoplastic brain tissues, I~II grade gliomas, grade III gliomas (anaplastic gliomas, AAs) and GBMs.

Our group showed that miR-21 was over expressed in 57 of 60 glioma samples and miR-21 was detected in the cytoplasm of the neoplastic cells of all the positive cases. MiR-21 displayed varying degrees of intensity in glioma with different grades and the positive rate increased with the ascending order of the WHO grade. There were 27 of 30 (90%) in WHO I and II gliomas, 15 of 15 (100%) in AAs and GBMs, whereas miR-21 was rarely detected in control brain tissues. The first indication of miR-21's aberrant expression came from the miRNA profiling of human glioblastoma. Compared to normal brain tissue, miR-21 relative expression was seven to eleven folds in low-grade astrocytomas, AAs and GBMs. Besides providing the consistent data to the previous study, it is important to note that miR-21 ISH was conducted at both the tissue level and the cellular level to indicate that miR-21 disregulation could be a marker to predict the outcome of glioma patients.

2.3 miR-21 regulated GBM cell growth in vitro and in vivo

To evaluate the significance of miR-21 overexpression in glioma cells, we used a loss-of-function antisense approach. An As-miR-21 oligonucleotide (ODN) was used to knock down miR-21 expression in U251 and LN229 cells. RT-realtime PCR results determined that the relative expression level of miR-21 in As-miR-21 ODN-treated U251 cell was 6.25% (P<0.01) and 12.5% for LN229 cells (P<0.01) compared with their control cells, respectively. In addition, LNA-based in situ hybridization showed that transfection of a scrambled ODN had no effect on miR-21 expression. In contrast, the cy3 red fluorescence signal in As-miR-21-transfected U251 cells was lower (Figure 1B). These data suggested that As-miR-21 can specifically inhibit the endogenous miR-21 expression in U251 and LN229 cells.

The GBM cell growth inihibitory effect (MTT assay) of decreased miR-21 reached maximum three days post transfection. G1 phase blockage was observed to indicate cell cycle distribution changed significantly after miR-21 inhibitory. Additionally, the Annexin V positive early phase apoptotic cells were significantly increased in cells transfected with AS-miR-21 as compared to that in parental cells and cells treated with scrambled ODN.

The in vitro experiments suggest that miR-21 is a potential target for therapy in GBM. To further confirm this, we performed a proof-of-principle experiment using a U251 glioma xenograft model and a lipofectamine-mediated gene therapy approach. The xenograft tumors volume suppression indicated that miR-21 contributed a lot to U251 GBM cell proliferation in vivo. Pathological examination found micro-vessel density indicated that was and evaluated miR-21 expression by in situ hybridization and cellular apoptosis by TUNEL assay.

Despite the apparently predominance of microRNA in cancer therapy, several problems have to be overcome for successful clinical application. They show a poor stability towards nuclease activity, low intracellular penetration and low bioavailability. Although chemical modifications were brought to the basic microRNA, their sensitivity to degradation and poor intracellular penetration is still hampering their widespread clinical applications. In fact, the major bottleneck in the development of miRNA strategy is the delivery of these macromolecules to the target cells, tissues or organs. Therefore the development of more efficient delivery systems is regarded as one of the most promising strategies to solve these pharmaceutical hurdles. Specifically, delivery vectors must be designed to effectively complex with nucleic acid molecules and aid in overcoming intracellular barriers such as endosomal escape and cytoplasmic vector dissociation. For that reason, improvements on effective delivery have progressed rapidly. Among the different approaches under study, dendrimers are attracting a great interest for their well defined structure and great versatility in their chemistry that offer a unique platform for the rational design of efficient antisense delivery systems.

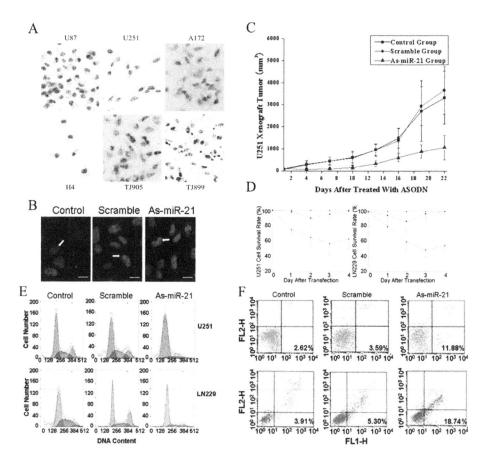

Fig. 1. The effect of miR-21 knockdown on U251 and LN229 GBM cell proliferation. (A) miR-21 was overexpressed in six glioma cells. (B) In situ examination of miR-21 expression in U251 cells. Arrows highlight miR-21 in situ expression in U251 cells. Bar¼20 mm. (C、 D) MTT cell proliferation assay. miR-21 knockdown in U251 and LN229 GBM inhibits cell proliferation in vitro and in vivo. (E) Cell-cycle profiles after PI staining. miR-21 knockdown induced G1 arrest in both U251 and LN229 GBM cells. (F). As-miR-21 and scramble ODN-transfected U251 and LN229 GBM cells were analyzed using FCM to determine cell-cycle status.

3. Polyamidoamine (PAMAM) dendrimers

Recently, a great deal of attention has been given to polyamidoamine (PAMAM) dendrimers; these are one of the most appropriate candidates for suitable carrier systems. PAMAM dendrimers represent an exciting new class of macromolecular architecture called dense star polymers. Unlike classical polymers, dendrimers have a high degree of molecular uniformity, a narrow molecular weight distribution, specific size and shape character [15]. The terminal amine groups of PAMAM dendrimers can be modified with different functionalities and can be linked with various biomolecules. These unique structural features of PAMAM dendrimers make them ideal nanoplatforms to conjugate biologically important substances.

3.1 PAMAM dendrimer in gene transfection

Gene therapy is a promising approach for the treatment of cancer because it enables the production of bioactive agents or the cessation of abnormal functions in the tumor cell. However, the success of gene therapy requires efficient and safe transfer systems because of the degradation of the delivered gene in the systemic circulation.

A variety of molecules including polymers, lipids, and peptides have been studied for their effectiveness as delivery vectors for DNA and RNA molecules. Successful delivery vectors must exhibit a combination of functional attributes. Polymeric carrier molecules should be cationic to complex with nucleic acids, possess a high buffering capacity, exhibit low cytotoxicity, and also contain chemically reactive groups that can be modified for the addition of targeting moieties or other groups.

As a non-viral gene delivery carrier, highly branched, dendritic polymers including poly(amidoamine) (PAMAM) have recently attracted interest as nucleic acid delivery vectors. Previous work has demonstrated that dendrimers can bind to DNA and RNA molecules and mediate modest cellular delivery of these nucleic acids. (PAMAM) dendrimers have attracted great interest due to their high efficacy in vitro gene delivery because of their branched structure. These dendritic polymers bear primary amine groups on their branched surface, which can bind DNA, compact it into polyplexes, and promote the cellular uptake of genes. Therefore, PAMAM dendrimers show high levels of transfection in a wide variety of cultured cells, especially in fractured form of G5 (commercially named SuperFect). Enhanced transfection efficiency has been reported by surface modification of PAMAM with L-arginine. Moreover, the primary amines located on the surface of PAMAM make it possible to conjugate suitable ligands, such as Transferrin, for efficient brain-targeting gene delivery.

Studies that focus on the cell entry mechanisms for several nonviral vectors, including PAMAM dendrimers [16]. The cationic surface charge imparted to the complex through high dendrimer–DNA charge ratios is required for subsequent interaction with the anionic glycoproteins and phospholipids that reside on the cell membrane surface. This interaction initiates the interior movement of the dendrimer–DNA complex into the cell cytosol, either by passive transport caused by membrane perturbations or by endocytosis. Complexes formed without an excess cationic surface charge do not mediate high gene transfection efficiency, which furnishes support for the importance of the initial electrostatic interaction between the complex and cell membrane. Studies following the incorporation of radiolabeled DNA and/or dendrimer components into cells established that the uptake in most cells was primarily via an active endocytosis mechanism. Cells preincubated with inhibitors of endocytosis (i.e. cytochalasin B and deoxyglucose) or cellular metabolism (i.e. sodium azide) reduced the uptake that corresponded to lower transgene expression, regardless of cell type.

These dendrimers as nanocarriers possess the following advantages: (1) neutral surface of the dendrimer for low cytotoxicity; (2) existence of cationic charges inside the dendrimer (not on the outer surface) resulting in highly organized compact nanoparticles, which can potentially protect nucleic acids from degradation. Noteworthy, surface modified QPAMAM-NHAc dendrimer demonstrated enhanced cellular uptake of siRNA when compared with the internally cationic QPAMAM-OH dendrimer (degree of quaternization 97%).

George's study shows PEG-G5 and PEG-G6 dendrimers, with PEG conjugation molar ratio at 8% (PEG to surface amine per PAMAM), can facilitate dramatic intramuscular gene delivery in neonatal mice [17]. Park's group concluded that di-arginine conjugation to PAMAM dendrimers can improve polyplex stability, ntra-nuclear localization, and transfection efficiency but also induce charge density- and generation-dependent cytotoxicity. Therefore, a novel strategy for highly densed arginine conjugation maintaining low cytotoxicity will be needed for the development of efficient gene delivery carriers [18].

3.2 PAMAM dendrimer as drug delivery system

Polymeric drug delivery can improve bioavailability and efficacy of therapeutics with intrinsically poor water solubility and high toxicity. Dendrimers, a class of highly branched polymers, are effective drug delivery vehicles due to their monodispersity and nanoscopic size. With each increase in dendrimer generation, the diameter increases linearly while the number of surface groups increases exponentially. These high density surface groups can be conjugated to drug molecules, targeting moieties and imaging agents, rendering dendrimers a versatile drug delivery platform. In addition, surface groups on dendrimers can be modified to modulate cytotoxicity and permeation across biological barriers.

During their synthesis, PAMAM dendrimers can be produced that are either anionic or cationic in nature, with "full generations" (ie. G1, G2) having amine terminal groups and "half generations" (ie, G0.5, G1.5) possessing carboxylic acid terminal groups. The size and charge of PAMAM dendrimers impact their cytotoxicity and transepithelial transport, with cationic dendrimers showing higher toxicity in vitro. Due to their intrinsically low cytotoxicity and appreciable transepithelial permeation characteristics across Caco-2 monolayers and everted rat intestinal sac models, anionic dendrimers show distinct advantages as vehicles for oral drug delivery, with higher generation dendrimers showing the greatest potential because of their large number of modifiable surface groups.

PAMAM has well-defined internal cavities and an open architecture, guest molecules can become directly encapsulated into the macromolecule interior through hydrophobic interactions. Drug-polymer conjugates are potential candidates for the selective delivery of anticancer agents to tumor tissue. The main advantages of conjugating drugs to polymeric carriers include an increase in water solubility of low soluble or insoluble drugs, and therefore, enhancement of drug bioavailability, protection of drug from deactivation and preservation of its activity during circulation, a reduction in antigenic activity of the drug leading to a less pronounced immunological body response, and the ability to provide passive or active targeting of the drug specifically to the site of its action.

Surface-modified dendrimers were predicted to enhance pilocarpine bioavailability [19]. The anticancer drugs adriamycin and methotrexate were encapsulated into PAMAM dendrimers (i.e. G=3 and 4) which had been modified with PEG monomethyl ether chains (i.e. 550 and 2000 Da respectively) attached to their surfaces. A similar construct involving PEG chains and PAMAM dendrimers was used to deliver the anticancer drug 5-fluorouracil. Encapsulation of 5-fluorouracil into G=4 increase in the cytotoxicity and permeation of dendrimers.

Dendrimers have ideal properties which are useful in targeted drug-delivery system. One of the most effective cell-specific targeting agents delivered by dendrimers is folic acid PAMAM dendrimers modified with carboxymethyl PEG5000 surface chains revealed reasonable drug loading, a reduced release rate and reduced haemolytic toxicity compared with the non-PEGylated dendrimer. A third-generation dendritic unimolecular micelle with indomethacin entrapped as model drug gives slow and sustained in vitro release, as compared to cellulose membrane control [20]. Controlled release of the Flurbiprofen could be achieved by formation of complex with amine terminated generation 4 (G4) PAMAM Dendrimers [21]. The results found that PEG-dendrimers conjugated with encapsulated drug and sustained release of methotrexate as compare to unencapsulated drug.

4. Multifunctional dendrimer nanodevices: In vitro and in vivo testing

4.1 Target gene therapy to rat C6 glioma cells rhrough folate receptor-PAMAM

Despite the progress in the PAMAM mediated gene delivery, few studies have investigated the suitability of PAMAM dendrimers for ASODN delivery in vivo, especially for brain gliomas. The purpose of the present study is to evaluate whether in vivo gene delivery by folate-PAMAM (G5) conjugates can inhibit the development of gliomas. We selected the EGFR gene as an antisense target and the rat C6 intracranial glioma model for the in vivo study. Synthetic foliated (FA-)PAMAM was complexed with EGFR ASODN, and then the gene transfection efficacy, dynamic uptake, and biological effects of the FA-PAMAM delivery system on C6 rat glioma cells were investigated both in vitro and in vivo. Our results showed that the FA-PAMAM dendrimer conjugates transported EGFR-ASODNs into glioma cells in vitro, and yielded a favorable therapeutic effect in vivo on administration by local perfusion. Therefore, FA-PAMAM may represent a potential delivery system for short oligonucleotides in glioma-targeted therapy [22].

We chose G5 PAMAM as the gene vector in the present study because its many surface amine groups enable efficient complex formation with ASODNs through charge-based interactions. Western blot analysis demonstrated the binding of G5 PAMAM to ASODNs, with an optimum ASODN/PAMAM ratio of 16:1. TEM analysis revealed that the complexes were >70 nm in size, and this small size likely enabled the efficient transfer of ASODNs to cells that we observed by flow cytometry. We used ASODNs directly labeled with fluorescent probes, such that flow cytometry directly reflected the uptake of the ASODN by the tumor. ASODN uptake mediated by PAMAM increased twofold in comparison with oligofectamine. The high uptake of ASODNs resulted in significant down-regulation of EGFR, suggesting that PAMAM mediated high efficiency transfection of C6 tumor cells with ASODNs. This high transfection efficiency can be attributed to not only the small size of the complexes, but also to the 'proton sponge' effect of PAMAM,31 in which the acidification of tertiary amino groups on PAMAM in the endosome increases the osmotic pressure within the endosome, leading to the release of ASODNs into cytoplasm.

However, while nonderivatized PAMAM achieves high efficiency transfection, its low targeting efficiency needs to be improved. One strategy to achieve this is the derivatization of PAMAM with ligands. Various ligands such as folic acid, transferring, and lactoferrin have been conjugated to PAMAM, thus enabling efficient gene targeting to tumors or brain. We chose folic acid as the functional ligand with which to modify PAMAM because of its low immunogenicity, unlimited availability, functional stability, defined conjugation chemistry, and a favorable nondestructive cellular internalization pathway.23 More importantly, the receptor for folic acid is a cell-proliferation protein that is overexpressed in many types of cancer cells.32 – 34 The expression levels of folate receptor in tumors have been reported to be 100 – 300 times higher than those observed in normal tissue.35 Although some ambiguity surrounds the expression level of the folate receptor in brain tumors,36 our results demonstrate that conjugation with folic acid enhanced the uptake of ASOND/PAMAM complexes by tumor cells and resulted in greater inhibition of EGFR expression in comparison with the native dendrimer. The in vivo study also demonstrates the superiority of FAPAMAM over either PAMAM or oligofectamine as a vector for mediating ASODN gene therapy. Dynamic contrast MRI scanning indicated significant suppression of tumor growth 2 weeks after C6 cell implantation (Fig. 2), which prolonged the survival time of rats in the FA-PAMAM-mediated therapeutic groups.

In the first place, we evaluated the efficiency of folate-PAMAM dendrimers conjugates (FA-PAMAM) for the in situ delivery of therapeutic antisense oligonucleotides (ASODN) that could inhibit the growth of C6 glioma cells. Folic acid was coupled to the surface amino groups of G5-PAMAM dendrimer (G5D) through a 1-[3-(dimethylamino)propyl]-3-ethylcarbodiimide bond, and ASODNs corresponding to rat epidermal growth factor receptor (EGFR) were then complexed with FA-PAMAM. At an ASODN to PAMAM ratio of 16:1, agarose electrophoresis indicated that antisense oligonucleotides were completely complexed with PAMAM or FA-PAMAM. The ASODN transfection rates mediated by FA-PAMAM and PAMAM were superior to oligofectamine, resulting in greater suppression of EGFR expression and glioma cell growth. Stereotactic injection of EGFR ASODN:FA-PAMAM complexes into established rat C6 intracranial gliomas resulted in greater suppression of tumor growth and longer survival time of tumor-bearing rats compared with PAMAM and oligofectamine-mediated EGFR-ASODN therapy. The current study demonstrates the suitability of folate-PAMAM dendrimer conjugates for efficient EGFR ASODN delivery into glioma cells, wherein they release the ASODN from the FA-PAMAM to knock down EGFR expression in C6 glioma cells, both in vitro and in vivo. FA-PAMAM may thus represent a novel delivery system for short oligonucleotides in glioma-targeted therapy.

4.2 Co-delivery of as-mir-21 and 5-fu by poly(amidoamine) dendrimer attenuates human glioma cell growth in vitro

The efficacy of conventional chemotherapy is limited owing to the low therapeutic index of many anticancer drugs, as well as intrinsic or acquired drug resistance. To circumvent these difficulties, novel therapeutic strategies have been developed, and one attractive strategy is the combination of gene therapy with chemotherapy.

MicroRNAs have been demonstrated to be deregulated in different types of cancer. miR-21 is a key player in the majority of cancers. Down-regulation of miR-21 in glioblastoma cells leads to repression of cell growth, increased cellular apoptosis and cell-cycle arrest, which can theoretically enhance the chemotherapeutic effect in cancer therapy.

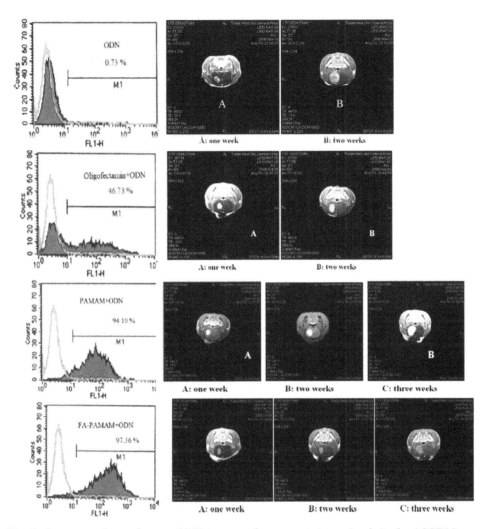

Fig. 2. Contrast-enhanced coronal MR images of representative animals in the ASODN, Oligofectamine/ASODN, PAMAM/ASODN, FA-PAMAM/ASODN group at 1, 2, and 3weeks after tumor xenograft. Four animals in PAMAM/ASODN and FA-PAMAM/ASODN reached the 3-week time point, preventing a valid statistical comparison at that interval. The tumor in this animal is smaller in diameter and less contrast-enhanced than the one in the animal without gene therapy.

With positively charged primary amino groups on the surface, the PAMAM dendrimer can feasibly interact with biomolecules to form complexes through charge-based interactions, and protect them from rapid degradation by cellular endo- and exonucleases. Thus, the PAMAM dendrimer may be suitable for gene transfer or oligonucleotide delivery. Besides, because PAMAM has well-defined internal cavities and an open architecture, guest molecules can become directly encapsulated into the macromolecule interior through hydrophobic interactions. In this study, the poly(amidoamine) (PAMAM) dendrimer was employed as a carrier to co-deliver antisense-miR-21 oligonucleotide (as-miR-21) and 5-fluorouracil (5-FU) to achieve delivery of as-miR-21 to human glioblastoma cells and enhance the cytotoxicity of 5-FU antisense therapy.

Taking advantage of hydrogen-bond interaction, we encapsulated 5-FU in the PAMAM nanoparticles simply by a membrane dialysis method. the encapsulation efficiency and loading efficiency of the drug were determined by UV spectroscopy to be 66.21 and 31.77%, respectively. Through their charge-based interactions, 5-FU-PAMAM could conjugate with as-miR-21. The co-delivery of as-miR-21 not only significantly improved the cytotoxicity and chemosensitivity of 5-FU and dramatically increased the apoptotic percentage of the U251 cells but also brought down the migration ability of the tumor cells. The inhibitory effect toward brain tumors was evaluated by MTT assay, and measurements of cell apoptosis and invasion using the human brain glioma cell line U251. PAMAM could be simultaneously loaded with 5-FU and as-miR-21, forming a complex smaller than 100 nm in diameter. Both the chemotherapeutant and as-miR-21 could be efficiently introduced into tumor cells. The co-delivery of as-miR-21 significantly improved the cytotoxicity of 5-FU and dramatically increased the apoptosis of U251 cells, while the migration ability of the tumor cells was decreased. These results suggest that our co-delivery system may have important clinical applications in the treatment of miR-21-overexpressing glioblastoma.

We report the anticancer potential of a combination of 5-FU treatment and antisense miR-21 technology using PAMAM dendrimers. PAMAM dendrimers, an available co-carrier of chemotherapeutant and as-miR-21, could effectively deliver 5-FU and as-miR-21 simultaneously, forming complexes smaller than 100 nm in diameter. The small size of the complexes facilitated their effective uptake by tumor cells, so the chemotherapeutant and as-miR-21 could be synchronously introduced to glioma cell for combined actions. The co-delivery of as-miR-21 significantly improved the cytotoxicity of 5-FU and dramatically increased the level of apoptosis of U251 cells; it also decreased the migration abilities of the tumor cells. Our results provide invaluable information regarding the future application of drug – polymer complexes combined with gene therapy for cancer treatments. Taken together, our findings suggest that the combination of 5-FU treatment and as-miR-21 might be a potential clinical strategy for cancer chemotherapy [23].

4.3 MicroRNA-21 inhibitor sensitizes human glioblastoma cells to taxol using PAMAM dendrimer

Chemotherapeutic drugs are fundamental in cancer management and are responsible for most cases of adjuvant treatment in patients with GBMs after surgical procedures. Recently, much attention has been focused on the use taxol on glioma, both in experimental studies and in clinical trails [24]. However, the median overall survival did not increase in patients treated by concurrent chemoradiotherapy.

The successful of anti-cancer treatment are often limited by the development of drug resistance. Consequently, further studies that could enhance the therapeutic effect of taxol should be encouraged.Recent work has highlighted the involvement of non-coding RNAs, microRNAs(miRNAs) in cancer development, and their possible involvement in the evolution of drug resistance has been proposed.

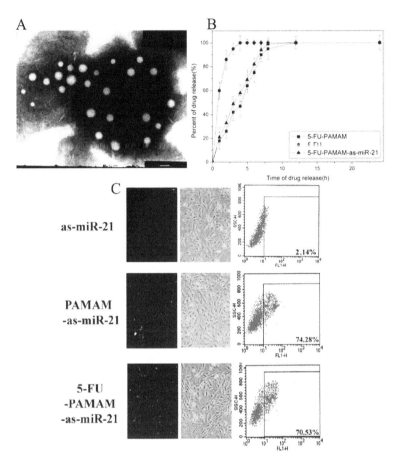

Fig. 3. Characterization of 5-FU/PAMAM/As-miR-21 complex. TEM image of 5-FU‑PAMAM‑as-miR-21 complex, N/P = 16. Magnification 58 000×, scale bar = 100 nm (A). Release profiles of 5-FU from PAMAMand PAMAM‑as-miR-21 complexes compared with free 5-FU (B). Cell uptake detected by flow cyctometry and fluorescent microscopy image of U251 cells after transfection with different complexes (C).

Substantial data indicate that the oncogene microRNA 21 (miR-21) is significantly elevated in glioblastoma multiforme (GBM) and regulates multiple genes associated with cancer cell proliferation, apoptosis, and invasiveness. Thus, miR-21 can theoretically become a target to enhance the chemotherapeutic effect in cancer therapy. So far, the effect of downregulating miR-21 to enhance the chemotherapeutic effect to taxol has not been studied in human GBM.

In this study, we combine taxol chemotherapy and miR-21 inhibitor treatment via polyamidoamine (PAMAM) dendrimers vector to evaluate the effects of combination therapy on suppression of glioma cells. The result indicated that the miR-21 inhibitor can decrease the proliferation of both U251 and LN229 cells and increase the cells' sensitivity to taxol treatment. The taxol concentration causing 50% growth inhibition (IC50) of U251 cells is 400 nmol/mL; whereas, in combination with the miR-21 inhibitor (20 μmol/L) the IC50

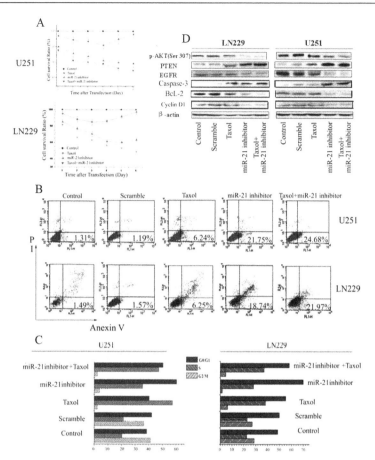

Fig. 4. Effect of the miR-21 inhibitor on the chemo-sensitivity of U251 and LN229 cells to taxol treatment. The growth of U251 and LN229 cells were inhibited by the miR-21 inhibitor, taxol only, and the indicated combinations. The cells were treated with the miR-21 inhibitor complexed to PAMAM for 6 h at 37°C. The medium was then replaced with media containing various concentrations of taxol. After 72 h of incubation, an MTT assay was performed. Absorbance at 570 nm was normalized to the control (untreated cells) to determine cell viability. Each value represents the mean ±SD from triplicate determinations. An aqueous solution of taxol (circles) and miR-21 inhibitor-loaded PAMAM (triangle) was incubated with human glioblastoma U251 and LN229 cells for six days. Druginduced decrease in cell numbers was measured using the MTT assay. The miR-21 inhibitor enhanced taxol induced apoptosis. Flow cytometry analyses of propidium iodide-stained cells were performed in triplicate (B). miR-21 inhibitor and taxol induce G1 and S phase arrest on cell cycle distribution. U251 and LN229 cells were treated with the miR-21 inhibitor and taxol alone or in combination, and cell cycle distributions were detected by Flow cytometry 48 h later (C). Evaluation of the expression of PTEN, EGFR, STAT3, and p-STAT3 in human glioblastoma LN229 and U251 cell lines. Western blot of protein extracts from cells treated with the miR-21 inhibitor or taxol, alone or combination (D). The expression of b-actin was examined to ensure uniform protein loading in all lanes.

was 60 nmol/mL. Taxol can also increase the efficacy of the miR-21 inhibitor. For example, combination treatment reduced cell viability to 20% compared with 86% viability for miR-21 inhibitor gene therapy alone. In LN229 cells, combination treatment with 20 μ mol/L of the miR-21 inhibitor reduced the IC50 of taxol from 820 to 160 nmol/L . It is worth noting that the miR-21 inhibitor additively interacted with taxol on U251cells and synergistically on LN229 cells.

Taxol treatment also increased the percentage of apoptotic cancer cells in miR-21 inhibitor transfected cells compared with control cells. Furthermore, treatment of the miR-21 inhibitor-transfected cells with the anti-cancer drugs taxol resulted in significantly reduced cell viability and invasiveness compared with control cells. These results indicated that the miR-21 plays an important role in the resistance of brain cancer cells to chemotherapeutic drugs. Therefore, miR-21 inhibitor gene therapy combined with taxol chemotherapy might represent a promising novel therapeutic approach for the treatment of glioblastoma.

Thus, the miR-21 inhibitor might interrupt the activity of EGFR pathways, independently of PTEN status. Meanwhile, the expression of STAT3 and p-STAT3 decreased to relatively low levels after miR-21 inhibitor and taxol treatment. The data strongly suggested that a regulatory loop between miR-21 and STAT3 might provide an insight into the mechanism of modulating EGFR/STAT3 signaling [25].

5. Conclusion

MiR-21 was one of the most frequently overexpressed miRNA in human glioblastoma (GBM) cell lines which can serve as a therapeutic target for glioblastoma. We validated that downregulation of miR-21 inhibited the growth of GBM cell lines and induced apoptosis. These effects were only partially dependent on PTEN, highlighting the existence of multiple, and possibly yet unknown, targets of miR-21. Inhibition of miR-21 also suppressed EGFR and Akt activity. These observations were confirmed in in vivo xenograft experiments that showed the potential clinical relevance of miR-21-targeting agents. Targeting miR-21 by antisense or small-molecule compounds may represent new targeted therapeutic strategies for human cancers, including gliomas.

PAMAM dendrimer has been reported to be good gene delivery candidate. Although the biological effects obtained from in vitro analysis of PAMAM and FA-PAMAM are approximate, our in vivo study implies that FAPAMAM is functionally effective for gene delivery into three-dimensional tissues. This may be due to folate-mediated targeting of ASODNs to folate receptor-expressing cells in solid tumors. Stereotactic administration, which enables FA-PAMAM-ASODNs to be injected directly into a tumor, may also produce better results than intravenous injection. Site-specific delivery remains the best choice to overcome gene delivery side effects and to increase its efficacy.

Next, we exhibit the anticancer potential of a combination of 5-FU treatment and antisense miR-21 technology using PAMAM dendrimers. PAMAM dendrimers, an available co-carrier of chemotherapeutant and as-miR-21, could effectively deliver 5-FU and as-miR-21 simultaneously, forming complexes smaller than 100 nm in diameter. The small size of the complexes facilitated their effective uptake by tumor cells, so the chemotherapeutant and as-miR 21 could be synchronously introduced to glioma cell for combined actions. The co-delivery of as-miR-21 significantly improved the cytotoxicity of 5-FU and dramatically increased the level of apoptosis of U251 cells; it also decreased the migration abilities of the tumor cells. Our results provide invaluable information regarding the future application of drug–polymer complexes combined with gene therapy for cancer treatments. Taken together, our findings suggest that the combination of 5-FU treatment and as-miR-21 might be a potential clinical strategy for cancer chemotherapy.

Furthermore, the miR-21 inhibitor could enhance the chemo-sensitivity of human glioblastoma cells to taxol via PAMAM dendrimer. A combination of miR-21 inhibitor and taxol could be an effective therapeutic strategy for controlling. The above data suggested that in both the PTEN mutant U251 cell line and the PTEN wild-type LN229 cells, miR-21 blockage could increase the chemosensitivity to taxol. It is worth noting that the miR-21 inhibitor additively interacted with taxol on U251cells and synergistically on LN229 cells. Thus, the miR-21 inhibitor might interrupt the activity of EGFR pathways, independently of PTEN status. The miR-21 inhibitor enhanced the chemo-sensitivity of human glioblastoma cells to taxol and combination of the miR-21 inhibitor and taxol could be an effective therapeutic strategy for suppressing the growth of GBM.

the growth of GBM by inhibiting STAT3 expression and phosphorylation.

6. Acknowledgements

This work was financially supported by the China National Natural Scientific Fund (51073118 and 30971136), the Tianjin Science and Technology Committee (09JCZDJC17600, 10JCYBJC12500), and a Program for New Century Excellent Talents in University (NCET-07-0615).

7. References

Minniti G, et al. (2009). Chemotherapy for glioblastoma: current treatment and future perspectives for cytotoxic and targeted agents. *Anticancer Res*, Vol.29, No.12, (2009 Dec) pp: 5171-84, ISSN: 0250-7005

Santos-Rebouças CB,et al (2010). MicroRNAs: macro challenges on understanding human biological functions and neurological diseases. *Curr Mol Med*. Vol.10, No.8, (2010 Nov) pp: 692-704, ISSN: 1566-5240

Kaneda Y. (2010). Update on non-viral delivery methods for cancer therapy: possibilities of a drug delivery system with anticancer activities beyond delivery as a new therapeutic tool. *Expert Opin Drug Deliv*. Vol.7, No.9, (2010 Sep), pp: 1079-93, ISSN: 1742-5247.

He L, Hannon GJ. (2004) MicroRNAs: small RNAs with a big role in gene regulation. *Nat Rev Genet*. Vol. 5, No. 7, (2004 Jul), pp: 522-31 , ISSN: 1471-0056

Bartel DP. (2004). MicroRNAs: genomics, biogenesis, mechanism, and function. *Cell*. Vol. 116, No. 2, (2004 Jan), pp: 281-97, ISSN: 2155-1790

Akbergenov R, et al (2006). Molecular characterization of geminivirus-derived small RNAs in different plant species. *Nucleic Acids Res*, Vol.34, (2006 Jan) pp: 462–471, ISSN: 0305-1048

Valeri N, et al (2009). Epigenetics, miRNAs, and human cancer: a new chapter in human gene regulation. *Mamm Genome*, Vol. 20, No. 9-10, (2009 Sep-Oct), pp: 573-80 , ISSN: 0938-8990

Selcuklu SD, Donoghue MT, Spillane C (2009). miR-21 as a key regulator of oncogenic processes. *Biochem Soc Trans*. Vol. 37, No. 4, (2009 Aug), pp: 918-25, ISSN: 0300-5127

Zhu S, et al (2007). MicroRNA-21 targets the tumor suppressor gene tropomyosin 1 (TPM1). *J Biol Chem*, Vol. 282, No.19, (2007 May), pp: 14328–14336, ISSN: 0021-9258

Asangani IA, et al (2008). MicroRNA-21 (miR-21) post-transcriptionally downregulates tumor suppressor Pdcd4 and stimulates invasion, intravasation and metastasis in colorectal cancer. *Oncogene*, Vol. 27, No. 15, (2008 Apr), pp: 2128–2136, ISSN: 0950-9232

Moore LM, Zhang W. Targeting miR-21 in glioma: a small RNA with big potential. Expert Opin Ther Targets. Vol. 14, No.11, (2010 Nov r), pp: 1247-57, ISSN: 1472-8222

Ciafre` SA, et al. Extensive modulation of a set of microRNAs in primary glioblastoma. *Biochem Biophys Res Commun* Vol. 334 , No.4 , (2005 Sep), pp: 1351–1358 , ISSN: 0006-291X

Meng F, et al (2007). MicroRNA-21 regulates expression of the PTEN tumor suppressor gene in human hepatocellular cancer. *Gastroenterology*, Vol. 133, No. 2, (2007 Aug), pp: 647–658, ISSN: 0016-5085

Malzkorn B, et al (2010). Identification and functional characterization of microRNAs involved in the malignant progression of gliomas. *Brain Pathol.* Vol.20, No.3, (2010 May), pp: 539-50, ISSN: 1015-6305

Baker JR Jr (2009). Dendrimer-based nanoparticles for cancer therapy. *Hematology Am Soc Hematol Educ Program.* pp: 708-19 , ISSN: 1520-4391

Eichman JD, et al (2000). The use of PAMAM dendrimers in the efficient transfer of genetic material into cells. *Pharm Sci Technolo Today*, Vol. 3, No. 7, (2000 Jul), pp: 232-245, ISSN: 1461-5347

Qi R, et al (2009). PEG-conjugated PAMAM dendrimers mediate efficient intramuscular gene expression. *AAPS J.* Vol. 11 , No. 3, (2009 Sep) pp: 395-405, ISSN: 1550-7416

Kim TI, et al (2009). Comparison between arginine conjugated PAMAM dendrimers with structural diversity for gene delivery systems. *J Control Release.* Vol. 136, No. 2, (2009 Jun) pp: 132-9, ISSN: 0168-3659

Tolia,G.T et al (2008). The role of dendrimers in drug delivery, Pharmaceut. Tech., Vol. 32, No.11, (2008 Nov) pp:88-98, ISSN:

Patri, A.K., Majoros and. Baker, J.R., (2002). Dendritic polymer macromolecular carriers for drug delivery, *Curr. Opin. Chem. Biol.* Vol. 6, No. 4, (2002 Aug) pp: 466-71, ISSN: 1367-5931

Asthana ,A.,et al, 2005 . Poly (amidoamine) (pamam) dendritic nanostructures for controlled site specific delivery of acidic anti-inflammatory active ingredient, *AAPS PharmSciTech.* Vol. 6 , No. 3, (2005 Oct) pp: E536-42, ISSN: 1530-9932

Kang C, et al (2010). Evaluation of folate-PAMAM for the delivery of antisense oligonucleotides to rat C6 glioma cells in vitro and in vivo. *J Biomed Mater Res A.* (2010 May), Vol. 93 , No. 2, pp: 585-94, ISSN: 1549-3296

Ren Y, et al (2010). Co-delivery of as-miR-21 and 5-FU by poly(amidoamine) dendrimer attenuates human glioma cell growth in vitro. *J Biomater Sci Polym Ed.* Vol. 21 , No. 3, (2010 Mar) pp: 303-14., ISSN: 0920-5063

Karmakar S, et al (2007). Combination of all- trans retinoic acid and taxol regressed glioblastoma T98G xenografts in nude mice. *Apoptosis*, Vol.12, No.11, (2007 Nov) pp: 2077 87, ISSN: 1360 8185.

Ren Y, et al (2010). MicroRNA-21 inhibitor sensitizes human glioblastoma cells U251 (PTEN-mutant) and LN229 (PTEN-wild type) to taxol. *BMC Cancer*. Vol. 10 , (2010 Jan) pp: 27, ISSN: 1471-2407

4

Nanomedicine Based Approaches to Cancer Diagonsis and Therapy

Roderick A. Slavcev, Shawn Wettig and Tranum Kaur
School of Pharmacy, University of Waterloo, Ontario
Canada

1. Introduction

Pharmaceutical nanoparticles were first described in 1970s, and the term "nanotechnology" is now commonly used to refer to the fabrication of new materials with nanoscale dimensions between 1 and 100 nm (Thrall 2004). Several types of nanometer scale systems such as nanoparticles, nanospheres, nanotubes, nanogels and molecular conjugates are being investigated (Lemieux et al. 2000;Liu et al. 2007;Ravi et al. 2004). The field of nanomedicine aims to use the properties and physical characteristics of nanomaterials which have been extensively investigated as novel intravascular or cellular probes for both diagnostic (imaging) and therapeutic purposes (drug/gene delivery). The sub-micron size of nanoparticle delivery systems confers distinct advantages as compared to large sized systems including targeted delivery, higher and deeper tissue penetrability, greater cellular uptake and greater ability to cross the blood-brain barrier (Kreuter et al. 1995;Vinogradov et al. 2002;Vogt et al. 2006). Therapeutic transgene(s) encoded by plasmid or chemically modified DNA can be dissolved, entrapped, chemically conjugated, encapsulated or adsorbed to the surface of nanoparticles. There are, broadly, two main types of nanosized particles with different inner structures: A. Nanoparticle/Nanosphere: Matrix composed of entangled oligomer or polymer units; and B. Nanocapsule: Reservoir consisting of a hydrophobic core surrounded by a polymer wall. Lipids can also be used to generate liposomes or micelles (discussed in detail later). These nanodevices can confer protection to the DNA against a variety of degradative and destabilizing factors, and enhance delivery efficiency to the cells while minimizing the toxic effects.

Nanoparticles are expected to play a critical role in the innovation and development of future cancer treatment modalities. Recent research has developed functional nanoparticles that are covalently linked to biological molecules such as peptides, proteins, nucleic acids, or small-molecule ligands (Alivisatos 2004;Chan et al. 2002;Michalet et al. 2005). Medical applications have also appeared, such as the use of superparamagnetic iron oxide nanoparticles as a contrast agent in the detection of lymph node prostate cancer (Harisinghani et al. 2003) and the use of polymeric nanoparticles for targeted gene delivery to tumor vasculatures (Hood et al. 2002). Target-specific drug/gene delivery and early diagnosis is currently a high priority R&D area, and one in which nanomedicine will inevitably make critical contributions. Current modalities of diagnosis and treatment of various diseases, especially cancer, have major limitations such as poor sensitivity or specificity and high drug toxicities respectively. The success of nanoparticle delivery systems will ultimately depend on the ability to efficiently deliver the gene of interest and express a therapeutic gene(s) in tumor cells in a targeted manner in order to mitigate toxicity. This chapter examines current existing nanoparticle-based gene therapy approaches to cancer treatment, and assesses their therapeutic utility.

2. Nanobased cancer treatment strategies

Most neoplasm's are derived from multiple mutations and rarely can be controlled through the targeting of a single mutation. The efficacy of gene therapy in tumor treatment will undoubtedly rely upon the simultaneous targeting of multiple cellular processes or the ability to invoke various antitumor responses. Current clinical trials in cancer exploit a variety of different treatment approaches. Tumor suppressor modalities compensate for a genetic mutation via gene transfer or replacement of an altered tumor suppressor gene (e.g. *p53*, *BRCA1*). Molecular chemotherapy, involves the transfer of a suicide gene (e.g. Herpes Simplex Virus-thymidine kinase [*HSV-tk*], CD::upp) targeted to specific tissues by extracellular tumor/tissue targeting strategies, and/or via tissue-specific expression. The delivered gene then makes the cell susceptible to a prodrug (e.g. gancyclovir, 5-FC) making tumor-specific expression critical. Tumor immunotherapy involves the gene transfer of cytokines (e.g. IL-2, IL-12) that impart antitumor immunomodulatory properties. Oncofactor inhibition strategies such as growth factor inhibition and oncogene inhibition (e.g. erb-B2 silencing) aim to prevent tumor progression by inhibiting key growth factors. Anti-angiogenesis therapy seeks to destroy the vasculature supplying the tumor in the hopes of starving it of essential nutrients to diminish or prevent its progression. Multi Drug Resistance associated genes strategies, involve knocking down gene associated with or conferring MDR, such as *PRP-4* and *survivin* to improve chemosensitivity. We will examine in detail each of these strategies.

2.1 Tumor suppressor gene therapy

As a critical player in cancer onset, *p53* has come to the forefront of oncological research and is now recognized to be the single most frequently inactivated gene in human cancers (Ning et al. 2011;Olivier et al. 2002;Olivier et al. 2010). The *p53* gene enforces a variety of anticancer functions by encouraging cells to arrest or die in the face of DNA damage, hypoxia, oxidative stress, excessive mitogenic stimuli or denuded telomers. In addition, the protein influences several biological functions such as involvement in cell cycle regulation, programmed cell death, senescence, differentiation and development, transcription, DNA replication, DNA repair and maintenance of genomic stability. Thus, it's not surprising that *p53* is regarded as the "*Guardian of the Genome*" in preventing human neoplasia (Lane 1992). P53 protein has emerged as a key tumor suppressor protein in cellular stress response pathways. The *p53* gene, mapped to chromosome 17p13.1, consists of 11 exons spanning over 20 kb of DNA encoding a 393 amino acid and 53 kDa nuclear protein. Its structure consists of an acidic N-terminus with a transactivation domain, a hydrophobic central DNA-binding core and a basic C-terminus with regulatory and oligomerization domains (Hainaut and Vahakangas 1997). Although greater than 90% of the isolated mutations in this gene have been localized to the DNA binding site of *p53*, coded by exons 5 to 8; some mutations have also been reported outside the evolutionary conserved regions (Hainaut and Hollstein

2000). The *p53* gene product is a sequence-specific nuclear transcription factor that binds to defined consensus sites within DNA as a tetramer and affects the transcription of its target genes. These target genes are involved in critical cell processes such as:
1. Growth arrest: P21, Gadd45 and 14-3-3σ.
2. DNA repair: *P53R2*.
3. Apoptosis: Bax, Bcl-xL, Fas, FasL, DR5/Killer, Apaf-1, Puma and Noxa.

The loss of *p53* function is of relevance to a broad array of cancer types, including 15–50% of breast cancer cases, 25–70% of metastatic prostate cancers, 25–75% of lung cancers, 33–100% of head and neck cancers and 60–80% advanced ovarian cancers (Ruley, 1996). Furthermore, the null mutation of the gene imparts strongly unfavorable prognosis when associated within human ovarian, lung, colon and breast cancer cases. *P53* also represses genes involved in tumor angiogenesis, and recent evidence suggests that tumor cells possessing a wild-type *p53* allele are more sensitive to chemotherapeutic agents and radiation than *p53* null mutants (Lowe et al. 1994). The pleiotropic abnormalities imparted by deficient *p53* in a significant fraction of human cancers make it one of the primary candidates for cancer gene therapy, whereby the effective expression or replacement of *p53* may re-establish cell growth control, restore appropriate responses to DNA-damaging agents (e.g. chemotherapy and radiotherapy) and preclude tumor angiogenesis. In human neoplasia's that express the wild-type protein, aberrations of p53 regulators, such as MDM2, account for p53 inhibition. For this reason, improved understanding of the p53 pathway should lead to better diagnosis and treatment of cancer in the future.

The *p53* gene therapeutic, Gendicine, is currently approved in China and its US counterpart, Advexin, has shown activity in number of clinical trials. In more conventional approaches a range of small drug like molecules targeting the *p53* mediated system have been developed and several are now in clinical trials. Of critical importance has been the development of small-molecule inhibitors of the p53–Mdm2 protein interaction such as the Nutlins (Vassilev 2004), which have shown activity against human xenografts in preclinical models. Therefore, designing small-molecule inhibitors of the *p53*-MDM2 protein-protein interaction is a promising strategy for the treatment of cancers retaining wild-type *p53* (Lauria et al. 2010). Advanced structural approaches have provided compelling support for the idea that some *p53* mutants can be targets for small molecules that would cause them to regain wild-type function (Joerger et al. 2006). Many adenoviral vectors with cancer specific conditional replication properties have been preclinically evaluated to date. Most promising among these are: i) the Ad dl1520 that possesses a deletion of the 55-kd E1B gene limiting growth to only *p53*-deficient tumor cells. This strategy has shown preclinical efficacy against *p53*-deficient nude mouse-human ovarian carcinomatosis xenografts (Vasey et al. 2002); and ii) the integrin-targeted Ad5-D24RGD and serotype 3 receptor-targeted Ad5/3-D24 that possesses a 24 bp deletion in the retinoblastoma binding site of E1A, conferring selective replication in cancer cells that are deficient in the Rb/p16 pathway.

2.2 Molecular chemotherapy

Suicide gene therapy/molecular chemotherapy is a new experimental form of cancer chemotherapy that is currently being evaluated in human trials (Bhaumik 2011; Onion et al. 2009;Xu et al. 2009). This approach involves intra-tumoral delivery of genes encoding enzymes that convert nontoxic prodrugs into toxic anti-metabolites. Two suicide genes that are being evaluated in the clinic are the *Escherichia coli* CD (*codA* cytosine deaminase) and

HSV-1 *tk* (thymidine kinase) genes, which confer sensitivity to 5-FC (5-flourocytosine) and GCV, respectively. The rationale behind the suicide gene therapy approach is that after "targeted" transfer of these genes to the tumor, only tumor and neighboring cells will be rendered sensitive to their cytotoxic action. A variety of tumor models have demonstrated that both the CD/5-FC (by inhibiting thymidylate synthase) and HSV-1 *tk*/GCV prodrug systems (by inhibiting DNA chain elongation) can enhance the efficacy of radiation therapy, resulting in significantly better tumor control and/or cure (Rogulski et al., 1997). Suicide gene therapy is a particularly attractive approach to the treatment of cancer as it is essentially a tumor-targeted chemotherapy. As such, the systemic toxicity commonly associated with, and a major limitation of, conventional chemotherapy is avoided. Using a pair of adenoviral vectors that express a CD/HSV-1 *tk* fusion gene without or with the wt human *p53* gene, it has been found that co-expression of *p53* did not enhance the cytotoxicity of CD/5-FC or HSV-1 *tk*/GCV suicide gene therapies using the SK-OV-3 and Hep3B tumor models *in vitro* or *in vivo* (Xie et al., 1999). This notion is consistent with the fact that CD/5-FC and HSV-1 *tk*/GCV suicide gene therapies have demonstrated effectiveness against a variety of tumors that lack functional *p53* (e.g., SK-OV-3, Hep3B, 9L, WiDr, U251, DU145, PC-3, C33A, and many others). Azatian et al. (Azatian et al. 2009) investigated the effectiveness of HSV-*tk* activation as gene therapy for gastroesophageal junction and gastric adenocarcinomas using a stress-inducible Grp78 promoter. The gastric adenocarcinoma cell line MKN-74/*tk* cells were completely killed when cultured with 1 µg/ml GCV for 10 days. Cell viability was also significantly lower under glucose starvation conditions when HSV-*tk* expression was regulated by the Grp78 promoter . Furthermore, non-viral approaches are being investigated for use in combination with suicide gene therapy for treatment of various carcinomas. Using transferrin lipoplexes, prepared from cationic liposomes and cholesterol, significant tumor reduction was achieved upon intratumoral delivery of HSV-*tk* or CD genes, followed by intraperitoneal injection of GCV or 5-FC, respectively (Neves et al. 2009). Enhanced apoptosis, the recruitment of NK cells, CD4 and CD8 T-lymphocytes and an increase in the levels of several cytokines/chemokines were observed within the tumors. These observations suggest that suicide gene therapy with lipoplexes modifies the tumor microenvironment, and leads to the recruitment of immune effector cells that can act as adjuvants in reducing the tumor size.

2.3 Immunomodulatory strategies

Tumor cells alter antigen presentation on their surface compromising recognition by the immune system and immunosurveillance evasion. Tumor immunotherapy strategies aim to boost the anti-tumor immune response by stimulating the cell-mediated arm of the immune system (Wojtowicz-Praga 1997). Gene therapy approaches to enhance immune responses include delivery of cytokines to the tumor, administration of tumor vaccines based on tumor-associated antigens (TAAs), upregulation of Major Histocompatibitlity Complexes (MHC)(Nabel et al. 1993) or co-stimulatory molecules, and inhibition of immunosuppressive molecules. Many cytokines activate the immune system, including interleukins (IL) 2, 4, 7, 12 and 18, interferon γ (IFN-γ), tumor necrosis factor α (TNF-α), and granulocyte–macrophage colony-stimulating factor (GM-CSF), which are among the most potent inducers of anti-tumor activity in a variety of preclinical studies. More recently, some exciting new cytokines have been characterized, such as IL-21, IL-23, IL-27, and their immunomodulatory and antitumor effects *in vitro* and *in vivo* suggest that they may have considerable promise for future immunotherapy protocols (Weiss et al. 2007). Recent studies using animal models have shown that genetically modified tumor cells expressing cytokines such as IL-2, IL-4, IL-6, IFN-γ or GM-CSF were capable of inducing an immune response against preexisting tumors (Connor et al. 1993). In preclinical models and clinical trials, cytokines have been delivered to melanoma lesions by intratumoral injection of naked DNA, recombinant viral vectors and transduced tumor cells and fibroblasts (Sun et al. 1998). Initial clinical trials evaluating the systemic delivery of IL-2 and TNF-α were complicated by significant systemic toxicity (Rosenberg 1999), thereby generating interest in gene transfer strategies that limit cytokine production to the tumor milieu. Preclinical studies employing TAAs to generate tumor vaccines have been promising, and seem to suggest that immunization with recombinant, virus-encoding TAAs can confer suppression of growth in pre-established tumors and the production of specific cytotoxic T lymphocyte responses. However, conversion to clinical trials has failed to show significant efficacy.

The cytokine IFN-γ has been shown to up-regulate MHC expression, antigen processing, antigen processing and presentation expression in many cell populations, including dendritic cells, B cells, macrophages, and endothelial cells, producing more potent antigen presenting cells (APCs), as IFN-γ can induce multiple gene expressions that are related to MHC processing and presentation. Dendritic cells (DCs) play a vital role in the initiation of immune response as professional antigen presenting cells to T cells promoting CD8+ T-cell-mediated cytotoxic responses. Reported research in animal studies indicates that vaccine immunity may represent a promising alternative therapy for cancer patients. However, broad clinical utility has yet to be achieved, owing to the low transfection efficiency of DCs (Chen et al. 2010b). Different formulations of liposomes have been designed to improve the uptake by DCs through different receptor-mediated routes. These formulations include liposomes prepared with mannosylated phosphatidylethanolamine (Man-PE), trimethyl ammonium propane, and phosphatidylserine targeted to mannose receptor (MR), negatively charged surface proteins and phosphatidylserine receptor (PSR) of DCs, respectively. Several other immunomodulatory clinical trials are under way with cytokines currently comprising 18.3% of immunotherapy clinical trials (http://www.wiley.com/legacy/wileychi/genmed/clinical/). Table 1 provides a list of various types of genes currently involved in various gene therapy clinical trials. A number of other monoclonal antibodies; namely EC90, Removab, and CNTO-95 which target FOLR1, EpCAM and α-integrin (CD51), respectively are in Phase I/II studies, and indicate that further clinical investigation in this area is warranted (Bell-McGuinn et al. 2011;Kowalski et al. 2010).

2.4 Oncofactor inhibition strategies
2.4.1 Growth factor inhibition

The epidermal growth factor receptor (EGFR) belongs to the proto-oncogene family, which consists of four structurally-related transmembrane receptors (i.e., EGFR, ErbB2, ErbB3, and ErbB4) and is a key therapeutic target in the treatment of many types of cancer. The most extensively studied growth factors are ErbB1 (Javle et al. 2010) and ErbB2 (Nihira 2003). These ErbB/EGF receptors are tyrosine kinases and play important physiologic roles in cell proliferation, survival, adhesion, motility, invasion, and angiogenesis. High expression of EGF receptor protein is observed in several types of cancer including breast, bladder, colon, lung and gastric cancers, making them potential targets for targeted therapies, which represent some of the most successful therapeutic approaches to date (Iqbal et al. 2011;Lai et al. 2009;Yarom and Jonker 2011).

Gene type	Gene Therapy Clinical Trials	
	Number	%
Adhesion molecule	10	0.6
Antigen	334	20.7
Antisense	13	0.8
Cell cycle	8	0.5
Cell protection/Drug resistance	19	1.1
Cytokine	317	18.5
Deficiency	136	7.9
Growth factor	128	7.5
Hormone	8	0.5
Marker	54	3.2
Oncogene regulator	11	0.6
Oncolytic virus	37	2.2
Porins, ion channels, transporters	12	0.7
Receptor	113	6.6
Replication inhibitor	74	4.3
Ribozyme	6	0.4
siRNA	11	0.6
Suicide	144	8.4
Transcription factor	28	1.6
Tumor suppressor	150	8.8
Viral vaccine	6	0.4
Others	26	1.5
Unknown	49	2.9
Total	1714	

Table 1. List of various types of genes presently involved in various gene therapy clinical trials (Source: http://www.wiley.com/legacy/wileychi/genmed/clinical/).

Gefitinib and Erlotinib are small molecules that exert their function by inhibiting the intracellular tyrosine kinase domain of EGFR. Recently, the southwest oncology group study S0413, a phase II trial of lapatinib was conducted as first-line therapy in patients with advanced or metastatic gastric cancer. Median (95% CI) time to treatment failure was 1.9 (1.6-3.1) months and overall survival (OS) was 4.8 (3.2-7.4) months. Lapatinib is well tolerated, with modest single-agent activity in advanced/metastatic gastric cancer patients. Potential molecular correlatives such as HER2, interleukin (IL)-8 and genomic polymorphisms IL-8, and vascular endothelial growth factor correlated with OS (Iqbal et al. 2011). Similarly, in other Phase II studies with single agent Gefitinib or Erlotinib only modest activity was observed. Gefitinib cytotoxic combinations are also currently under examination (Wagner et al. 2007). Further, very recently it was observed that direct covalent coupling of antibodies to glutaraldehyde activated nanoparticles is an appropriate method to achieve cell-type specific drug carrier systems based on polymeric nanoparticles that have potential to be applied for targeted chemotherapy in EGFR positive cancer (Aggarwal et al. 2011).

Trastuzumab (trade name Herceptin) is the first anticancer drug generated by Genentech, Inc. whose use as a treatment for breast cancer patients is decided based on the status of the HER2 gene amplification/HER2 protein over-expression. The development and standardization of an HER2 test was a key strategy in clinical development of this drug, since appropriate selection of patients with HER2 over-expression was critical for success. This also highlights the important and evolving era of personalized and targeted therapies. In the clinic, the success of imatinib (Gleevec®, STI571) and trastuzumab, both firsts of their kind, spurred further development of new, second-generation drugs that target kinases in cancer. Further, these targeted drugs combined with chemotherapeutic drugs are found effective and well tolerated in nanoparticle based drug delivery (e.g. albumin-bound paclitaxel combined with carboplatin and trastuzumab or as trastuzumab-dextran iron oxide nanoparticles) for the treatment of cancer (Conlin et al. 2010).

2.4.2 Signal transduction (P13K/AKT/mTOR pathway) inhibition

Phosphoinositide 3-kinase (PI3K) is a major signaling component downstream of growth factor receptor tyrosine kinases (RTKs). PI3K catalyzes the production of the lipid second messenger phosphatidylinositol-3,4,5-triphosphate (PIP3) at the cell membrane. PIP3 in turn contributes to the recruitment and activation of a wide range of downstream targets, including the serine-threonine protein kinase Akt (also known as protein kinase B). The PI3K-Akt-mTOR signaling pathway regulates many normal cellular processes including cell proliferation, survival, growth, and motility — processes that are critical for tumorigenesis. Components of this pathway are frequently abnormal in a variety of tumors, making them an attractive target for anti-cancer therapy. In contrast to *p53* and other tumor-suppressor pathways, the PI3K pathway is activated in cancer, making this an optimal target for therapy as it is easier to inhibit activation events than to replace lost tumor-suppressor function. Studies have demonstrated that phosphorylative activation via the mTOR pathway results in increased G1 cell cycle progression, cell survival, and tumor cell proliferation (Campbell et al. 2004;Vega et al. 2006). The mTOR pathway has been shown in preclinical studies to play a role in the carcinogenesis of breast, ovary and prostate as well as gastrointestinal malignancies. Novel analogs of rapamycin (temsirolimus, everolimus, and deforolimus), which have improved pharmaceutical properties, have been designed for oncology indications. Clinical trials of these analogs have already validated the importance of mTOR inhibition as a novel treatment strategy for several malignancies (Gibbons et al. 2009).

2.4.3 Oncogene inhibition

Gene therapy has also been employed in a reversed approach, namely by inhibition of oncogenes. The use of vectors to express anti-sense (ODN), ribozymes or small interfering RNAs (siRNA) to silence a variety of oncogenes has enabled genetic loss-of-function studies in tissue culture systems. Gene expression can be disrupted at the transcriptional (triplex DNA) or translational (antisense DNA or short inference RNA) level (Braasch et al. 2002). In the triplex DNA-based antigene approach, transcription is disrupted by the binding of a triplex-forming oligonucleotide at the promoter region of a target gene. In the antisense strategy, the oligonucleotide (ON) molecule corresponding to a target gene is delivered inside a cell where it binds to its complementary, targeted messenger RNA (mRNA), to produce a partially double-stranded ON/mRNA complex. Extensive work in this area has already led to one antisense ON product approved for local therapy of cytomegalovirus retinitis (Vitravene) and nearly twenty others in late-stage clinical trials (Cheung et al. 2010).

Silencing of specific mRNA using double stranded RNA oligonucleotides represents one of the newest technologies for suppressing a specific gene product. Small interfering RNA (siRNA) are 21 nucleotides long, double stranded RNA fragments that are identical in sequence to the target mRNA. Silencing of specific gene targets, such as cancer-associated mutations in oncogenes and their amplification in tumors therefore represents promising therapeutic approach in treating cancer, and strategies focusing on classic oncogenes (such as *bcl-2*, *ras* and *HER-2/neu*) have been extensively explored in esophageal, breast, ovarian and other carcinomas. Other candidate targets may include genes associated with cell proliferation, metastasis, angiogenesis, and drug resistance. Very recently, Liang et al., (2011) showed that DNA vector-based Stat3-specific RNA interference (si-Stat3) blocks Stat3 signalling which was delivered by hydroxyapatite nanoparticles and suppresses mouse prostate tumor growth *in vivo*. In this study, the Stat3 downstream genes Bcl-2, VEGF and cyclin D1 were also strongly downregulated in the tumor tissues that also displayed significant increases in Bax expression and Caspase3 activity (Liang et al. 2011). While the application of antisense technology to the treatment of human cancer is conceptually straightforward, selection of appropriate gene targets is an important parameter in the potential success of siRNA cancer therapies (Ashihara 2010), and in practice there are many complicated, mechanistically based questions that must be considered. Importantly, folding of target RNAs or their association with specific proteins in the cell often prevents the ON molecules from binding to their targets. In addition, silencing of such genes must not affect the functions of normal cells.

2.5 Anti-angiogenic therapy

The ability of solid tumors to grow locally, and subsequently disseminate to distant organs, is dependent upon the formation of new blood vessels (Azad et al. 2008) and involves angiogenic factors such as vascular endothelial growth factor (VEGF). VEGF plays an important role in the proliferation of cancer cells, angiogenesis and vascular permeability in peritoneal dissemination. BevacizumAb, the only United States Food and Drug Administration (FDA)-approved anti-VEGF agent, is a monoclonal antibody that inhibits the binding of VEGF to VEGF receptors. CBO-P11, a cyclo-peptide, has proven to specifically bind to receptors of VEGF and may be used as targeting ligand for tumor angiogenesis. Deshayes et al., (2011) investigated the conjugation of CBO-P11 on the surface of poly(vinylidene fluoride) nanoparticles using the copper(I)-catalyzed Huisgen 1,3-dipolar cycloaddition known as a "click" reaction. Nanoparticles were found to be spherical, dense, monodisperse and stable. No cytotoxicity was observed after four days of incubation demonstrating the biocompatibility of nanoparticles. Fluorescence highlighted the specific interaction of these functionalized nanoparticles for VEGF receptors, suggesting that the targeting peptide bioactivity was retained (Deshayes et al. 2011). Therapies based on mAb targeting and blocking of vascular endothelial growth factor, such as that conferred by the monoclonal bevacizumAb, have clearly demonstrated remarkable antitumor efficacy, although the mechanism of action here is not well understood. Combined treatment of bevacizumAb with Sorafenib (a small molecular inhibitor of several tyrosine protein kinases such as VEGFR and PDGFR) resulted in partial response or disease stabilization for ≥ 4 months (median, 6 months; range, 4 to 22+ months) in 22 (59%) of 37 assessable patients with advanced solid tumors .

Matrix metalloproteases (MMPs) are a family of more than 20 zinc and calcium dependent enzymes that degrade all major basement membrane and extracellular matrix components. These enzymes also promote tumor invasion and metastasis, regulating host defense mechanisms and normal cell function. They are well adapted to serve as signaling conduits in the tumor-stromal microenvironment given their crucial roles in the complex processes of tissue invasion, blood vessel homeostasis, and metastasis. Specifically, MMP-1, MMP-2 and MMP-9 mRNA expression in multivariate analyses has been correlated with a well-characterized clinical significance in solid tumors but have no such role in effusions, suggesting the clinical role of MMP is limited to solid lesions. MMP inhibitors (MMPIs) are expected to be useful for the treatment of diseases such as cancer, osteoarthritis, and rheumatoid arthritis. A vast number of MMPIs have been developed in recent years. With the failure of these inhibitors in clinical trials, more efforts have been directed to the design of specific inhibitors with different Zn-binding groups (Tu et al. 2008).

2.6 Multidrug resistance inhibition/gene transfer strategies

Cancer cells counter the influx of a chemotherapeutic by draining the drug from cells, deactivating the protein that transports the drug across cell walls, restoring DNA breaks, or developing some other mechanism to deactivate the drug. Multidrug resistance continues to be a major problem in the management of cancer and knockdown of drug resistance associated genes such as MDR1 (ABCB1), survivin, and pre-mRNA processing factor-4 (PRP-4) has been attempted in cancer cell lines. PRP-4 belongs to the serine/threonine protein kinase family, plays a role in pre-mRNA splicing and cell mitosis whereas survivin, a member of the inhibitor of apoptosis family of proteins, is implicated in both apoptosis inhibition and cell cycle control. Recently, Chen et al., (2010) developed two nanoparticle formulations, cationic liposome-polycation-DNA (Whitmore et al. 1999) and anionic liposome-polycation-DNA (LPD-II), for systemic co-delivery of doxorubicin (Dox) and a therapeutic small interfering RNA (siRNA) to multiple drug resistance (Hesdorffer et al. 1998) tumors. In this study, they have provided four strategies to overcome drug resistance. First, the investigators formed the LPD nanoparticles with a guanidinium-containing cationic lipid, i.e. N,N-distearyl-N-methyl-N-2-(N'-arginyl) aminoethyl ammonium chloride, which can induce reactive oxygen species, down-regulate MDR transporter expression, and increase Dox uptake. Second, to block angiogenesis and increase drug penetration, the authors have further formulated LPD nanoparticles to co-deliver vascular endothelial growth factor siRNA and Dox. An enhanced Dox uptake and a therapeutic effect were observed when combined with vascular endothelial growth factor siRNA in the nanoparticles. Third, to avoid P-glycoprotein-mediated drug efflux, they further designed another delivery vehicle, LPD-II, which showed much higher entrapment efficiency of Dox than LPD. Finally, the authors delivered a therapeutic siRNA to inhibit MDR transporter. Three daily intravenous injections of therapeutic siRNA and Dox (1.2 mg/kg) co-formulated in either LPD or LPD-II nanoparticles showed a significant improvement in tumor growth inhibition (Chen et al. 2010a). Numerous other similar studies highlights a potential clinical use for these multifunctional nanoparticles with an effective delivery property and a function to overcome drug resistance in cancer.

3. Delivery systems

Over the past 20 years, a variety of techniques have been developed for encapsulating both conventional drugs (such as anticancer drugs and antibiotics) and new genetic drugs (plasmid DNA containing therapeutic genes, antisense oligonucleotides and small interfering RNA) within nanoparticles. Nanoparticle delivery systems for gene delivery possess useful inherent attributes, including a diameter of approximately 100 nm or less, a high drug-to-lipid ratio (in the case of lipid based systems), excellent retention of the encapsulated drug, and a long (> 6 h) circulation lifetime. These properties permit nanoparticles to protect their contents during circulation, prevent contact with healthy normal tissues, and accumulate at sites of disease.

3.1 Viral and non-viral delivery systems
A major impediment to the successful application of gene therapy for the treatment of a range of diseases is not a paucity of therapeutic genes, but the lack of an efficient non-toxic gene delivery system. Gene delivery is generally accomplished using one of two categories of delivery vector: 1) Viral delivery vectors derived from engineered retrovirus, adenovirus, herpesvirus, lentivirus or hybrid retro/adeno virus), and 2) Non-viral (synthetic) vectors comprised of polymers and lipids, naked DNA, plasmid-protein conjugates.   Other (physical as opposed to chemical) methods include microneedle coating, gene gun, and ultrasound/microbubble-mediated gene delivery.

Viral vectors account for nearly 75% of all clinical trials conducted thus far (http://www.wiley.co.uk/genetherapy/ clinical). These vectors are essentially viruses that have been genetically modified to remove any replication/pathogenic genes, and instead encode a gene of interest (Hesdorffer et al. 1998). This strategy preserves the viruses highly efficient ability to infect cells, while eliminating/attenuating toxicity. The most commonly used viral vectors are retroviral, adenoviral, adeno-associated viral and herpes simplex viral-based (Young et al. 2006). Although Vitravene, an antisense oligonucleotide-based product, is the only gene delivery product approved so far by US-FDA, there are several other products in late stages of clinical trials. Gendicine, an adenovirus encoding the *p53* gene, developed by SiBiono GeneTech Co., Ltd., was recently approved by China's state Food and Drug Administration, for the treatment of head and neck squamous cell carcinoma. Virus-based treatments tend to maximize efficiency of gene transfer, often at the cost of safety, while non-viral options generally capitalize on a higher safety profile, but usually at the expense of Gene of Interest (GOI) expression efficiency. Many viruses including retroviruses, adenoviruses, herpes simplex viruses, adeno-associated viruses (AAV) and pox viruses have been modified to eliminate their toxicity, maintain their high gene transfer capability and long term gene expression.

However, despite these advantages, there are currently major limitations to the use of viruses as gene delivery vectors. These include the limited carrying capacity of transgenic materials (i.e. size of plasmid) since the packaging capacity of viral vectors (usually up to 5 kb) is constrained; the potential for oncogenesis due to chromosomal integration or activation of oncogenes/inactivation of oncogene regulators; the generation of infectious viruses due to recombination; and concerns regarding instability that challenge production and storage.

The potentially hazardous nature of viral vectors has been observed in a number of gene therapy-related patient mortalities in various clinical trials. Patient complications to date have included the rejection of DNA carriers, resulting in immune response that have led to already one death, Jesse Gelsinger, who died in 1999 from a rare metabolic disorder during a gene-therapy clinical trial at the University of Pennsylvania (Branca 2005;Ledford 2007;Stolberg 1999;Wilson 2010). DNA constructs need to be optimized to carry minimal immunogenic components without compromising both efficient and long-term transgene expression. In this context, technology employing minimal immunological defined gene expression technology (MIDGE) represents a promising future alternative to conventional plasmids in terms of biosafety, improved gene transfer, potential bioavailability, minimal size and low immunogenicity associated with these chemically engineered miniDNA vectors. MIDGEs are non-viral, lcc (linear covalently closed) miniplasmids synthesized *in vitro* via a patented chemical modification of linear open (lo). These plasmids confer the advantage of a minimal coding sequence that relieves complications from expression of additional unwanted genes and CpG motifs that have a 20-fold higher occurrence in bacterial cells. MIDGE lcc plasmid transfection expression was reported to increase luciferase transgene expression from 2.5 to 17 fold *ex vivo* compared to circular covalently closed (ccc), isogenic forms in a tissue-dependent manner (Schakowski et al. 2007) . In addition, the mean numbers of MIDGE vector molecules per cell was also found to be significantly higher, suggesting that linear lcc plasmids transfect cells more efficiently. MIDGE technology has already been applied, with promising results, to the development of a Leishmania DNA vaccine and a colon carcinoma treatment. Here, therapy was based on IL-2 delivery to specific tumor cell lines *ex vivo*, and revealed 2 to 4 fold higher relative transgene expression compared to the ccc control (Schakowski et al. 2001). In combination, the existing studies employing lcc DNA systems suggest that lcc DNA is superior to lo DNA in transfection efficiency, and to ccc DNA in transgene expression. Purified TelN (closely related to Tel) was previously reported to generate lcc plasmids *in vitro* in (*pal*-related) *telRL*-dependent manner and was shown to successfully deliver EGFP to human embryonal kidney cells *in vitro*, as well as IL-12 in an untargeted manner to inhibit metastasis formation in B16F10C57BL/6 melanoma model mice *in vivo* (Heinrich et al. 2002).

At present, our laboratory is involved in design, and construction of bacteriophage-encoded recombination systems to generate linear covalently closed (lcc) DNA mini-vectors. Conditional expression recombinase systems *in vivo* in *E. coli* provide a one step production system for step minivectors from specialized parental plasmids. The exploitation of this recombination system allows us to generate lcc miniplasmids that should have a preferential safety profile, preventing viable vector-chromosome, single recombination products in mammalian cells. In theory, the integration of covalently closed linear exogenous DNA into double-stranded (ds) DNA breaks is unlikely due to the unavailability of terminal ends, and a vector single recombination event into a target chromosome should theoretically result in the disruption of the chromosome, killing the cell (see Figure 1).

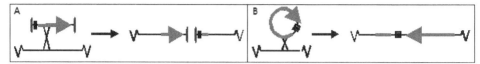

Fig. 1. Plasmid Integration Events: A miniplasmid that undergoes a single recombination event with the host chromosome should be rare due to the removal of all elements except the gene of interest. Any integration events by: A. A lcc miniplasmid should result in chromosomal disruption that is likely lethal and cannot be replicated or segregated; B. A ccc miniplasmid can integrate without disrupting the host chromosome.

Non-viral gene delivery is emerging as a realistic alternative to the use of viral vectors with the potential to have a significant impact on clinical therapies. Synthetic vectors provide flexibility in formulation design and can be tailored to the size and topology of the DNA cargo and the specific route of vector administration, and can be delivered selectively to a specific tissue type through the incorporation of a targeting ligand. Compared to viral vectors, synthetic vectors are potentially less immunogenic, relatively easy to produce in clinically relevant quantities, and are associated with fewer safety concerns (Liu and Huang 2002). As a result of these advantages, their use has rapidly moved from transfection of cell cultures to clinical cancer gene therapy applications.

Synthetic vectors designed for parenteral administration encompass a wide range of formulations. These include unmodified (naked) DNA, which is designed for direct intra-tissue injection, cationic polymer–DNA complexes, cationic lipid–DNA complexes, and cationic polymer–lipid–DNA ternary complexes (lipopolyplexes), which are mostly aimed at systemic administration.

3.1.1 Naked DNA
The simplest employed method of transgene delivery is the injection of naked DNA. It shows very little dissemination and transfection at distant sites following delivery and can be re-administered multiple times into mammals (including primates) without inducing an antibody response against itself (i.e., no anti-DNA antibodies generated) (Wolff and Budker, 2005). The simplicity of this approach is offset by serious limitations such as inefficient uptake of the therapeutic gene into the target cells and rapid clearance of the DNA from the circulation. Direct *in vivo* gene transfer with naked DNA was first demonstrated by efficient transfection of myofibers following injection of mRNA or pDNA into skeletal muscle (Wolff JA, 1990). This novel approach was heralded as a superior method of *in vivo* transfection and its application was later advanced to confer high level expression in hepatocytes in mice by the rapid injection of naked DNA in large volumes into the tail vein (Zhang et al., 1999). This hydrodynamic tail vein (HTV) procedure has proven very useful not only to gene expression studies, but also more recently for the delivery of siRNA (Lewis et al., 2002; McCaffrey et al., 2002). Ultrasound-mediated eruption of polyethyleneglycol (PEG)-modified liposomes loaded with naked plasmid-DNA is also a feasible and efficient technique for gene delivery (Negishi et al. 2010).

3.1.2 Cationic liposomes

Cationic liposomes are one of the most efficient, and among the most widely used non-viral vector systems. They are composed of positively charged lipid bilayers that can be complexed to DNA through electrostatic interactions resulting in complexes, termed lipoplexes. The application of cationic liposomes to gene therapy was first described in 1987 by Felgner (Felgner et al. 1987). The lipoplexes are generally composed of a positively charged lipidic component (see Figure 2), such as dioleylpropyltrimethylammonium chloride, dioleoyl triethylammonium propane (DOTAP), or dimethylaminoethane carbamoyl cholesterol (DC-Chol), that is capable of complexing and condensing the DNA (Giatrellis et al. 2009). Most lipoplex formulations include a "helper" lipid, such as dioleoylphosphatidyl-ethanolamine (DOPE, as seen in Figure 2), or cholesterol that provides added stability to the lipoplexes and enhances DNA release from endosomal compartments. While transfection activity of lipoplexes is shown to vary depending on their DNA/cationic lipid ratio, it is necessary for them to be positively charged to interact with the negatively charge cell membranes and exhibit transfection activity. Lipoplex uptake occurs through endosome formation (via a number of mechnisms including caveosomes, clathrin dependent, etc.), followed by disruption of the endosomal membrane by fusion with, or incorporation of the lipoplex lipids resulting in DNA release.

The advantages of liposomes in delivery system designs include their simplicity in preparation, ability to complex relatively large amounts of DNA, versatility for use with any size or type of DNA/RNA, ability to transfect non-dividing cells and overall stability (Dutta et al. 2010). In addition, lipids are non-immunogenic allowing for repeated administration without adverse immunologic reaction(Barron et al. 1999). The primary disadvantages of lipoplex delivery vectors include low tumor transfection efficiency and lack of tumor specificity.

In order to enhance gene transfection, based upon structure-activity relationship, various gemini surfactants (Gemini surfactants consist of two hydrophobic chains and two polar headgroups linked chemically by a spacer group) have been designed. In order to enhance gene transfection based upon structure-activity relationship, various gemini surfactants have been designed, synthesized and tested for gene delivery in our laboratory (Donkuru et al. 2010;Wang and Wettig 2011;Wettig et al. 2007a;Wettig et al. 2007b;Wettig and Verrall 2001). Recent reports have shown that obstacles can be overcome by exploiting receptor-mediated endocytosis for highly efficient internalization of ligands naturally employed by eukaryotic cells. Advances along this line include the conjugation of mAbs ("immunoliposomes"), ligands such as growth factors, or hormones to liposomes to confer targeting capability. Nanoparticle based anti-cancer gene/drug delivery first reached clinical trial in mid 1980s and the first nanomedicine Doxil® (liposomal encapsulated doxorubicin) was marketed in 1995. Other example of liposome-mediated drug delivery include daunorubicin (Daunoxome), which is also currently being marketed as liposome delivery systems. Numerous new nanoparticle based cancer gene therapy systems are under development.

3.1.3 Polyplexes

Polyplexes differ from lipoplexes in that they are comprised of charged complexes of plasmid DNA and a cationic polymer, such as poly-L-lysine (PLL), polyethylenimine, polyamidoamine (starburst) dendrimers, and chitosan with a net positive charge (See Figure 2). Cationic polymers differ from cationic lipids primarily in that they do not contain a hydrophobic moiety and are completely soluble in water. A wide variety of cationic polymers that transfect cells *in vitro* have been characterized (Midoux et al., 2008). A key determinant of polyplex gene transfer efficiency is the positive (on amine nitrogen atoms in the polymer) to negative charge ratio or the related negative to positive (N/P) ratio. Given their polymeric nature, cationic polymers can be synthesized in different lengths, with different geometry (linear versus branched), and with substitutions or additions of functional groups with relative ease and flexibility, which opens the way to extensive structure/function relationship studies.

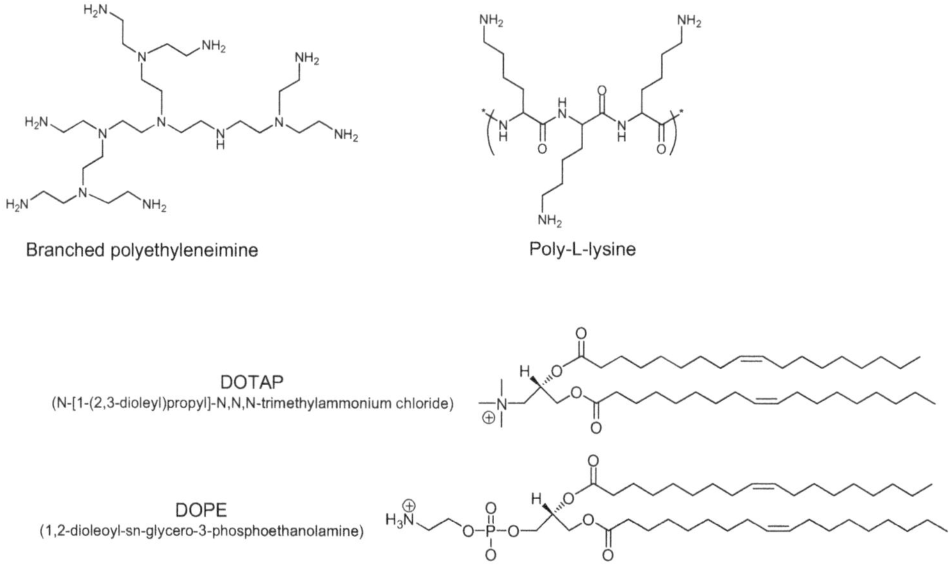

Branched polyethyleneimine   Poly-L-lysine

DOTAP
(N-[1-(2,3-dioleyl)propyl]-N,N,N-trimethylammonium chloride)

DOPE
(1,2-dioleoyl-sn-glycero-3-phosphoethanolamine)

Fig. 2. Examples of commonly used lipids (DOPE and DOTAP) and polymers (PEI and poly-L-lysine) in gene therapy.

Polymer-based nanoparticles are now widely used for gene and drug delivery and targeted therapy. One of the most widely applied cationic polymers used for DNA transfections is polyethyleneimine (Choosakoonkriang et al. 2003). DNA complexation with PEI, has not been found to result in an alteration of DNA conformation, remaining essentially in the B form, and the utility of PEI as a gene delivery vector has been demonstrated in numerous studies (Jere et al. 2009;Moore et al. 2009). High molecular weight PEI has been shown to be one of the most successful polymeric vectors due to the large number of protonatable amine groups that result in an enhanced ability to escape from the endosome following uptake by the cell via the so-called "proton sponge" effect. This benefit is contrasted by the high level of cellular toxicity also imparted by the number of amine groups within the polymer. Attempts to overcome this increased level of toxicity have involved using low molecular weight PEI; however, transfection efficiencies are directly correlated with decreases in molecular weight while the tendency to aggregate can increase with decreasing polymer molecular weight. Another successful strategy has involved the shielding of the polyethylenimine/DNA core with a shell of polyethylene glycol (PEG). This approach results in the formation of a dense hydrophilic outer surface of the complexes, reducing hydrophobic interactions with serum proteins and components of the reticulo-endothelial system (RES). In addition to decreasing toxicity of the polyplexes, this strategy also confers increased biocirculation times and therefore, further increases transfection efficiencies. [Please see van Vlerken et al. 2007 for a recent review of PEG modification of nanocarriers]. The presence of the terminal alcohol groups in this PEG outer shell also provides sites for further modification that have been conjugated to various types of targeting ligands, including glycoprotein, transferring, carbohydrates, folate and epidermal growth factors, facilitating tissue-specific gene delivery (Guo and Lee 1999;Han et al. 1999;Lai et al. 2009). Such complexes have been found to mediate efficient gene transfer into tumor cell lines in a receptor-dependent and cell-cycle-dependent manner. While the modifications described here have resulted in significant improvements in both the transfection efficiencies and toxicity profiles of polycation-based transfection vectors, a number of questions relating to mechanisms of endosome escape (Tros, I et al. 2010), structure-activitiy relationships, pharmacokinetics, and *in-vitro* vs *in-vivo* application remain (Jere et al. 2009). Overall, while proving to be a very promising strategy toward gene therapy design, polyplex systems still require much further testing and improvement prior to entering clinical trials (Midoux et al., 2008).

3.1.4 Lipopolyplexes

Lipopolyplexes (lipid-polymer-DNA complexes or LPDs) combine plasmid DNA with both a cationic polymer and liposomes via electrostatic interactions. In general, these vectors are compact particles that exhibit superior colloidal stability, reduced cytotoxicity, and provide elevated transfection efficiency compared to either polyplexes or lipoplexes alone. The cationic polymer may be covalently linked to the liposomes (e.g. lipopolylysine) or be non-covalently incorporated into a ternary lipid–polymer–DNA complex by a charge-mediated self-assembly process. The polycation component facilitates the optimal condensation of plasmid DNA, whereas lipidic components, to which targeting ligands can be attached, further stabilize the vector formulation and mediate the efficient endosomal escape of the vector following cellular internalization. LPD particles prepared using protamine as the cationic polymer and DOTAP/Chol cationic liposomes have been reported to inhibit tumor growth following i.v. administration in mice (Whitmore et al. 1999). Both *in vitro* and *in vivo* studies have demonstrated improved outcomes of (liposomes/protamine/DNA) LPD-mediated gene transfer over conventional liposomes (El-Aneed 2004) . It is believed that the small size of LPD (100 to 250 nm, which is almost three to five times less than conventional lipoplexes) will facilitate endocytosis and increase the *in vivo* circulating half life.

4. Challenges in nanoparticle based gene therapy

To facilitate efficient gene expression, delivered plasmid DNA must initially circumnavigate various barriers to cellular and nuclear entry as seen in Figure 3. The lipoplex/polyplex must first be internalized by the cell membrane,for which there are many different possible routes including receptor mediated endocytosis, pinocytosis and phagocytosis (Godbey and Mikos 2001). Receptor-mediated endocytosis or clathrin-dependent internalization is the most common of these and can be exploited to engineer polyplexes to express attached ligands to facilitate this process (Morille et al. 2008).

Pinocytosis is the process by which cells internalize liquids which contain suspended or soluble particles. Untargeted polyplexes that interact with the cell membrane electrostatically may be internalized via this pathway . Phagocytosis is another possible method of internalization involving the ingestion of larger particles greater than 0.5 µm in diameter.

Targeting and internalization of microspheres to phagocytic cells *in vivo* can be achieved through size exclusion. It is important to note that internalization mechanisms may also be largely dependent on the cell type, the vector used, and the process parameters of that a particular vector system (Duncan et al. 2006). On the cellular level, many complexes become buried in the endolysosomal compartment or are degraded in the cytoplasm. After internalization occurs, the lipoplex/polyplex is believed to be most commonly contained within an endocytic vesicle after which it is transferred to late endosomes and lysosomes. In these compartments the pH rapidly changes to the range of 4.5–6, and in order for successful transfection to occur the DNA must find a way to escape from these structures and reach the nucleus as DNA that remains in these cellular compartments is readily degraded (Pack et al. 2005). The final obstacle in the DNA vector's journey is the double bilayer membrane surrounding the nucleus, or nuclear membrane. While small molecules may gain access to the nucleus directly through its network of pores, larger molecules must be internalized by specific nuclear import proteins. This process is largely dependent on the size of the DNA and its conformation. As such, in the absence of specialized enhancer sequences, nuclear import of plasmids is limited to actively dividing cells undergoing mitosis.

In gene therapy studies, nuclear localization signal (NLS) peptides have been investigated as facilitators of nuclear transport with the aim of enhancing transgene expression. In order to improve overall transfection specificity and efficiency it is necessary to optimize intracellular trafficking of the DNA complex as well as the performance after systemic administration (Schatzlein 2001). Properties of vector such as size, shape, and surface characteristics can also have a major impact on its pharmacokinetic properties and delivery efficiency. For most nanoparticles, it is unknown what size and/or charge of nanoparticles could lead to defects in DNA transcription and chromosomal damage and aberration. However, there are indications that certain types of nanoparticles are capable of causing DNA damage, where the composition and the coating of nanoparticles are likely the key factors imparting genotoxic effects.

With respect to systematic *in vivo* applications, nanocarrier approaches face additional hurdles. First, despite advances in using PEG or other hydrophilic polymers for extracellular stability to prolong their circulation in the blood stream, a large fraction of the injected dose of nanoparticles accumulates in the liver and is taken up by hepatic phagocytes. Second, due to the vascular endothelial barrier, nanoparticles can only reach certain tissues such as the liver, spleen, and some types of tumors as a result of enhanced permeability and retention (an effect due to the presence of fenestrated endothelium in tumor blood vessels i.e passive targeting) effect, where the nanoparticles tend to accumulate in tumor tissues much more than in normal tissues. However, nanoparticles cannot, or rarely access, parenchymal cells in most normal tissues as they are simply excluded by the endothelial barrier. Thus, many potential disease targets cannot at present be addressed by existing nanocarrier approaches.

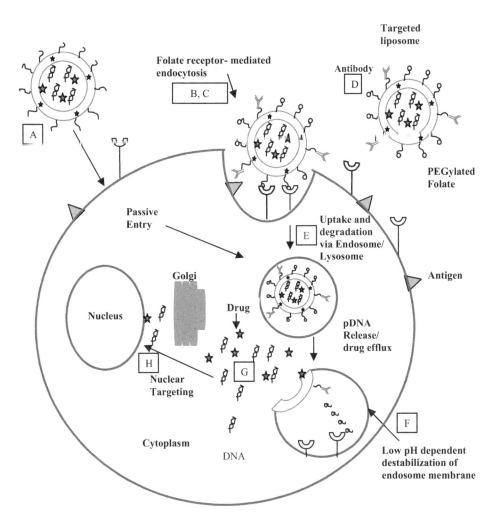

Fig. 3. A schematic generalized diagram of folate receptor/ non-receptor mediated non-viral delivery system: The tethers connecting the folate to the lipid headgroups consist of 250 Å long polyethyleneglycol spacers. Condensation/ complexation of DNA-based therapeutics with DNA delivery vector; (B, C) Non-specific adsorption to cell membrane and cellular internalization via non-receptor mediated (passive entry) or folate-receptor (folate tittered PEGylated liposome's shown in yellow balls and encapsulated drugs as red stars) mediated endocytosis pathway; (D) Monoclonal antibody-antigen complex mediated endocytosis pathway; (E) Uptake and degradation via endosome, lysosome; (F) Low pH dependent destabilization of endosome membrane; (G) Cytoplasmic release of plasmid DNA and drug efflux; (H) Nuclear targeting via nuclear localization signals, transcription and transgene expression.

4.1 Targeted nanomedicine

Construction of organ-targeted gene delivery vectors is a promising route to improve the safety and efficacy of nanomedicine based cancer gene therapy. There are a variety of 'vector targeting' strategies, that can be accomplished using transcriptional targeting, transductional targeting, or ideally, a combination of these. While transcriptional targeting refers to the use of gene regulatory elements (promoters and enhancers) to restrict gene expression to specific cells, transductional targeting refers to the delivery of DNA to specific cells. Targeted gene expression has been analyzed using tissue-specific promoters (breast-, prostate-, and melanoma-specific promoters) and disease-specific promoters (carcinoembryonic antigen, HER-2/neu, Myc-Max response elements, DF3/MUC). The addition of a ligand (i.e., folate, transferrin, RGD peptide, among others) to the nanoparticle surface, thus targeting the DNA to cells *in vivo* has been demonstrated quite successfully. Folate-receptor-targeted liposomes have proven effective in delivering doxorubicin *in vivo* and have been found to bypass multidrug resistance in cultured tumor cells (Immordino et al. 2006). Hong et al., (2010) exploited the possibility of combination of the functions of passive and active targeting by transferring-PEGlyated nanoparticles (Tf-PEG-NP), as well as sustained drug release in tumor by PEGylated drug for most efficient tumor targeting and anti-tumor effects enhancement. Such Tf-PEG-NP loaded with PEGylated drug conjugates could be one of the promising strategies in nanomedicine to deliver anti-tumor drugs to tumor (Hong et al. 2010). Further enhancement of the therapeutic index may also be achieved by overcoming barriers both at cellular and nuclear levels. In gene therapy studies, nuclear localization signal peptides have been investigated as facilitators of nuclear transport with the aim of enhancing transgene expression. Selective tumor targeting with minimal toxicity using folate modified, incorporating nuclear localization signal represents a popular approach. In recent years, Poly(ε-caprolactone)/poly(ethylene glycol) (PCL/PEG) copolymers which are biodegradable and amphiphilic, are also emerging as a potential nanoplatform for anticancer agent delivery (Gou et al. 2011).

5. Nanobased cancer diagnosis approaches

Current problems and unmet needs in translational oncology include (i) advanced technologies for tumor imaging and early detection, (ii) new methods for accurate diagnosis and prognosis, (iii) strategies to overcome the toxicity and adverse side effects of chemotherapy drugs, and (iv) basic discovery in cancer biology leading to new knowledge for treating aggressive and lethal cancer phenotypes such as bone metastasis. Advances in these areas will undoubtedly form the major cornerstones for a future medical practice of personalized oncology. Cancer detection, diagnosis, and therapy will be tailored to each individual's tumor molecular profile and used in predictive oncology, whereby genetic/molecular markers will play an essential role in the prediction of disease development, progression, and clinical outcomes.

The probability of a successful treatment modality increases dramatically if tumor cells can be selectively removed before they evolve to their mature stages and metastases production. As such, novel and more sensitive diagnostic tools like metallic and semiconducting nanoparticles are being developed with the aim of improving the early and noninvasive detection of rising malignancies and the accuracy of tumor tissue localization. Paramagnetic nanoparticles, quantum dots, nanoshells and nanosomes represent some of these new technologies, used for diagnostic purposes (See Figure 4). Compared to conventional materials, inorganic nanomaterials provide several advantages such as simple preparative processes and precise control over their shape, composition and size. These systems provide promising potential not only in diagnostics, but also as delivery systems for therapeutic agents and are discussed in detail below.

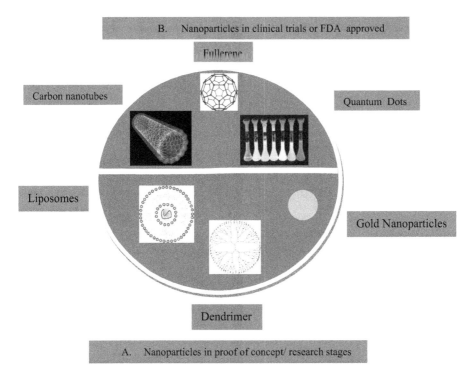

Fig. 4. Nanoparticles used in cancer diagnosis and treatment. Liposomes contain amphiphilic molecules, which have hydrophobic and hydrophilic groups that self-assemble in water. Gold nanoparticles are solid metal particles that are conventionally coated with drug molecules, proteins, or oligonucleotides. Quantum dots consist of a core-and-shell structure (e.g., CdSe coated with zinc and sulfide with a stabilizing molecule and a polymer layer coated with a protein). Fullerenes (typically called "buckyballs" because they resemble Buckminster Fuller's geodesic dome) and carbon nanotubes have only carbon-to-carbon bonds.

5.1 Quantum dots

Quantum Dots (QDs) are a unique class of light emitting semiconductor nanoparticles ranging from 2-10 nanometers in diameter and are becoming highly popular for biological imaging due to their high intensity and stable fluorescence profile (most QDs are approximately 10-20× brighter than organic dyes). QDs usually consist of a CdSe core surrounded by a inorganic shell composed of ZnS (Pinaud et al. 2010). For biological imaging applications, they are given hydrophilic coatings of PEG or multiple carboxylate groups.

Compared to the commercially available organic dyes and fluorescent proteins used in medical imaging, QDs provide many advantages (Park et al. 2009;Pic et al. 2010;Rogach and Ogris 2010;Yong et al. 2009). The first and foremost important feature is the long-term photostability of QD imaging probes, which opens the possibility of investigating the dynamics of cellular processes over time, such as continuously tracking cell migration, differentiation, and metastasis. In addition, QD emission wavelengths are size-tunable and extend from visible to near infrared (NIR) (650 nm to 950 nm), to take advantage of the improved tissue penetration depth and reduced background fluorescence at these wavelengths. For example, CdSe/ZnS QDs of approximately 2 nm in diameter produce a blue emission, while QDs approximately 7 nm in diameter emit red light. While fluorescence imaging is often limited by the poor transmission of visible light through biological tissue, there is a NIR optical window in most biological tissue that is suitable for deep tissue optical imaging, where only a few organic dyes emit brightly in this region and generally suffer from photobleaching. In contrast, the novel optical properties of QDs allow the synthesis of bright and stable fluorescent labels that emit in the near infra red spectrum by adjusting their size and composition.

Surface functionalization using peptides, proteins and antibodies, confers the ability of QDs to provide high biological compatibility and capacity to target and image tumors in living subjects through the rapid readout of fluorescence imaging. Moreover, QDs allow imaging of deeper tissues and is also used to image lymph nodes and blood vessels in tissues. A key property for *in vivo* imaging is the unusual QD Stokes shift (measured by the distance between excitation and emission peaks), which can be as large as 300-400nm depending on the wavelength of the excitation light, which can be used to further improve the detection sensitivity. Organic dye signals with a small stoke shift are often buried by strong tissue autofluorescene, whereas QD signal with large Stokes shift are clearly detectable above the background. Unlike traditional dyes which usually show a broad emission band, QDs exhibit narrow sharp emission peaks and broadband absorption, which are ideal for multiplexed multicolor imaging. QDs are thus able to increase the number of labels that can be used simultaneously in a single system. The effective brightness per probe particle is also superior with quantum dots as evidenced by their large molar absorption cross-sections which are a consequence of their nanometer size and composition. Different from "soft" organic nanoparticles (e.g., polymers, micelles, liposomes), inorganic nanomaterials with rigid cores usually show inefficient extravasation inside tumors. A number of reports suggest that QDs tend to stay within the tumor vasculatures without getting into the interstitial space or tumor cells, reducing the nonspecific tumor cell labeling in angiogenesis imaging (Liu and Peng 2010). The long term photostability and superior brightness of QDs make them appealing for live animal targeting and imaging. These properties have made QDs a topic of intensive interest in cancer biology, molecular imaging, and molecular profiling.

The ability to functionalize as well as control the surface of quantum dots with specific linkers and multi-functional molecules is critical for nanoparticle-based gene therapy. Currently, QDs are used both as a transfection vector as well as a fluorescence label in RNA interference research. Quantum dot conjugates have been successfully used for targeted silencing of bcr/abl gene by RNA interference in human myelogenous leukemia K562 cells (Zhao et al. 2010). In addition, Derfus et al., (2007) using PEGlyated quantum dot core as a scaffold, and conjugating siRNA and tumor-homing peptides (F3) to functional groups on the particle's surface found that the homing peptide was required for targeting internalization by tumor cells, and that siRNA cargo could be co-attached without affecting the function of the peptide (Derfus et al. 2007). Using an EGFP model system, the role of conjugation chemistry was also investigated, with siRNA attached to the particle by disulfide cross-linkers showing greater silencing efficiency than when attached by a non-reducible thioether linkage. Delivery of these F3/siRNA-QDs to EGFP-transfected HeLa cells and release from their endosomal entrapment led to significant knockdown of EGFP signal. By designing the siRNA sequence against a therapeutic target (e.g., oncogene) instead of EGFP, this technology may be ultimately adapted to simultaneously treat and image metastatic cancer. These nanoprobes could be used for both active and passive targeting. Therefore, in future research, QDs can be seen as multi-functional platforms focusing on targeted delivery, high transfection efficiency, and multi-modal imaging/tracking and treatment of cancer as shown in Figure 5.

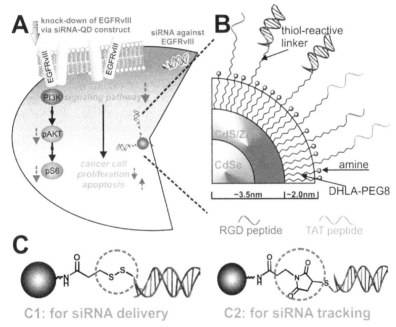

Fig. 5. (A): Quantum dots as a multi-functional nanoplatform to deliver siRNA and to elucidate of EGFR knockdown effect of PI3K signaling pathway in brain tumor cells. (B): Detailed structural information of multifunctional siRNA-QDs: CdSe as core with ZnS capping along with thiol reactive linker for siRNA conjugation as well as RGD peptides as shown in red and TAT peptides as shown in green. In order to make QD constructs water-soluble and suitable for conjugating with siRNA, hydrophobic ligands are displaced with a dihydrolipoic acid (DHLA) derivatized with an amine terminated polyethylene glycol (PEG) spacer. (C): Two different strategies for the siRNA-QD conjugate. (C1) Linker for attaching siRNA to QDs through a disulfide linkage which are easily reduced within the cells to release the siRNA. (C2) Linker for covalently conjugating siRNA to QDs which enable tracking of siRNA-QDs within the cells. (Taken from: Jung et al. 2010).

However, there have been some QD concentration dependent toxicity and distribution concerns. QDs have been shown to remain in liver, lymph nodes and bone marrow of mice for 1 month after tail injection, despite of its low affinity to cells and tissues (Ballou et al. 2004;Ballou et al. 2009). Recently, the hydrophilic QDs (diameter <10 nm) have attracted more attention for *in vivo* applications, due to the rapid renal clearance of QDs, minimizing the potential toxicity to the system (Park et al. 2009). Recently, Peng and co-workers developed InAs/InP/ZnSe core/shell/shell QDs with high quantum yield (76%) of NIR fluorescence, ultrasmall hydrodynamic sizes (< 10 nm), and the biocompatibility desired for *in vivo* applications (Liu and Peng 2010). These novel QDs have obviously lower intrinsic toxicity compared to commercial Cd-containing NIR emitting QDs and showed significantly improved circulation half-life with reduced RES uptake. NIR-emitting QDs demonstrate exceptional brightness and fluorescent quantum yields. Also, once capped with a chemically stable shell, QDs can exhibit remarkable photostability, providing continuous fluorescent singles for long-term imaging applications. Other types of novel QDs with entirely different compositions and photoluminescence mechanism such as silicon QDs and carbon dots have also emerged as potential probes in bioimaging applications. Further, typical fluorescence images of a single QD shows changes in emission intensity. The intensity time trace illustrates the random alternation between "on" and "off" states, which is known as blinking and it is a signature feature of an individual QD. Also, reducing size of QDs has proven difficult because of decreased colloidal stability and increased nonspecific interactions. Other major limitations include reproducibility in production, proper control of surface functionality, bulky surface coatings (PEG, multiple antibodies, ampiphilic molecules) which leads to restrictions on studying spatially confined, crowded regions of the cell and may also perturb the behavior of the labeled molecules. Quantum dots are not yet approved for use in humans and much more research is needed in future for this growing field.

5.2 Carbon nanotubes

Molecular imaging exploits the specific recognition of labeled probes to their biological targets in conventional imaging techniques to monitor biological processes at the molecular level with improved specificity and sensitivity. Conventional clinical cancer imaging techniques, such as X-ray, CT and MRI, do not possess sufficient spatial resolution for early detection of the disease. Positron emission tomography (PET) is a highly sensitive and accurate imaging technology that relies on changes in tissue biochemistry and metabolism. It is the most valuable means we have so far to identify early-stage alterations in molecular biology, often before there is any morphologic change. Nevertheless, fluoro-desoxy-glucose (FDG), the most commonly used PET tracer in clinical oncology (more than 95% of the molecular imaging procedures make use of FDG at present), is not a specific tracer for malignant diseases but for increased metabolism. Therefore, it is imperative to develop new tools for early cancer diagnosis.

CNTs have been explored in almost every single cancer treatment modality, including drug delivery, lymphatic targeted chemotherapy, thermal therapy, photodynamic therapy, and gene therapy. Based on their structure, CNTs can be classified into two general categories: single-walled (SWNTs), which consist of one layer of cylinder graphene (diameter 0.4-2 nm) and multi-walled (MWNTs), which contain several concentric graphene sheets (diameter 2-100 nm). CNTs have unique physical and chemical properties such as high aspect ratio, ultralight weight, high mechanical strength, high electrical conductivity, and high thermal conductivity (Ji et al. 2010). Carbon nanotubes are the strongest and stiffest materials yet discovered in terms of tensile strength and elastic modulus respectively. As CNTs are intrinsically not water soluble, modification through chemical functionalization can increases the solubility of carbon nanotubes in aqueous solutions.

Imaging functionalities and therapeutics can be incorporated on the same nanoparticle for multifunctional cancer imaging and treatment. SWNT-paclitaxel (PTX) conjugates also showed higher efficacy in suppressing tumor growth than clinical Taxol alone in a murine 4T1 breast cancer model, owing to prolonged blood circulation time and enhanced permeability and retention (EPR) in the tumor (Feazell et al. 2007). Besides, with very high surface area per unit weight, SWNTs provide higher capacity of drug loading, compared to that reported for conventional liposomes and dendrimer drug carriers. Doxorubicin, a commonly used cancer chemotherapy drug, can be loaded on the surface of PEGylated SWNTs with remarkably high loading, up to 4 g of drug per 1 g of nanotube, owing to the ultrahigh surface area of SWNTs. Further, the intrinsic stability and structural flexibility of CNTs may prolong the circulation time as well as improve the bioavailability of drug molecules conjugated to them. Surface-enhanced Raman spectroscopy of carbon nanotubes opens up a method of protein microarray with detection sensitivity down to 1 fmol/L. *In vitro* and *in vivo* toxicity studies reveal that highly water soluble and serum stable nanotubes are biocompatible, nontoxic, and potentially useful for biomedical applications. However, nonfunctionalized nanotubes are toxic to cells and animals and therefore one has to be cautious about the safety aspects of CNTs. If well functionalized, nanotubes may be excreted mainly through the biliary pathway in feces.

Carbon nanotube-based drug delivery has shown promise in various *in vitro* and *in vivo* experiments including delivery of small interfering RNA (siRNA), paclitaxel and doxorubicin (Liu et al. 2009). Multiwalled PEGylated carbon nanotubes are found to be successful, effective and do not alter particle sizes and zeta potentials of carbon nanotubes after PEGylation (Ilbasmis-Tamer et al. 2010). In addition, the propensity to absorb the body transparent NIR radiation also envisages photothermal and photoacoustic therapy using nanotubes.

5.3 Gold and other nanoparticles for cancer diagnosis

Thermal ablation therapy is one the most promising of methods in cancer treatment but is limited by incomplete tumor destruction and damage to adjacent normal tissues. Current radiofrequency ablation techniques require invasive needle placement and are limited by accuracy of targeting. Use of nanoparticles has refined noninvasive thermal ablation of tumors, and several nanomaterials have been used for this purpose. These include gold nanomaterials, iron nanoparticles, magnetic nanoparticles, carbon nanotubes and affisomes (thermosensitive liposomes). Heating of the particles can be induced by magnets, lasers, ultrasound, photodynamic therapy and low-power X-rays. The clinical trials include studies of designed nanoparticles such as the thermosensitive liposomal doxorubicin (Thermodox®) as a novel activated therapy using radiofrequency ablation (Wang and Thanou 2010). As gold nanoparticles have evolved other gold structures have also been suggested. Nanorods, with the appropriate PEG stealth layer, are being developed as an improved means of hyperthermia. By attaching monoclonal antibodies (mAbs), which can recognize a specific cancer cell, to gold nanoparticles or nanorods are also used in cancer detection. Gold nanoparticles conjugated to anti-epidermal growth factor receptor (El-Sayed et al. 2006) mAbs specifically and homogeneously bind to the surface of the cancer cells with 600% greater affinity than to the noncancerous cells. This specific and homogeneous binding is found to give a relatively sharper surface plasma resonance (Hinz et al. 2006) absorption band with a red shifted maximum compared to that observed when added to the noncancerous cells . Surface plasma resonance scattering imaging or SPR absorption spectroscopy generated from antibody conjugated gold nanoparticles may be useful in molecular biosensor techniques for the diagnosis and investigation of cancer cells *in vivo* and *in vitro*.

These inorganic nanoparticles represent a different class of nanoparticles that are usually much smaller, 5–40 nm and they do not have the flexibility observed in liposomes and polymeric nanoparticles. Inorganic nanoparticles have made their appearance in cancer therapy during the last decades in a number of applications. The main type of inorganic nanoparticles – the iron oxide nanoparticles, has been used for imaging tumor (Wang and Thanou 2010). The main advantage of magnetic nanoparticles is their ability to be visualised by Magnetic Resonance (MR) imaging. Additionally, iron oxide nanoparticles can be guided to target sites (i.e. tumor) using external magnetic field and they can be also heated to provide hypethermia for cancer therapy. Yu et al. reported thermally cross-linked superparamagnetic iron oxide nanoparticles that could carry a Cy5.5 near infra-red probe (dual imaging) and doxorubicin for the imaging and treatment of cancer. The nanoparticles substantially diminished tumor size and provided the proof of concept that they can combine several modalities for maximum antitumor effect (Yu et al. 2010). Magnetic nanoparticles have been used in the development of dual purpose probes for the *in vivo* transfection of siRNA. The iron nanoparticles deliver siRNA at the same time as imaging their own accumulation in tumor sites. Hence, multifunctional nanoparticles have emerged that are capable of cancer targeting and simultaneous cancer imaging and therapy.

Metal nanoshells are another class of nanoparticles with tunable optical resonances. Metal nanoshells consist of a spherical dielectric core nanoparticle, in this case silica, which is surrounded by a thin metal shell, such as gold. These particles possess a highly tunable plasmon resonance, a resonant phenomenon whereby light induces collective oscillations of conductive metal electrons at the nanoshell surface. Nanoshells derived from gold provide an attractive system for imaging applications owing to the established ease of preparation, chemical inertness, good biocompatibility, and surface functionalization. Further, nanoparticle based near infrared imaging (NIR) is steadily presenting itself as a powerful diagnostic technique with the real potential to serve as a minimally invasive, nonionizing method for sensitive, deep tissue diagnostic imaging that are not prone to the rapid photobleaching and instability of their organic counterparts. NIR laser treatment of the bulk tissue selectively heats and destroys the nanoshell-laden tumor regions within the tissue, while leaving surrounding tissue intact. Nanoshells are currently evaluated in a number of clinical settings after a 5-year period of intensive preclinical development. Such development of nanoshells included the combination of nanoshells with cancer antibodies. Anti-HER2 antibody conjugated onto nanoshells provides the potential of combining antibody therapy with imaging and hyperthermia. NIR dye-encapsulating nanoparticles also demonstrate improved optical performances compared to unencapsulated organic fluorophores. Specifically, the encapsulation shields the dye molecules from unfavorable environmental influences that normally hinder fluorescence signals, thereby enhancing quantum yields, emission brightness, and fluorescent lifetime. While, at present, these NIR nanoparticulates appear to be superior in terms of optical performances, they are marred by their heavy metal composition and high propensity for toxicity. It is therefore reasonable to be concerned about the ineffectual clearance and long-term accumulation in untargeted organs and tissues of these particulates for *in vivo* use.

6. Conclusion

With the understanding of the genetic origins of certain cancers, an entirely new approach to the treatment of this disease has evolved, employing nanoparticle-based gene therapy. Numerous nanoparticle based cancer gene therapy strategies are already in clinical trials. The key to the success of any new therapeutic is to maximize safety without compromising efficacy, which has led to growing interest in non-viral gene delivery systems (such as liposomes) over the viral gene delivery systems. Grafting biorecognition molecules (ligands, antibodies) onto the nanoparticles (i.e active targeting) aims to improve targeting by specific cell uptake and using hydrophilic polymer coating, PEG, which aims to further enhance biocompatibility. To overcome other challenges of gene therapy, such as escape from endosome and other nuclear and cytosolic barriers, next generation vectors are being designed with use of gene regulatory elements (promoters and enhancers) to restrict gene expression to specific cells, along with nuclear localization signal peptides for nuclear targeting.

There has been substantial interest in dual purpose nanoparticle based gene therapy for both diagnostic (imaging) and therapeutic purposes (drug/gene delivery). Newer technologies for cancer detection/diagnosis using metallic and semiconducting nanoparticles are also under intense investigation. These nanoparticles for *in vivo* application targeting cancer are amenable to different size structures and possess tunable properties. Quantum dots possess unique size- and composition- dependent optical and electrical properties. In addition to quantum dots, carbon nanotubes, paramagnetic nanoparticles, nanoshells and nanosomes represent just a few of these novel technologies, used for both diagnostic and delivery purposes.

The imminent research challenge facing investigators moving forward is the expansion of the knowledge and understanding of the chemical and physical properties associated with these nanoparticle systems toward the design of superior cancer therapy modalities that maximize efficiency of treatment, while maintaining a superior safety profile.

7. References

Aggarwal,S., Yadav,S. and Gupta,S. (2011) EGFR targeted PLGA nanoparticles using gemcitabine for treatment of pancreatic cancer. *J. Biomed. Nanotechnol.* 7, 137-138.

Alivisatos,P. (2004) The use of nanocrystals in biological detection. *Nat. Biotechnol.* 22, 47-52.

Ashihara,E. (2010) [RNA interference for cancer therapies]. *Gan To Kagaku Ryoho.* 37, 2033-2041.

Azad,N.S., Posadas,E.M., Kwitkowski,V.E., Steinberg,S.M., Jain,L., Annunziata,C.M., Minasian,L., Sarosy,G., Kotz,H.L., Premkumar,A., Cao,L., McNally,D., Chow,C., Chen,H.X., Wright,J.J., Figg,W.D. and Kohn,E.C. (2008) Combination targeted therapy with sorafenib and bevacizumab results in enhanced toxicity and antitumor activity. *J. Clin. Oncol.* 26, 3709-3714.

Azatian,A., Yu,H., Dai,W., Schneiders,F.I., Botelho,N.K. and Lord,R.V. (2009) Effectiveness of HSV-tk suicide gene therapy driven by the Grp78 stress-inducible promoter in esophagogastric junction and gastric adenocarcinomas. *J. Gastrointest. Surg.* 13, 1044-1051.

Ballou,B., Ernst,L.A., Andreko,S., Fitzpatrick,J.A., Lagerholm,B.C., Waggoner,A.S. and Bruchez,M.P. (2009) Imaging vasculature and lymphatic flow in mice using quantum dots. *Methods Mol. Biol.* 574, 63-74.

Ballou,B., Lagerholm,B.C., Ernst,L.A., Bruchez,M.P. and Waggoner,A.S. (2004) Noninvasive imaging of quantum dots in mice. *Bioconjug. Chem.* 15, 79-86.

Barron,L.G., Uyechi,L.S. and Szoka,F.C., Jr. (1999) Cationic lipids are essential for gene delivery mediated by intravenous administration of lipoplexes. *Gene Ther.* 6, 1179-1183.

Bell-McGuinn,K.M., Matthews,C.M., Ho,S.N., Barve,M., Gilbert,L., Penson,R.T., Lengyel,E., Palaparthy,R., Gilder,K., Vassos,A., McAuliffe,W., Weymer,S., Barton,J. and Schilder,R.J. (2011) A phase II, single-arm study of the anti-alpha5beta1 integrin antibody volociximab as monotherapy in patients with platinum-resistant advanced epithelial ovarian or primary peritoneal cancer. *Gynecol. Oncol.* [Epub ahead of print]-doi:10.1016/j.ygyno.2010.12.362.

Bhaumik,S. (2011) Advances in Imaging Gene-Directed Enzyme Prodrug Therapy. *Curr. Pharm. Biotechnol.* 12 (4):497-507.

Braasch,D.A. and Corey,D.R. (2002) Novel antisense and peptide nucleic acid strategies for controlling gene expression. *Biochemistry.* 41, 4503-4510.

Branca,M.A. (2005) Gene therapy: cursed or inching towards credibility? *Nat. Biotechnol.* 23, 519-521.

Campbell,I.G., Russell,S.E., Choong,D.Y., Montgomery,K.G., Ciavarella,M.L., Hooi,C.S., Cristiano,B.E., Pearson,R.B. and Phillips,W.A. (2004) Mutation of the PIK3CA gene in ovarian and breast cancer. *Cancer Res.* 64, 7678-7681.

Chan,W.C., Maxwell,D.J., Gao,X., Bailey,R.E., Han,M. and Nie,S. (2002) Luminescent quantum dots for multiplexed biological detection and imaging. *Curr. Opin. Biotechnol.* 13, 40-46.

Chen,Y., Bathula,S.R., Li,J. and Huang,L. (2010a) Multifunctional nanoparticles delivering small interfering RNA and doxorubicin overcome drug resistance in cancer. *J. Biol. Chem.* 285, 22639-22650.

Chen,Y.Z., Yao,X.L., Tabata,Y., Nakagawa,S. and Gao,J.Q. (2010b) Gene carriers and transfection systems used in the recombination of dendritic cells for effective cancer immunotherapy. *Clin. Dev. Immunol.* 2010, 565-643.

Choosakoonkriang,S., Lobo,B.A., Koe,G.S., Koe,J.G. and Middaugh,C.R. (2003) Biophysical characterization of PEI/DNA complexes. *J. Pharm. Sci.* 92, 1710-1722.

Conlin,A.K., Seidman,A.D., Bach,A., Lake,D., Dickler,M., D'Andrea,G., Traina,T., Danso,M., Brufsky,A.M., Saleh,M., Clawson,A. and Hudis,C.A. (2010) Phase II trial of weekly nanoparticle albumin-bound paclitaxel with carboplatin and trastuzumab as first-line therapy for women with HER2-overexpressing metastatic breast cancer. *Clin. Breast Cancer.* 10, 281-287.

Connor,J., Bannerji,R., Saito,S., Heston,W., Fair,W. and Gilboa,E. (1993) Regression of bladder tumors in mice treated with interleukin 2 gene-modified tumor cells. *J. Exp. Med.* 177, 1127-1134.

Derfus,A.M., Chen,A.A., Min,D.H., Ruoslahti,E. and Bhatia,S.N. (2007) Targeted quantum dot conjugates for siRNA delivery. *Bioconjug. Chem.* 18, 1391-1396.

Deshayes,S., Maurizot,V., Clochard,M.C., Baudin,C., Berthelot,T., Esnouf,S., Lairez,D., Moenner,M. and Deleris,G. (2011) "Click" Conjugation of Peptide on the Surface of Polymeric Nanoparticles for Targeting Tumor Angiogenesis. *Pharm. Res.*

Donkuru,M., Badea,I., Wettig,S., Verrall,R., Elsabahy,M. and Foldvari,M. (2010) Advancing nonviral gene delivery: lipid- and surfactant-based nanoparticle design strategies. *Nanomedicine. (Lond).* 5, 1103-1127.

Duncan,R., Ringsdorf,H. and Satchi-Fainaro,R. (2006) Polymer therapeutics--polymers as drugs, drug and protein conjugates and gene delivery systems: past, present and future opportunities. *J. Drug Target.* 14, 337-341.

Dutta,T., Jain,N.K., McMillan,N.A. and Parekh,H.S. (2010) Dendrimer nanocarriers as versatile vectors in gene delivery. *Nanomedicine.* 6, 25-34.

El-Aneed,A. (2004) An overview of current delivery systems in cancer gene therapy. *J. Control Release.* 94, 1-14.

El-Sayed,I.H., Huang,X. and El-Sayed,M.A. (2006) Selective laser photo-thermal therapy of epithelial carcinoma using anti-EGFR antibody conjugated gold nanoparticles. *Cancer Lett.* 239, 129-135.

Feazell,R.P., Nakayama-Ratchford,N., Dai,H. and Lippard,S.J. (2007) Soluble single-walled carbon nanotubes as longboat delivery systems for platinum(IV) anticancer drug design. *J. Am. Chem. Soc.* 129, 8438-8439.

Felgner,P.L., Gadek,T.R., Holm,M., Roman,R., Chan,H.W., Wenz,M., Northrop,J.P., Ringold,G.M. and Danielsen,M. (1987) Lipofection: a highly efficient, lipid-mediated DNA-transfection procedure. *Proc. Natl. Acad. Sci. U. S. A.* 84, 7413-7417.

Giatrellis,S., Nikolopoulos,G., Sideratou,Z. and Nounesis,G. (2009) Calorimetric study of the interaction of binary DMTAP/DOTAP cationic liposomes with plasmid DNA. *J. Liposome Res.* 19, 220-230.

Gibbons,J.J., Abraham,R.T. and Yu,K. (2009) Mammalian target of rapamycin: discovery of rapamycin reveals a signaling pathway important for normal and cancer cell growth. *Semin. Oncol.* 36 Suppl 3:S3-S17., S3-S17.

Godbey,W.T. and Mikos,A.G. (2001) Recent progress in gene delivery using non-viral transfer complexes. *J. Control Release.* 72, 115-125.

Gou,M., Wei,X., Men,K., Wang,B., Luo,F., Zhao,X., Wei,Y. and Qian,Z. (2011) PCL/PEG Copolymeric Nanoparticles: Potential Nanoplatforms for Anticancer Agent Delivery. *Curr. Drug Targets.* [Epub ahead of print].

Guo,W. and Lee,R.L. (1999) Receptor-targeted gene delivery via folate-conjugated polyethylenimine. *AAPS. PharmSci.* 1, E19.

Hainaut,P. and Hollstein,M. (2000) p53 and human cancer: the first ten thousand mutations. *Adv. Cancer Res.* 77, 81-137.

Hainaut,P. and Vahakangas,K. (1997) p53 as a sensor of carcinogenic exposures: mechanisms of p53 protein induction and lessons from p53 gene mutations. *Pathol. Biol. (Paris).* 45, 833-844.

Han,J., Lim,M. and Yeom,Y.I. (1999) Receptor-mediated gene transfer to cells of hepatic origin by galactosylated albumin-polylysine complexes. *Biol. Pharm. Bull.* 22, 836-840.

Harisinghani,M.G., Barentsz,J., Hahn,P.F., Deserno,W.M., Tabatabaei,S., van de Kaa,C.H., de la,R.J. and Weissleder,R. (2003) Noninvasive detection of clinically occult lymph-node metastases in prostate cancer. *N. Engl. J. Med.* 19;348, 2491-2499.

Heinrich,J., Schultz,J., Bosse,M., Ziegelin,G., Lanka,E. and Moelling,K. (2002) Linear closed mini DNA generated by the prokaryotic cleaving-joining enzyme TelN is functional in mammalian cells. *J. Mol. Med.* 80, 648-654.

Hesdorffer,C., Ayello,J., Ward,M., Kaubisch,A., Vahdat,L., Balmaceda,C., Garrett,T., Fetell,M., Reiss,R., Bank,A. and Antman,K. (1998) Phase I trial of retroviral-mediated transfer of the human MDR1 gene as marrow chemoprotection in patients undergoing high-dose chemotherapy and autologous stem-cell transplantation. *J. Clin. Oncol.* 16, 165-172.

Hinz,T., Buchholz,C.J., van der,S.T., Cichutek,K. and Kalinke,U. (2006) Manufacturing and quality control of cell-based tumor vaccines: a scientific and a regulatory perspective. *J. Immunother.* 29, 472-476.

Hong,M., Zhu,S., Jiang,Y., Tang,G., Sun,C., Fang,C., Shi,B. and Pei,Y. (2010) Novel anti-tumor strategy: PEG-hydroxycamptothecin conjugate loaded transferrin-PEG-nanoparticles. *J. Control Release.* 141, 22-29.

Hood,J.D., Bednarski,M., Frausto,R., Guccione,S., Reisfeld,R.A., Xiang,R. and Cheresh,D.A. (2002) Tumor regression by targeted gene delivery to the neovasculature. *Science.* 296, 2404-2407.

Ilbasmis-Tamer,S., Yilmaz,S., Banoglu,E. and Degim,I.T. (2010) Carbon nanotubes to deliver drug molecules. *J. Biomed. Nanotechnol.* 6, 20-27.

Immordino,M.L., Dosio,F. and Cattel,L. (2006) Stealth liposomes: review of the basic science, rationale, and clinical applications, existing and potential. *Int. J. Nanomedicine.* 1, 297-315.

Iqbal,S., Goldman,B., Fenoglio-Preiser,C.M., Lenz,H.J., Zhang,W., Danenberg,K.D., Shibata,S.I. and Blanke,C.D. (2011) Southwest Oncology Group study S0413: a phase II trial of lapatinib (GW572016) as first-line therapy in patients with advanced or metastatic gastric cancer. *Ann. Oncol.* [Epub ahead of print] doi:-10.1093/annonc/mdr021.

Javle,M.M., Shroff,R.T., Xiong,H., Varadhachary,G.A., Fogelman,D., Reddy,S.A., Davis,D., Zhang,Y., Wolff,R.A. and Abbruzzese,J.L. (2010) Inhibition of the mammalian target of rapamycin (mTOR) in advanced pancreatic cancer: results of two phase II studies. *BMC. Cancer.* 10:368., 368.

Jere,D., Jiang,H.L., Arote,R., Kim,Y.K., Choi,Y.J., Cho,M.H., Akaike,T. and Cho,C.S. (2009) Degradable polyethylenimines as DNA and small interfering RNA carriers. *Expert. Opin. Drug Deliv.* 6, 827-834.

Ji,S.R., Liu,C., Zhang,B., Yang,F., Xu,J., Long,J., Jin,C., Fu,D.L., Ni,Q.X. and Yu,X.J. (2010) Carbon nanotubes in cancer diagnosis and therapy. *Biochim. Biophys. Acta.* 1806, 29-35.

Jiang,N., Wang,J., Wang,Y., Yan,H. and Thomas,R.K. (2005) Microcalorimetric study on the interaction of dissymmetric gemini surfactants with DNA. *J. Colloid Interface Sci.* 284, 759-764.

Joerger,A.C., Ang,H.C. and Fersht,A.R. (2006) Structural basis for understanding oncogenic p53 mutations and designing rescue drugs. *Proc. Natl. Acad. Sci. U. S. A.* 103, 15056-15061.

Kaur,T., Slavcev,R.A. and Wettig,S.D. (2009) Addressing the challenge: current and future directions in ovarian cancer therapy. *Curr. Gene Ther.* 9, 434-458.

Kowalski,M., Entwistle,J., Cizeau,J., Niforos,D., Loewen,S., Chapman,W. and MacDonald,G.C. (2010) A Phase I study of an intravesically administered immunotoxin targeting EpCAM for the treatment of nonmuscle-invasive bladder cancer in BCGrefractory and BCG-intolerant patients. *Drug Des Devel. Ther.* 4:313-20., 313-320.

Kreuter,J., Alyautdin,R.N., Kharkevich,D.A. and Ivanov,A.A. (1995) Passage of peptides through the blood-brain barrier with colloidal polymer particles (nanoparticles). *Brain Res.* 674, 171-174.

Lai,M.D., Yen,M.C., Lin,C.M., Tu,C.F., Wang,C.C., Lin,P.S., Yang,H.J. and Lin,C.C. (2009) The effects of DNA formulation and administration route on cancer therapeutic efficacy with xenogenic EGFR DNA vaccine in a lung cancer animal model. *Genet. Vaccines. Ther.* 7, 2.

Lane,D.P. (1992) Cancer. p53, guardian of the genome. *Nature.* 358, 15-16.

Lauria,A., Tutone,M., Ippolito,M., Pantano,L. and Almerico,A.M. (2010) Molecular modeling approaches in the discovery of new drugs for anti-cancer therapy: the investigation of p53-MDM2 interaction and its inhibition by small molecules. *Curr. Med. Chem.* 17, 3142-3154.

Ledford,H. (2007) Death in gene therapy trial raises questions about private IRBs. *Nat. Biotechnol.* 25, 1067.

Lemieux,P., Vinogradov,S.V., Gebhart,C.L., Guerin,N., Paradis,G., Nguyen,H.K., Ochietti,B., Suzdaltseva,Y.G., Bartakova,E.V., Bronich,T.K., St-Pierre,Y., Alakhov,V.Y. and Kabanov,A.V. (2000) Block and graft copolymers and NanoGel copolymer networks for DNA delivery into cell. *J. Drug Target.* 8, 91-105.

Liang,Z.W., Guo,B.F., Li,Y., Li,X.J., Li,X., Zhao,L.J., Gao,L.F., Yu,H., Zhao,X.J., Zhang,L. and Yang,B.X. (2011) Plasmid-based Stat3 siRNA delivered by hydroxyapatite nanoparticles suppresses mouse prostate tumor growth in vivo. *Asian J. Androl.* [Epub ahead of print], doi:10.1038/aja.2010.167.

Liu,F. and Huang,L. (2002) Development of non-viral vectors for systemic gene delivery. *J. Control Release.* 78, 259-266.

Liu,Y., Miyoshi,H. and Nakamura,M. (2007) Nanomedicine for drug delivery and imaging: a promising avenue for cancer therapy and diagnosis using targeted functional nanoparticles. *Int. J. Cancer.* 120, 2527-2537.

Liu,Z. and Peng,R. (2010) Inorganic nanomaterials for tumor angiogenesis imaging. *Eur. J. Nucl. Med. Mol. Imaging.* 37 Suppl 1, S147-S163.

Liu,Z., Tabakman,S., Welsher,K. and Dai,H. (2009) Carbon Nanotubes in Biology and Medicine: In vitro and in vivo Detection, Imaging and Drug Delivery. *Nano. Res.* 2, 85-120.

Lowe,S.W., Bodis,S., McClatchey,A., Remington,L., Ruley,H.E., Fisher,D.E., Housman,D.E. and Jacks,T. (1994) p53 status and the efficacy of cancer therapy in vivo. *Science.* 266, 807-810.

Michalet,X., Pinaud,F.F., Bentolila,L.A., Tsay,J.M., Doose,S., Li,J.J., Sundaresan,G., Wu,A.M., Gambhir,S.S. and Weiss,S. (2005) Quantum dots for live cells, in vivo imaging, and diagnostics. *Science.* 307, 538-544.

Moore,N.M., Sheppard,C.L. and Sakiyama-Elbert,S.E. (2009) Characterization of a multifunctional PEG-based gene delivery system containing nuclear localization signals and endosomal escape peptides. *Acta Biomater.* 5, 854-864.

Morille,M., Passirani,C., Vonarbourg,A., Clavreul,A. and Benoit,J.P. (2008) Progress in developing cationic vectors for non-viral systemic gene therapy against cancer. *Biomaterials.* 29, 3477-3496.

Nabel,G.J., Nabel,E.G., Yang,Z.Y., Fox,B.A., Plautz,G.E., Gao,X., Huang,L., Shu,S., Gordon,D. and Chang,A.E. (1993) Direct gene transfer with DNA-liposome complexes in melanoma: expression, biologic activity, and lack of toxicity in humans. *Proc. Natl. Acad. Sci. U. S. A.* 90, 11307-11311.

Negishi,Y., Endo-Takahashi,Y., Suzuki,R., Maruyama,K. and Aramaki,Y. (2010) [Development of gene delivery system into skeletal muscles by bubble liposomes and ultrasound]. *Yakugaku Zasshi.* 130, 1489-1496.

Neves,S., Faneca,H., Bertin,S., Konopka,K., Duzgunes,N., Pierrefite-Carle,V., Simoes,S. and Pedroso de Lima,M.C. (2009) Transferrin lipoplex-mediated suicide gene therapy of oral squamous cell carcinoma in an immunocompetent murine model and mechanisms involved in the antitumoral response. *Cancer Gene Ther.* 16, 91-101.

Nihira,S. (2003) Development of HER2-specific humanized antibody Herceptin (trastuzumab). *Nippon Yakurigaku Zasshi.* 122, 504-514.

Ning,X., Sun,Z., Wang,Y., Zhou,J., Chen,S., Chen,D. and Zhang,H. (2011) Docetaxel plus trans-tracheal injection of adenoviral-mediated p53 versus docetaxel alone in patients with previously treated non-small-cell lung cancer. *Cancer Gene Ther.* [Epub ahead of print], doi:10.1038/cgt.2011.15.

Olivier,M., Eeles,R., Hollstein,M., Khan,M.A., Harris,C.C. and Hainaut,P. (2002) The IARC TP53 database: new online mutation analysis and recommendations to users. *Hum. Mutat.* 19, 607-614.

Olivier,M., Hollstein,M. and Hainaut,P. (2010) TP53 mutations in human cancers: origins, consequences, and clinical use. *Cold Spring Harb. Perspect. Biol.* 2, a001008.

Onion,D., Patel,P., Pineda,R.G., James,N. and Mautner,V. (2009) Antivector and tumor immune responses following adenovirus-directed enzyme prodrug therapy for the treatment of prostate cancer. *Hum. Gene Ther.* 20, 1249-1258.

Pack,D.W., Hoffman,A.S., Pun,S. and Stayton,P.S. (2005) Design and development of polymers for gene delivery. *Nat. Rev. Drug Discov.* 4, 581-593.

Park,J.H., Gu,L., von,M.G., Ruoslahti,E., Bhatia,S.N. and Sailor,M.J. (2009) Biodegradable luminescent porous silicon nanoparticles for in vivo applications. *Nat. Mater.* 8, 331-336.

Patil,S.D., Rhodes,D.G. and Burgess,D.J. (2005) DNA-based therapeutics and DNA delivery systems: a comprehensive review. *AAPS. J.* 7, E61-E77.

Pic,E., Pons,T., Bezdetnaya,L., Leroux,A., Guillemin,F., Dubertret,B. and Marchal,F. (2010) Fluorescence imaging and whole-body biodistribution of near-infrared-emitting quantum dots after subcutaneous injection for regional lymph node mapping in mice. *Mol. Imaging Biol.* 12, 394-405.

Pinaud,F., Clarke,S., Sittner,A. and Dahan,M. (2010) Probing cellular events, one quantum dot at a time. *Nat. Methods.* 7, 275-285.

Ravi,K.M., Hellermann,G., Lockey,R.F. and Mohapatra,S.S. (2004) Nanoparticle-mediated gene delivery: state of the art. *Expert. Opin. Biol. Ther.* 4, 1213-1224.

Rogach,A.L. and Ogris,M. (2010) Near-infrared-emitting semiconductor quantum dots for tumor imaging and targeting. *Curr. Opin. Mol. Ther.* 12, 331-339.

Rosenberg,S.A. (1999) A new era of cancer immunotherapy: converting theory to performance. *CA Cancer J. Clin.* 49, 70-3, 65.

Schakowski,F., Gorschluter,M., Buttgereit,P., Marten,A., Lilienfeld-Toal,M.V., Junghans,C., Schroff,M., Konig-Merediz,S.A., Ziske,C., Strehl,J., Sauerbruch,T., Wittig,B. and Schmidt-Wolf,I.G. (2007) Minimal size MIDGE vectors improve transgene expression in vivo. *In Vivo.* 21, 17-23.

Schakowski,F., Gorschluter,M., Junghans,C., Schroff,M., Buttgereit,P., Ziske,C., Schottker,B., Konig-Merediz,S.A., Sauerbruch,T., Wittig,B. and Schmidt-Wolf,I.G. (2001) A novel minimal-size vector (MIDGE) improves transgene expression in colon carcinoma cells and avoids transfection of undesired DNA. *Mol. Ther.* 3, 793-800.

Schatzlein,A.G. (2001) Non-viral vectors in cancer gene therapy: principles and progress. *Anticancer Drugs.* 12, 275-304.

Sinha,N. and Yeow,J.T. (2005) Carbon nanotubes for biomedical applications. *IEEE Trans. Nanobioscience.* 4, 180-195.

Stolberg,S.G. (1999) The biotech death of Jesse Gelsinger. *N. Y. Times Mag.* 136-150.

Sun,Y., Jurgovsky,K., Moller,P., Alijagic,S., Dorbic,T., Georgieva,J., Wittig,B. and Schadendorf,D. (1998) Vaccination with IL-12 gene-modified autologous melanoma cells: preclinical results and a first clinical phase I study. *Gene Ther.* 5, 481-490.

Thrall,J.H. (2004) Nanotechnology and medicine. *Radiology.* 230, 315-318.

Tros,d., I, Sun,Y. and Duzgunes,N. (2010) Gene delivery by lipoplexes and polyplexes. *Eur. J. Pharm. Sci.* 40, 159-170.

Tu,G., Xu,W., Huang,H. and Li,S. (2008) Progress in the development of matrix metalloproteinase inhibitors. *Curr. Med. Chem.* 15, 1388-1395.

van Vlerken,L.E., Vyas,T.K. and Amiji,M.M. (2007) Poly(ethylene glycol)-modified nanocarriers for tumor-targeted and intracellular delivery. *Pharm. Res.* 24, 1405-1414.

Vasey,P.A., Shulman,L.N., Campos,S., Davis,J., Gore,M., Johnston,S., Kirn,D.H., O'Neill,V., Siddiqui,N., Seiden,M.V. and Kaye,S.B. (2002) Phase I trial of intraperitoneal injection of the E1B-55-kd-gene-deleted adenovirus ONYX-015 (dl1520) given on days 1 through 5 every 3 weeks in patients with recurrent/refractory epithelial ovarian cancer. *J. Clin. Oncol.* 20, 1562-1569.

Vassilev,L.T. (2004) Small-molecule antagonists of p53-MDM2 binding: research tools and potential therapeutics. *Cell Cycle.* 3, 419-421.

Vega,F., Medeiros,L.J., Leventaki,V., Atwell,C., Cho-Vega,J.H., Tian,L., Claret,F.X. and Rassidakis,G.Z. (2006) Activation of mammalian target of rapamycin signaling pathway contributes to tumor cell survival in anaplastic lymphoma kinase-positive anaplastic large cell lymphoma. *Cancer Res.* 66, 6589-6597.

Vinogradov,S.V., Bronich,T.K. and Kabanov,A.V. (2002) Nanosized cationic hydrogels for drug delivery: preparation, properties and interactions with cells. *Adv. Drug Deliv. Rev.* 54, 135-147.

Vogt,A., Combadiere,B., Hadam,S., Stieler,K.M., Lademann,J., Schaefer,H., Autran,B., Sterry,W. and Blume-Peytavi,U. (2006) 40 nm, but not 750 or 1,500 nm, nanoparticles enter epidermal CD1a+ cells after transcutaneous application on human skin. *J. Invest Dermatol.* 126, 1316-1322.

Wagner,U., du,B.A., Pfisterer,J., Huober,J., Loibl,S., Luck,H.J., Sehouli,J., Gropp,M., Stahle,A., Schmalfeldt,B., Meier,W. and Jackisch,C. (2007) Gefitinib in combination with tamoxifen in patients with ovarian cancer refractory or resistant to platinum-taxane based therapy--a phase II trial of the AGO Ovarian Cancer Study Group (AGO-OVAR 2.6). *Gynecol. Oncol.* 105, 132-137.

Wang,H. and Wettig,S.D. (2011) Synthesis and aggregation properties of dissymmetric phytanyl-gemini surfactants for use as improved DNA transfection vectors. *Phys. Chem. Chem. Phys.* 13, 637-642.

Wang,M. and Thanou,M. (2010) Targeting nanoparticles to cancer. *Pharmacol. Res.* 62, 90-99.

Weiss,J.M., Subleski,J.J., Wigginton,J.M. and Wiltrout,R.H. (2007) Immunotherapy of cancer by IL-12-based cytokine combinations. *Expert. Opin. Biol. Ther.* 7, 1705-1721.

Wettig,S.D., Badea,I., Donkuru,M., Verrall,R.E. and Foldvari,M. (2007a) Structural and transfection properties of amine-substituted gemini surfactant-based nanoparticles. *J. Gene Med.* 9, 649-658.

Wettig,S.D. and Verrall,R.E. (2001) Thermodynamic Studies of Aqueous m-s-m Gemini Surfactant Systems. *J. Colloid Interface Sci.* 235, 310-316.

Wettig,S.D., Wang,C., Verrall,R.E. and Foldvari,M. (2007b) Thermodynamic and aggregation properties of aza- and imino-substituted gemini surfactants designed for gene delivery. *Phys. Chem. Chem. Phys.* 9, 871-877.

Whitmore,M., Li,S. and Huang,L. (1999) LPD lipopolyplex initiates a potent cytokine response and inhibits tumor growth. *Gene Ther.* 6, 1867-1875.

Wilson,R.F. (2010) The death of Jesse Gelsinger: new evidence of the influence of money and prestige in human research. *Am. J. Law Med.* 36, 295-325.

Wojtowicz-Praga,S. (1997) Reversal of tumor-induced immunosuppression: a new approach to cancer therapy. *J. Immunother.* 20, 165-177.

Xu,F., Li,S., Li,X.L., Guo,Y., Zou,B.Y., Xu,R., Liao,H., Zhao,H.Y., Zhang,Y., Guan,Z.Z. and Zhang,L. (2009) Phase I and biodistribution study of recombinant adenovirus vector-mediated herpes simplex virus thymidine kinase gene and ganciclovir administration in patients with head and neck cancer and other malignant tumors. *Cancer Gene Ther.* 16, 723-730.

Yarom,N. and Jonker,D.J. (2011) The role of the epidermal growth factor receptor in the mechanism and treatment of colorectal cancer. *Discov. Med.* 11, 95-105.

Yong,K.T., Hu,R., Roy,I., Ding,H., Vathy,L.A., Bergey,E.J., Mizuma,M., Maitra,A. and Prasad,P.N. (2009) Tumor targeting and imaging in live animals with functionalized semiconductor quantum rods. *ACS Appl. Mater. Interfaces.* 1, 710-719.

Young,L.S., Searle,P.F., Onion,D. and Mautner,V. (2006) Viral gene therapy strategies: from basic science to clinical application. *J. Pathol.* 208, 299-318.

Yu,M.K., Park,J., Jeong,Y.Y., Moon,W.K. and Jon,S. (2010) Integrin-targeting thermally cross-linked superparamagnetic iron oxide nanoparticles for combined cancer imaging and drug delivery. *Nanotechnology.* 21, 415102.

Zhao,Y., Zhao,L., Zhou,L., Zhi,Y., Xu,J., Wei,Z., Zhang,K.X., Ouellette,B.F. and Shen,H. (2010) Quantum dot conjugates for targeted silencing of bcr/abl gene by RNA interference in human myelogenous leukemia K562 cells. *J. Nanosci. Nanotechnol.* 10, 5137-5143.

5

Toxicity of Polymeric-Based Non-Viral Vector Systems for Pulmonary siRNA Application

Andrea Beyerle[1,2], Thomas Kissel[2] and Tobias Stoeger[1,2]
[1]Comprehensive Pneumology Center, Institute of Lung Biology and Disease
Helmholtz Zentrum, München
[2]Department of Pharmaceutics and Biopharmacy, Philipps-University Marburg
Germany

1. Introduction

Nanomedicine has the potential of clinical benefit by combination of engineering technologies and materials (Schatzlein, 2006). Development of nanometre scaled therapeutics which provides new and improved properties by specifically targeting the site of action and causing low level of side effects would be a big challenge to treat patients with severe and live-threatening diseases like cancer. Gene therapy provides a new way to treat patients and a lot of effort is made to improve the clinical benefit. But current gene therapy is still experimental and has not proven success in the clinics. Nevertheless there is a need for new approaches to treat „undruggable" disease sites and there are some clinical trials ongoing which using RNA inference (RNAi) as therapeutic mechanism (Table 1).

2. Gene silencing by siRNAs

2.1 RNA interference

RNA interference (RNAi), the Nobel Prize winning mechanism for gene silencing (Fire *et al.*, 1998), raises nowadays increasing attention of many researchers as a new way to treat life-threatening diseases like cancer (Akhtar, 2006) or other genetic disorders like cystic fibrosis (Griesenbach and Alton, 2009) or viral infection as respiratory syncytial virus (RSV) (Ge *et al.*, 2004) and as an in vitro research tool to investigate mechanisms which are involved in those diseases. Small interfering RNA (siRNA) duplexes of 19-23 base pairs could trigger sequence specific gene silencing in mammalian cells (Caplen *et al.*, 2001; Elbashir *et al.*, 2001; Hannon and Rossi, 2004; Meister *et al.*, 2004; Mello and Conte, 2004). The siRNAs are double stranded molecules, consisting of a guide strand that is perfectly complementary to a target mRNA and a passenger strand. Core components of this siRNA-mediated post-transcriptional silencing include the RNAse III enzyme Dicer and its co-factor transactivating response RNA-binding protein (TRBP) along with the Argonaute family of proteins, in particular Argonaute 2 (Ago 2) (Meister *et al.*, 2004), which is the catalytic engine of the RNA induced silencing complex (RISC). Dicer converts dsRNA into 21-25 nucleotide duplexes with 3′ 2nt overhangs. The siRNA is incorporated into one or more of the Argonaute proteins in RISC for sequence specific target degradation or translational inhibition (Tuschl *et al.*, 1999). In general, perfect or near perfect base pairing between the siRNA guide strand and the target mRNA is required for Ago2 cleavage to occur. In

Company	siRNA	Target	Disease/ Disorder	Status	Administration / Formulation	Remarks
Acuity Pharmaceuticals (Opko Health)	Bevasiranib (Cand5)	VEGF	AMD, DME	Phase II	intravitreal injection, free siRNA	-
Alnylam Pharmaceuticals	ALN-RSV-01 ALN-RSV-02	RSV Pediatric RSV	RSV Pediatric RSV	Phase IIb	aerosolized siRNA, free siRNA	-
	ALN-VSP02	KSP and VEGF	Liver cancer	Phase I	i.v., free siRNA	-
Silence Therapeutics	Atu027	PKN3	Advanced solid cancer	Phase I	i.v., free siRNA	-
Sirna Therapeutics (Calando Pharmaceuticals)	CALAA-01	RRM2	Solid tumor cancer	Phase I	i.v., Cyclodextrin-adamantan-PEG-transferrin nanocomplex.	-
Sirna Therapeutics (TransDerm Inc.)	TD101	PC keratin K6a	Pachyonychia congenita	Phase Ib	Injection into a callus on the bottom of one foot, free siRNA	-
Sirna Therapeutics	AGN211745 (Sirna-027)	VEGFR1	AMD, CNV & AMD	Phase II	intravitreal injection, free siRNA	-
Quarks Pharmaceuticals	I5NP (QPI-1002)	p53	Delayed graft function, Kidney transplantation	Phase I Phase II	i.v., free siRNA	-
	QPI-1007	Caspase 2	Chronic optic nerve atrophy Non-Arteritic Anterior Ischemic Optic Neuropathy	Phase I	intravitreal injection, free siRNA	-
Tekmira Pharmaceuticals Corporation	PRO-040201	APOB	Hyperchol-esterol-emia	Phase I	i.v., liposomal formulation	study has been terminated due to potential for immune stimulation to interfere with further dose escalation

Silenseed Ltd	siG12D LODER (Local Drug EluteR)	KRAS G12D	Pancreatic cancer	Phase I	miniature biodegradable polymeric matrix, placed in the tumor using an endoscopic ultrasound biopsy needle	-

source: http://clinicaltrials.ifpma.org/no_cache/en/search-trials-ongoing/all/index.htm,

Table 1. Summary of ongoing clinical trials for siRNA delivery,
abbreviations used: AMD: age related macular degeneration; APOB: apolipoprotein B; CNV: choroidale neovascularization; DME: diabetic macular edema; i.v.: intravenous; KSP: kinesin spindle protein; PC: pachyonychia congenital; PKN3: protein kinase N3; RRM2: ribonucleotide reductase M2 polypeptide; RSV: respiratory syntical virus; VEGF: vascular endothelial growth factor

laboratory work and in clinical trials siRNAs are most often chemically synthesized, bypassing the Dicer cleavage step for entry into RISC and avoiding any immune responses and toxicity which is described for long double stranded RNAs (dsRNAs) (Behlke, 2008).
RNAi has widely been used in drug development and several phase I and II clinical trials (Table 1) are ongoing. However, for therapeutic applications still some concerns and challenges need to be overcome, e.g. off-target effects, innate immune response and most importantly specific delivery into the cytoplasm of target cells.

3. Small interfering RNAs (siRNA)

siRNAs are very attractive for therapy because they are easily designed and synthesized, and their versatility allows simultaneous use of multiple siRNAs or change of sequences to accommodate virus mutations. The negative charge of siRNA and their size of around 14 kDa make it difficult to cross the cell membrane without any carrier. There are various delivery strategies under investigation, which includes nanoparticular systems consisting of polymers and/or lipids of different compositions and with or without any conjugation like antibodies or ligands for achieving the most specific way to the target side of action. Davis et al. showed 2008 first evidence for RNAi mechanism of action in human with their self-assembling, cyclodextrin polymer-based nanoparticle system (CALAA-01) targeting the riboucleotide reductase subunit 2 (RRM2) which could be used for therapy of different types of cancers (Heidel et al., 2007; Davis, 2009; Davis et al., 2010). At the same time Zimmermann, MacLachlan and colleagues reported successful siRNA delivery using a different approach for delivery (Zimmermann et al., 2006). They introduced so-called stable nucleic acid lipid particles (SNALP) generated by ethanol dilution technique and showed for the first time in non-human primate a successful targeting of ApoB in the liver (Soutschek et al., 2004; Morrissey et al., 2005; Zimmermann et al., 2006). Ge and co-workers (Ge et al., 2004) used PEI 25 kDa to complex and protect siRNA specific to influenza virus genes and they showed successful reduction of influenza virus infection in mice. Alton et al. gave first evidence for successful gene therapy by using a lipid-based system to delivery CFTR DNA in cystic fibrosis patients (Alton et al., 1999). Thus, gene therapy approaches still need improvements regarding specific targeting and successful delivery of the nucleic acid but clinical trials are ongoing and preclinical testing are conducted for different kind of diseases (Table 1).

4. Non-viral vector systems for siRNA delivery

RNA interference (RNAi) based therapeutics represent a fundamentally new way to treat human disease by addressing targets that are otherwise "undruggable" with existing medicines (Novina and Sharp, 2004; de Fougerolles et al., 2007). The goal of RNAi-based therapy represents the activation of selective mRNA cleavage for efficient gene silencing. There are two possibilities to harness the endogenous pathway: either i) by using viral vector to express short hairpin RNA (shRNA) that resembles miRNA precursors, or (ii) by introducing siRNAs that mimic Dicer cleavage product into the cytoplasm. Synthetic siRNAs utilize the naturally occurring RNAi pathway in a manner that is consistent and predictable, thus making them particularly attractive as therapeutics. Since they enter RNAi pathway later, siRNAs are less likely to interfere with gene regulation by endogenous miRNAs (Jackson et al., 2003; Grimm et al., 2006). The most important characteristics for effective design and selection of siRNAs are potency, specificity, and nuclease stability. Two types of off-target effects need to be avoided or minimized: i) silencing of genes sharing partial homology to the siRNA and ii) immune stimulation induced by recognition of certain siRNAs by the innate immune system. The activation of the innate immune systems by siRNA could be induced by recognition of dsRNAs by the serine/threonine protein kinase receptor (PKR) (Schlee et al., 2006). This pathway is normally triggered by dsRNAs that are more than 30 nucleotides long, but at higher concentrations also siRNAs may be able to activate this pathway resulting in global translational blockade and cell death. The potential to activate toll-like receptors (TLRs) in the endosomal compartment is more likely to occur after siRNA delivery due to recognition of specific nucleotide sequence motifs (e.g. GU) by TLRs. TLR activation could trigger the production of type I interferons and pro-inflammatory cytokines, and induce nuclear factor kappa B (NF-kB) activation (Hornung et al., 2005; Judge et al., 2005). For example, the presence of 2'-O-methyl modifications within the siRNA duplex could abrogate the binding to TLR7 in endosomes and abolish immunostimulatory response. In addition, these modifications also reduce sequence-dependent off-target silencing and may be particularly beneficial in enhancing siRNA target specificity (Judge et al., 2006; Robbins et al., 2008; Robbins et al., 2009).

Due to increasing mortality and morbidity caused by several lung diseases, RNAi strategies have attracted particular attention and the lung as target organ provides an attractive tool because of the accessibility via non-invasive routes, e.g. nasal or pulmonary applications. The clinical success of siRNA-mediated interventions critically depends upon the safety and efficacy of the delivery methods and agents. Naked siRNAs are degraded in human plasma with a half-life of minutes (Layzer et al., 2004; Choung et al., 2006). Thus, the search for optimized nanocarriers to deliver siRNA is still under intensive investigation. The negative charge and chemical degradability of siRNA under physiologically relevant conditions make its delivery a major challenge (Gary et al., 2007). Depending on their origin, two types of positively charged carriers could be distinguished: i) lipid–based and ii) polymeric-based carrier systems. Both systems provided several advantages to deliver siRNA. Liposome formation agents like Lipofectamine 2000 (Dalby et al., 2004; Santel et al., 2006) and cardiolipin analogues (Chien et al., 2005; Pal et al., 2005) have been successfully used for the delivery of siRNA. Negatively charged nucleic acids and positively charged lipids spontaneously form nanoparticles, known as lipoplexes, of 50-200 nm in diameter (Sitterberg *et al.*, 2010). Interaction with serum components represents one of the major hurdles that influence the performance when used systemically (Zuhorn *et al.*, 2007). Recently, lipid-mediated delivery of siRNA against apolipoprotein B (ApoB) has been used to target ApoB mRNA to the (Soutschek *et al.*, 2004; Zimmermann *et al.*, 2006). The in vivo use of cationic lipids especially by i.v. administration presents significant problems as these reagents can be quite toxic. Despite problems with i.v. use, cationic lipids are employed for i.p. injection (Verma *et al.*, 2003; Flynn *et al.*, 2004; Miyawaki-Shimizu *et al.*, 2006), for CNS injection (Hassani *et al.*, 2005; Luo *et al.*, 2005) or in topical epithelial surface application (Maeda *et al.*, 2005; Palliser *et al.*, 2006) and intratracheal (Griesenbach *et al.*, 2006). Toxicity varies with the precise chemical composition of the lipids employed dose, and the delivering route. Variations in chemical composition can have a large impact on the functional properties of cationic lipid mixtures (Spagnou et al., 2004), and lipoplex/liposomal preparations have been devised with decreased toxicity that are more compatible with i.v. administration. Liposomes can be modified with ligands such as folate or small peptides, which assist with delivery and help target specific cell types or tissues (Meyerhoff, 1999; Dubey *et al.*, 2004). Through the use of neutral polyethylene glycol-substituted surfaces and other approaches, liposomes can be stabilized and made more "stealthy" showing reduced clearance and improved pharmacokinetics (Oupicky *et al.*, 2002; Moghimi and Szebeni, 2003). These kinds of lipid nanoparticles have been successfully used to deliver antisense oligonucleotides and siRNAs in vivo (Braasch *et al.*, 2003; Chien *et al.*, 2005).

Similar to the lipid-based non viral vector systems, the positive charges of polycations allow an efficient interaction with siRNAs to form so-called polyplexes, which can bind onto cell plasma membrane and be endocytosed. In contrast to the lipid-based systems that rely on the fusogenic property of the liposomes to mediate endosomal escape, polymeric carriers such as poly(ethylene imine) (PEI) use the so-called "proton-sponge" effect to enhance endosomal release of endocytosed polyplexes (Boussif *et al.*, 1995; Behr, 1997; Akinc *et al.*, 2005; Demeneix and Behr, 2005; Nel *et al.*, 2009). According to this mechanism, the deprotonated amines with different pK_a values confer a buffer effect over a wide range of pH. This buffering may protect the siRNA from degradation in the endosomal compartment during maturation of the early endosomes to late endosomes and their subsequent fusion with the lysosomes. The buffering property also allows the polycation to escape from the endosome. At lower pH the buffering capacity causes an influx of chloride ions and water into the endosomes, which burst due to osmotic pressure and facilitating intracellular release of PEI - siRNA polyplexes. PEI has been used for many years to facilitate nucleic acid delivery (Boussif *et al.*, 1995; Demeneix and Behr, 2005). However, due to toxicity and variable performance it has not found generalized acceptance as a delivery tool for either antisense oligonucleotides or siRNAs. Nevertheless, PEI can be used as a prototype for formulation of more complex particles with improved properties (Kim and Kim, 2009).

5. PEI-based non-viral vector systems

Polyethylene imine (PEI) is a simple repetition of the 43 Da CH_2-CH_2-NH ethylene imine motifs. It can be synthesized from ethylene imine (aziridine) via ring opening polymerization or by hydrolysis of poly(2-ethyl-2-oxazolium), leading to branched or linear polymeric backbones, respectively (Godbey *et al.*, 1999). PEI represents one of the most comprehensive investigated cationic polymer for gene delivery in vitro and in vivo (Godbey *et al.*, 1999; Fischer *et al.*, 2002; Brus *et al.*, 2004; Neu *et al.*, 2005; Gary *et al.*, 2007). PEI 25 kDa serves as gold standard for in vitro transfection experiments (Godbey *et al.*, 2000). The mechanism of cell entry and action for gene delivery is intensively analyzed. To enhance the endosomal release of endocytosed polyplexes PEI uses the so-called "proton-sponge" effect (Boussif *et al.*, 1995; Behr, 1997) Due to the high buffer capacity of PEI amino groups in PEI molecules will be protonated at lower pHs like in the endosomal-lysosomal environment, additional chloride influx into the vesicles increases the osmolarity and the vesicles begin to swell and under the increased osmotic pressure the vesicle will be disrupted and the nucleic acid protected from PEI will be released into the cytoplasm (Godbey *et al.*, 1999; Akinc *et al.*, 2005; Nel *et al.*, 2009). PEI has been used for many years to facilitate nucleic acid delivery (Demeneix and Behr, 2005). However, due to toxicity and variable performance a lot of research is undertaken to reduce the toxicity of PEI and maintain or improve the efficacy and specificity by modification PEI backbone and/or conjugation of hydrophilic molecules like polyethylene glycol (PEG) (Petersen *et al.*, 2002a; Petersen *et al.*, 2002b), disulfide linkages (Breunig *et al.*, 2008), or for specific targeting molecules like transferrin, galactose, TAT-peptide, RGD-motifs (Ogris *et al.*, 1999; Kunath *et al.*, 2003a; Kunath *et al.*, 2003b; Kleemann *et al.*, 2005). Other approaches are reduction of the molecular weight of PEI 25 kDa or purification of PEI 25 kDa via gel filtration (Boeckle *et al.*, 2004; Urban-Klein *et al.*, 2005; Werth, 2006; Fahrmeir *et al.*, 2007) or using instead of the branched PEI 25 kDa the linear form PEI22kDa (Breunig *et al.*, 2005). Thomas and colleagues showed that full deacylation of linear PEI dramatically improves the efficacy but on cost of increased cytotoxicity due to increased numbers of protonatable nitrogens in the PEI molecule (Thomas *et al.*, 2005).

6. Modifications of PEI

Modifications of PEI with the hydrophilic poly(ethylene glycol) (PEG) reduces dramatically the cytotoxicity of PEI 25 kDa but in part on cost of efficacy and increased immunomodulatory and proinflammatory effects (Kichler *et al.*, 2002; Petersen *et al.*, 2002b; Mao *et al.*, 2005; Glodde *et al.*, 2006; Beyerle *et al.*, 2010a; Beyerle *et al.*, 2010b). PEG provides polyplexes with improved solubility, lower surface charge, diminished aggregation, lower cytotoxicity, and possibly improved "stealth effect" in the bloodstream.

Glodde et al. synthesized a series of PEG-PEI copolymers and found that the molecular weight of PEG was found to be the major determinant of polyplex size, via its influence on particle aggregation and polyplex stability (Glodde *et al.*, 2006). Transfection efficiency was correlated to polyplex stability and low molecular weight PEI 2 kDa grafted with PEG showed higher activity than their counterparts with high molecular weight PEI 25 kDa (Williams *et al.*, 2006). In contrast, Petersen and Mao showed good transfection efficiencies for PEI 25 kDa - PEG copolymers with high molecular weight PEG and low numbers of grafting on PEI backbone compare to low molecular weight PEG with high grafting numbers on PEI 25 kDa (Mao *et al.*, 2005; Merkel *et al.*, 2009; Beyerle *et al.*, 2011a).

Grayson and colleagues investigated the siRNA transfection efficacy of different PEI polymers (branched 800 Da, branched 25 kDa and linear 22 kDa) in HeLa derivative cell line (Grayson *et al.*, 2006). They showed that the siRNA delivery and activity was mainly dependent on the biophysical and structural characteristics of the polyplexes and only

25 kDa PEI was able to effective deliver siRNA. The authors explained the high activity of PEI25kDa/siRNA with good stability of polyplexes, small size, and positively surface charge, but nevertheless the cytotoxicity was highest for PEI 25 kDa.

Succinylated PEI polymers for complexation of siRNA were introduced by Wagner and colleagues which showed 10-fold lower toxicity and higher knockdown efficacy compare to pure PEI polyplexes (Zintchenko *et al.*, 2008).

7. Toxicity of PEI-based non-viral vector systems

Synthetic polymers and nanomaterials display selective phenotypic effects in cells and in the body that affect signal transduction mechanisms involved in inflammation, differentiation, proliferation, and apoptosis. When physically mixed or covalently conjugated with cytotoxic agents, bacterial DNA or antigens, polymers can drastically alter specific genetically controlled responses to these agents (Kabanov, 2006). These effects, in part, result from cooperative interactions of polymers and nanomaterials with plasma cell membranes and trafficking of polymers and nanomaterials to intracellular organelles. Cells and whole organism responses to these materials can be phenotype or genotype dependent. In selected cases, polymer agents can bypass limitations to biological responses imposed by the genotype, for example, phenotypic correction of immune response by polyelectrolytes. Overall, these effects are relatively benign as they do not result in cytotoxicity or major toxicities in the body. Collectively, however, these studies support the need for thoroughly assessing pharmacogenomic effects of polymer materials to maximize clinical outcomes and understand the pharmacological and toxicological effects of polymer formulations of biological agents, i.e. polymer genomics. In addition, it is well described in the literature that cationic nanoparticles disrupt lipid bilayers (Hong *et al.*, 2006; Leroueil *et al.*, 2008), induce oxidative stress inside the cell as a result of cell-type interplay and cause in some cases acute lung inflammation when administered intratracheally (Tan and Huang, 2002; Beyerle *et al.*, 2010b; Beyerle *et al.*, 2011a and Beyerle *et al.*, 2011c). Intensive efforts will have to focus on the issue of cytotoxicity to obtain more insight in the exact mechanisms behind, which are multidimensional and largely depend on the application route as well as the formulation that is delivered. Therefore, tissue specific toxicity profiles are still needed and represent a great implement in improving non-viral delivery systems.

8. General toxicity

Hornung et al. described that any rupture or leakage of the endosomal or lysosomal membrane will release cathepsin B, which leads to an inflammasome activation associated with IL-1 production and apoptosis (Hornung *et al.*, 2008). Beyerle et al. found that application PEI/siRNA complexes caused release of proinflammatory cytokines like IL-6, G-CSF, TNF-a, IP-10 in murine lung cell lines (Beyerle *et al.*, 2010a; Beyerle *et al.*, 2010b; Beyerle *et al.*, 2011a and Beyerle *et al.*, 2011c). Cytokine release upon PEI/nucleic acid polyplex treatment has been also described by Gautam and Kawakami et al. (Gautam *et al.*, 2001; Kawakami *et al.*, 2006). Cubillos-Ruis and co-workers investigated linear PEI/siRNA complexes for antitumor immunity and identified linear PEI as TLR 5 agonist of mouse and human. They found that linear PEI/siRNA complexes induced a pattern of inflammatory cytokines which are triggered in vivo by flagellin in a TLR5 dependent manner (Cubillos-

Ruiz *et al.*, 2009). Thus, for in vivo use a lot of effort should be made to avoid the high proinflammatory effects caused by the rupture or leakage of the endosome caused by PEI. Godbey classified PEI-mediated toxicity in an immediate toxicity, associated with free PEI and a delayed form, connected with cellular processing of PEI/DNA polyplexes (Godbey *et al.*, 2001). To form stable and protective PEI nucleic acid polyplexes an excess of PEI polymer is needed, 60-80% PEI remains in a free form after nucleic acid escape and is mainly attributed to PEI toxicity. The high positively charged PEI molecule is able to disrupt cell membranes, disruption of the endosome is on one hand favourable with respect to the intended cytoplasmatic delivery, but on the other hand disruption of other cell membranes (e.g., lysosomal membranes, mitochondrial membrane, plasma membrane) is not favourable as it will cause stress responses or even apoptotic or necrotic cell death. In this context it has been shown that PEI causes apoptosis in an unspecific manner in all kinds of cells (Beyerle *et al.*, 2010a; Merkel *et al.*, 2011) which should be avoided with regard to human use. Therefore, a purification approach of the PEI polymer before and after complexation with nucleic acid is one possibility to reduce PEI-related toxicity (Boeckle *et al.*, 2004; Werth, 2006; Fahrmeir *et al.*, 2007).

9. Lung toxicity

Espescially, when regarding the lung as target organ the activation of the inflammosome should be avoided. Lung targeting could in general be achieved by systemic delivery or pulmonary delivery. Pulmonary delivery enhances siRNA retention in the lungs, lowers the dose of siRNA required for efficient delivery, and therefore implicates reduced systemic toxic effects, and due to lower nuclease activity in the lung siRNA stability is increased. RNAi can be used to treat or prevent diseases affecting the lungs, such as lung cancer (Li and Huang, 2006; Tong, 2006; Jere *et al.*, 2008; Ren *et al.*, 2009; Zamora-Avila *et al.*, 2009), various types of respiratory infectious diseases (Ge *et al.*, 2004; Fulton *et al.*, 2009; DeVincenzo *et al.*, 2010), airway inflammatory diseases (Lee and Chiang, 2008; Seguin and Ferrari, 2009), and cystic fibrosis (Pison *et al.*, 2006).

Beyerle and co-workers investigated the effects of PEGylation on cytotoxicity and cell-compatibility of different PEG-PEI copolymers in murine lung cell lines and found a clear structure-function relationship (Fig. 1).

The higher the degree of PEGylation on PEI25kDa with low molecular weight PEG, the stronger was the reduction of cytotoxicity and oxidative stress, but the proinflammatory potential of PEI remained high (Beyerle *et al.*, 2010b). The same group evaluated the pulmonary toxicity of PEI/siRNA complexes and found at day three after intratracheal delivery still high numbers of neutrophils and high levels of proinflammatory cytokines in the airspace of polyplex treated mice (Beyerle *et al.*, 2011a and Beyerle *et al.*, 2011c). The higher inflammatory potential but lower toxicity of PEI modifications is still an issue to be overcome when targeting pulmonary diseases. There is an urgent need to balance the efficacy and toxicity of such nucleic acid carriers.

10. Toxicogenomics of PEI-based non-viral vector systems

Toxicogenomic and genotoxic information of non-viral vector systems is rare, but of great concern when nowadays focusing personalized medicine. Gene delivery systems should be

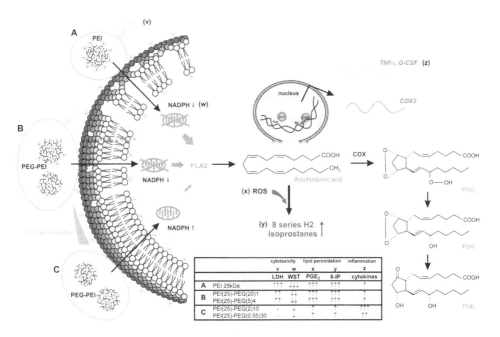

		cytotoxicity		lipid peroxidation		inflammation
		v	w	x	y	z
		LDH	WST	PGE$_2$	8-IP	cytokines
A	PEI 25kDa	↑↑↑	↓↓↓	↑↑↑	↑↑↑	↑
B	PEI(25)-PEG(20)1	↑↑	↓↓	↑↑↑	↑↑↑	↑
	PEI(25)-PEG(5)4	↑↑	↓↓	↑↑↑	↑↑↑	↑↑↑
C	PEI(25)-PEG(2)10	-	↓	↑	↑	↑↑
	PEI(25)-PEG(0.55)30	-	↓	↑	↑	↑↑

Fig. 1. Structure-function-relationships of PEG-PEI copolymers
Overview of the structure-function relationships of PEG modified PEI copolymers (B-C) in comparisonto PEI 25kDa (A) with regard to cytotoxic (v,w), oxidative stress (x,y) and proinflammatory responses (z). Arrows represent the up- or downregulation of the investigated molecules.

able to pass through biological membranes/barriers and transfer the desired information to target sites with minimal impact on the integrity of the target cell or tissue (Forrest and Pack, 2002; Omidi et al., 2008). Viral vectors possess high efficacy accompanied by stimulation of the immune systems which is a limitation of these systems to deliver nucleic acids and human use. Therefore, non-viral vector systems should overcome these adverse side effects and represent safer and more efficient alternatives with improved bioavailability and reduced cellular toxicity in the clinics (Akhtar et al., 2000; Somia and Verma, 2000; Panyam and Labhasetwar, 2003). It has been shown that cationic polymers and lipid-based transfection reagents could elicit cellular gene expression changes and complexation with siRNA increased these changes (Omidi et al., 2003; Omidi et al., 2005; Fedorov et al., 2006; Hollins et al., 2007; Tagami et al., 2007; Tagami et al., 2008). Beyerle et al. analyzed the expression changes of genes related to cytotoxicity, inflammation and oxidative stress in a pathway focused qRT-PCR array system upon treatment with different PEI-PEG copolymers in murine lung epithelial cells (LA-4 cell line) and could show that PEGylated PEI copolymers altered the gene expression profile on cost of upregulation of genes involved in inflammatory and oxidative stress processes while PEI 25 kDa mainly induced genes related to cytotoxicity and apoptosis (Beyerle et al., 2010a). In addition, the potential of PEI and PEI-PEG copolymers to induce DNA damage and therefore their genotoxic potential was investigated in a lung epithelial cell line derived from the MutaMouse, but no indication for genotoxicity of PEI 25 kDa and PEI-PEG copolymers was observed (Beyerle *et al.*, 2011b). These investigations showed that PEI uptake causes cellular oxidative stress which affects the cytoplasmatic compartment with subsequent gene expression responses, but PEI not necessarily penetrate the nuclear membrane and cause DNA damage.

11. Conclusion

In conclusion, for development of safe and efficient non-viral vector systems a lot of investigations are needed before enter clinical trials. In our book chapter we mainly focused on PEI-related polymers for siRNA delivery to the lungs and gave an overview of the ongoing research in this field with a great focus on toxicity. To improve the toxicity profile of such carriers for pulmonary application one of the biggest challenge is to overcome the inflammatory response besides reduction of the overall cytotoxicity. Future studies should implement basic toxicity testing like evaluation of cytotoxicity (cell viability, LDH release, erythrocytes aggregation, apoptosis), inflammation (cytokine release, gene regulation, in vivo analysis of relevant tissues and cells or liquids), oxidative stress (lipid mediators, GSH levels) before extensively improving the efficacy of such carriers.

12. References

Akhtar, S. (2006). Non-viral cancer gene therapy: beyond delivery. *Gene Ther* 13, 739-740.

Akhtar, S., Hughes, M. D., Khan, A., Bibby, M., Hussain, M., Nawaz, Q., Double, J., and Sayyed, P. (2000). The delivery of antisense therapeutics. *Adv Drug Deliv Rev* 44, 3-21.

Akinc, A., Thomas, M., Klibanov, A. M., and Langer, R. (2005). Exploring polyethylenimine-mediated DNA transfection and the proton sponge hypothesis. *J Gene Med* 7, 657-663.

Alton, E. W., Stern, M., Farley, R., Jaffe, A., Chadwick, S. L., Phillips, J., Davies, J., Smith, S. N., Browning, J., Davies, M. G., Hodson, M. E., Durham, S. R., Li, D., Jeffery, P. K., Scallan, M., Balfour, R., Eastman, S. J., Cheng, S. H., Smith, A. E., Meeker, D., and Geddes, D. M. (1999). Cationic lipid-mediated CFTR gene transfer to the lungs and nose of patients with cystic fibrosis: a double-blind placebo-controlled trial. *Lancet* 353, 947-954.

Behlke, M. A. (2008). Chemical modification of siRNAs for in vivo use. *Oligonucleotides* 18, 305-319.

Behr, J. (1997). The proton sponge: A trick to enter cells the viruses did not exploit. *Chimica* 51, 34-36.

Beyerle, A., Braun, A., Banerjee, A., Ercal, N., Eickelberg, O., Kissel, T., and Stoeger, T. (Biomaterials 2011c, in press). Inflammtory response to pulmonary application of PEI-based siRNA nanocarriers in mice.

Beyerle, A., Braun, A., Merkel, O., Koch, F., Kissel, T., and Stoeger, T. (2011a). Comparative in vivo study of poly(ethylene imine)/siRNA complexes for pulmonary delivery in mice. *J Control Release.* 151(1):51-6.

Beyerle, A., Irmler, M., Beckers, J., Kissel, T., and Stoeger, T. (2010a). Toxicity pathway focused gene expression profiling of PEI-based polymers for pulmonary applications. *Mol Pharm* 7, 727-737.

Beyerle, A., Long, A. S., White, P., Kissel, T. H., and Stoeger, T. (2011b). Poly(ethylene imine) nanocarriers do not induce mutations nor oxidative DNA damage in vitro in MutaMouse FE1 cells. *Mol Pharm.* 8(3):976-81

Beyerle, A., Merkel, O., Stoeger, T., and Kissel, T. (2010b). PEGylation affects cytotoxicity and cell-compatibility of poly(ethylene imine) for lung application: structure-function relationships. *Toxicol Appl Pharmacol* 242, 146-154.

Boeckle, S., von Gersdorff, K., van der Piepen, S., Culmsee, C., Wagner, E., and Ogris, M. (2004). Purification of polyethylenimine polyplexes highlights the role of free polycations in gene transfer. *J Gene Med* 6, 1102-1111.

Boussif, O., Lezoualc'h, F., Zanta, M. A., Mergny, M. D., Scherman, D., Demeneix, B., and Behr, J. P. (1995). A versatile vector for gene and oligonucleotide transfer into cells in culture and in vivo: polyethylenimine. *Proc Natl Acad Sci U S A* 92, 7297-7301.

Braasch, D. A., Jensen, S., Liu, Y., Kaur, K., Arar, K., White, M. A., and Corey, D. R. (2003). RNA interference in mammalian cells by chemically-modified RNA. *Biochemistry* 42, 7967-7975.

Breunig, M., Hozsa, C., Lungwitz, U., Watanabe, K., Umeda, I., Kato, H., and Goepferich, A. (2008). Mechanistic investigation of poly(ethylene imine)-based siRNA delivery: disulfide bonds boost intracellular release of the cargo. *J Control Release* 130, 57-63.

Breunig, M., Lungwitz, U., Liebl, R., Fontanari, C., Klar, J., Kurtz, A., Blunk, T., and Goepferich, A. (2005). Gene delivery with low molecular weight linear polyethylenimines. *J Gene Med* 7, 1287-1298.

Brus, C., Petersen, H., Aigner, A., Czubayko, F., and Kissel, T. (2004). Physicochemical and biological characterization of polyethylenimine-graft-poly(ethylene glycol) block copolymers as a delivery system for oligonucleotides and ribozymes. *Bioconjug Chem* 15, 677-684.

Caplen, N. J., Parrish, S., Imani, F., Fire, A., and Morgan, R. A. (2001). Specific inhibition of gene expression by small double-stranded RNAs in invertebrate and vertebrate systems. *Proc Natl Acad Sci U S A* 98, 9742-9747.

Chien, P. Y., Wang, J., Carbonaro, D., Lei, S., Miller, B., Sheikh, S., Ali, S. M., Ahmad, M. U., and Ahmad, I. (2005). Novel cationic cardiolipin analogue-based liposome for efficient DNA and small interfering RNA delivery in vitro and in vivo. *Cancer Gene Ther* 12, 321-328.

Choung, S., Kim, Y. J., Kim, S., Park, H. O., and Choi, Y. C. (2006). Chemical modification of siRNAs to improve serum stability without loss of efficacy. *Biochem Biophys Res Commun* 342, 919-927.

Cubillos-Ruiz, J. R., Engle, X., Scarlett, U. K., Martinez, D., Barber, A., Elgueta, R., Wang, L., Nesbeth, Y., Durant, Y., Gewirtz, A. T., Sentman, C. L., Kedl, R., and Conejo-Garcia, J. R. (2009). Polyethylenimine-based siRNA nanocomplexes reprogram tumor-associated dendritic cells via TLR5 to elicit therapeutic antitumor immunity. *J Clin Invest* 119, 2231-2244.

Dalby, B., Cates, S., Harris, A., Ohki, E. C., Tilkins, M. L., Price, P. J., and Ciccarone, V. C. (2004). Advanced transfection with Lipofectamine 2000 reagent: primary neurons, siRNA, and high-throughput applications. *Methods* 33, 95-103.

Davis, M. E. (2009). The first targeted delivery of siRNA in humans via a self-assembling, cyclodextrin polymer-based nanoparticle: from concept to clinic. *Mol Pharm* 6, 659-668.

Davis, M. E., Zuckerman, J. E., Choi, C. H., Seligson, D., Tolcher, A., Alabi, C. A., Yen, Y., Heidel, J. D., and Ribas, A. (2010). Evidence of RNAi in humans from systemically administered siRNA via targeted nanoparticles. *Nature* 464, 1067-1070.

de Fougerolles, A., Vornlocher, H. P., Maraganore, J., and Lieberman, J. (2007). Interfering with disease: a progress report on siRNA-based therapeutics. *Nat Rev Drug Discov* 6, 443-453.

Demeneix, B., and Behr, J. P. (2005). Polyethylenimine (PEI). *Adv Genet* 53, 217-230.

DeVincenzo, J., Lambkin-Williams, R., Wilkinson, T., Cehelsky, J., Nochur, S., Walsh, E., Meyers, R., Gollob, J., and Vaishnaw, A. (2010). A randomized, double-blind, placebo-controlled study of an RNAi-based therapy directed against respiratory syncytial virus. *Proc Natl Acad Sci U S A* 107, 8800-8805.

Dubey, P. K., Mishra, V., Jain, S., Mahor, S., and Vyas, S. P. (2004). Liposomes modified with cyclic RGD peptide for tumor targeting. *J Drug Target* 12, 257-264.

Elbashir, S. M., Harborth, J., Lendeckel, W., Yalcin, A., Weber, K., and Tuschl, T. (2001). Duplexes of 21-nucleotide RNAs mediate RNA interference in cultured mammalian cells. *Nature* 411, 494-498.

Fahrmeir, J., Gunther, M., Tietze, N., Wagner, E., and Ogris, M. (2007). Electrophoretic purification of tumor-targeted polyethylenimine-based polyplexes reduces toxic side effects in vivo. *J Control Release* 122, 236-245.

Fedorov, Y., Anderson, E. M., Birmingham, A., Reynolds, A., Karpilow, J., Robinson, K., Leake, D., Marshall, W. S., and Khvorova, A. (2006). Off-target effects by siRNA can induce toxic phenotype. *Rna* 12, 1188-1196.

Fire, A., Xu, S., Montgomery, M. K., Kostas, S. A., Driver, S. E., and Mello, C. C. (1998). Potent and specific genetic interference by double-stranded RNA in Caenorhabditis elegans. *Nature* 391, 806-811.

Fischer, D., von Harpe, A., Kunath, K., Petersen, H., Li, Y., and Kissel, T. (2002). Copolymers of ethylene imine and N-(2-hydroxyethyl)-ethylene imine as tools to study effects of polymer structure on physicochemical and biological properties of DNA complexes. *Bioconjug Chem* 13, 1124-1133.

Flynn, M. A., Casey, D. G., Todryk, S. M., and Mahon, B. P. (2004). Efficient delivery of small interfering RNA for inhibition of IL-12p40 expression in vivo. *J Inflamm (Lond)* 1, 4.

Forrest, M. L., and Pack, D. W. (2002). On the kinetics of polyplex endocytic trafficking: implications for gene delivery vector design. *Mol Ther* 6, 57-66.

Fulton, A., Peters, S. T., Perkins, G. A., Jarosinski, K. W., Damiani, A., Brosnahan, M., Buckles, E. L., Osterrieder, N., and Van de Walle, G. R. (2009). Effective treatment of respiratory alphaherpesvirus infection using RNA interference. *PLoS One* 4, e4118.

Gary, D. J., Puri, N., and Won, Y. Y. (2007). Polymer-based siRNA delivery: perspectives on the fundamental and phenomenological distinctions from polymer-based DNA delivery. *J Control Release* 121, 64-73.

Gautam, A., Densmore, C. L., and Waldrep, J. C. (2001). Pulmonary cytokine responses associated with PEI-DNA aerosol gene therapy. *Gene Ther* 8, 254-257.

Ge, Q., Filip, L., Bai, A., Nguyen, T., Eisen, H. N., and Chen, J. (2004). Inhibition of influenza virus production in virus-infected mice by RNA interference. *Proc Natl Acad Sci U S A* 101, 8676-8681.

Glodde, M., Sirsi, S. R., and Lutz, G. J. (2006). Physiochemical properties of low and high molecular weight poly(ethylene glycol)-grafted poly(ethylene imine) copolymers and their complexes with oligonucleotides. *Biomacromolecules* 7, 347-356.

Godbey, W. T., Barry, M. A., Saggau, P., Wu, K. K., and Mikos, A. G. (2000). Poly(ethylenimine)-mediated transfection: a new paradigm for gene delivery. *J Biomed Mater Res* 51, 321-328.

Godbey, W. T., Wu, K. K., and Mikos, A. G. (1999). Poly(ethylenimine) and its role in gene delivery. *J Control Release* 60, 149-160.

Godbey, W. T., Wu, K. K., and Mikos, A. G. (2001). Poly(ethylenimine)-mediated gene delivery affects endothelial cell function and viability. *Biomaterials* 22, 471-480.

Grayson, A. C., Doody, A. M., and Putnam, D. (2006). Biophysical and structural characterization of polyethylenimine-mediated siRNA delivery in vitro. *Pharm Res* 23, 1868-1876.

Griesenbach, U., and Alton, E. W. (2009). Gene transfer to the lung: lessons learned from more than 2 decades of CF gene therapy. *Adv Drug Deliv Rev* 61, 128-139.

Griesenbach, U., Kitson, C., Escudero Garcia, S., Farley, R., Singh, C., Somerton, L., Painter, H., Smith, R. L., Gill, D. R., Hyde, S. C., Chow, Y. H., Hu, J., Gray, M., Edbrooke, M., Ogilvie, V., MacGregor, G., Scheule, R. K., Cheng, S. H., Caplen, N. J., and Alton, E. W. (2006). Inefficient cationic lipid-mediated siRNA and antisense oligonucleotide transfer to airway epithelial cells in vivo. *Respir Res* 7, 26.

Grimm, D., Streetz, K. L., Jopling, C. L., Storm, T. A., Pandey, K., Davis, C. R., Marion, P., Salazar, F., and Kay, M. A. (2006). Fatality in mice due to oversaturation of cellular microRNA/short hairpin RNA pathways. *Nature* 441, 537-541.

Hannon, G. J., and Rossi, J. J. (2004). Unlocking the potential of the human genome with RNA interference. *Nature* 431, 371-378.

Hassani, Z., Lemkine, G. F., Erbacher, P., Palmier, K., Alfama, G., Giovannangeli, C., Behr, J. P., and Demeneix, B. A. (2005). Lipid-mediated siRNA delivery down-regulates exogenous gene expression in the mouse brain at picomolar levels. *J Gene Med* 7, 198-207.

Heidel, J. D., Yu, Z., Liu, J. Y., Rele, S. M., Liang, Y., Zeidan, R. K., Kornbrust, D. J., and Davis, M. E. (2007). Administration in non-human primates of escalating intravenous doses of targeted nanoparticles containing ribonucleotide reductase subunit M2 siRNA. *Proc Natl Acad Sci U S A* 104, 5715-5721.

Hollins, A. J., Omidi, Y., Benter, I. F., and Akhtar, S. (2007). Toxicogenomics of drug delivery systems: Exploiting delivery system-induced changes in target gene expression to enhance siRNA activity. *J Drug Target* 15, 83-88.

Hong, S., Leroueil, P. R., Janus, E. K., Peters, J. L., Kober, M. M., Islam, M. T., Orr, B. G., Baker, J. R., Jr., and Banaszak Holl, M. M. (2006). Interaction of polycationic polymers with supported lipid bilayers and cells: nanoscale hole formation and enhanced membrane permeability. *Bioconjug Chem* 17, 728-734.

Hornung, V., Bauernfeind, F., Halle, A., Samstad, E. O., Kono, H., Rock, K. L., Fitzgerald, K. A., and Latz, E. (2008). Silica crystals and aluminum salts activate the NALP3 inflammasome through phagosomal destabilization. *Nat Immunol* 9, 847-856.

Hornung, V., Guenthner-Biller, M., Bourquin, C., Ablasser, A., Schlee, M., Uematsu, S., Noronha, A., Manoharan, M., Akira, S., de Fougerolles, A., Endres, S., and Hartmann, G. (2005). Sequence-specific potent induction of IFN-alpha by short interfering RNA in plasmacytoid dendritic cells through TLR7. *Nat Med* 11, 263-270.

Jackson, A. L., Bartz, S. R., Schelter, J., Kobayashi, S. V., Burchard, J., Mao, M., Li, B., Cavet, G., and Linsley, P. S. (2003). Expression profiling reveals off-target gene regulation by RNAi. *Nat Biotechnol* 21, 635-637.

Jere, D., Xu, C. X., Arote, R., Yun, C. H., Cho, M. H., and Cho, C. S. (2008). Poly(beta-amino ester) as a carrier for si/shRNA delivery in lung cancer cells. *Biomaterials* 29, 2535-2547.

Judge, A. D., Bola, G., Lee, A. C., and MacLachlan, I. (2006). Design of noninflammatory synthetic siRNA mediating potent gene silencing in vivo. *Mol Ther* 13, 494-505.

Judge, A. D., Sood, V., Shaw, J. R., Fang, D., McClintock, K., and MacLachlan, I. (2005). Sequence-dependent stimulation of the mammalian innate immune response by synthetic siRNA. *Nat Biotechnol* 23, 457-462.

Kabanov, A. V. (2006). Polymer genomics: an insight into pharmacology and toxicology of nanomedicines. *Adv Drug Deliv Rev* 58, 1597-1621.

Kawakami, S., Ito, Y., Charoensit, P., Yamashita, F., and Hashida, M. (2006). Evaluation of proinflammatory cytokine production induced by linear and branched polyethylenimine/plasmid DNA complexes in mice. *J Pharmacol Exp Ther* 317, 1382-1390.

Kichler, A., Chillon, M., Leborgne, C., Danos, O., and Frisch, B. (2002). Intranasal gene delivery with a polyethylenimine-PEG conjugate. *J Control Release* 81, 379-388.

Kim, W. J., and Kim, S. W. (2009). Efficient siRNA delivery with non-viral polymeric vehicles. *Pharm Res* 26, 657-666.

Kleemann, E., Neu, M., Jekel, N., Fink, L., Schmehl, T., Gessler, T., Seeger, W., and Kissel, T. (2005). Nano-carriers for DNA delivery to the lung based upon a TAT-derived peptide covalently coupled to PEG-PEI. *J Control Release* 109, 299-316.

Kunath, K., Merdan, T., Hegener, O., Haberlein, H., and Kissel, T. (2003a). Integrin targeting using RGD-PEI conjugates for in vitro gene transfer. *J Gene Med* 5, 588-599.

Kunath, K., von Harpe, A., Fischer, D., and Kissel, T. (2003b). Galactose-PEI-DNA complexes for targeted gene delivery: degree of substitution affects complex size and transfection efficiency. *J Control Release* 88, 159-172.

Layzer, J. M., McCaffrey, A. P., Tanner, A. K., Huang, Z., Kay, M. A., and Sullenger, B. A. (2004). In vivo activity of nuclease-resistant siRNAs. *Rna* 10, 766-771.

Lee, C. C., and Chiang, B. L. (2008). RNA interference: new therapeutics in allergic diseases. *Curr Gene Ther* 8, 236-246.

Leroueil, P. R., Berry, S. A., Duthie, K., Han, G., Rotello, V. M., McNerny, D. Q., Baker, J. R., Jr., Orr, B. G., and Holl, M. M. (2008). Wide varieties of cationic nanoparticles induce defects in supported lipid bilayers. *Nano Lett* 8, 420-424.

Li, S. D., and Huang, L. (2006). Targeted delivery of antisense oligodeoxynucleotide and small interference RNA into lung cancer cells. *Mol Pharm* 3, 579-588.

Luo, M. C., Zhang, D. Q., Ma, S. W., Huang, Y. Y., Shuster, S. J., Porreca, F., and Lai, J. (2005). An efficient intrathecal delivery of small interfering RNA to the spinal cord and peripheral neurons. *Mol Pain* 1, 29.

Maeda, Y., Fukushima, K., Nishizaki, K., and Smith, R. J. (2005). In vitro and in vivo suppression of GJB2 expression by RNA interference. *Hum Mol Genet* 14, 1641-1650.

Mao, S., Shuai, X., Unger, F., Wittmar, M., Xie, X., and Kissel, T. (2005). Synthesis, characterization and cytotoxicity of poly(ethylene glycol)-graft-trimethyl chitosan block copolymers. *Biomaterials* 26, 6343-6356.

Meister, G., Landthaler, M., Patkaniowska, A., Dorsett, Y., Teng, G., and Tuschl, T. (2004). Human Argonaute2 mediates RNA cleavage targeted by miRNAs and siRNAs. *Mol Cell* 15, 185-197.

Mello, C. C., and Conte, D., Jr. (2004). Revealing the world of RNA interference. *Nature* 431, 338-342.

Merkel, O. M., Beyerle, A., Beckmann, B. M., Zheng, M., Hartmann, R. K., Stoger, T., and Kissel, T. H. (2011). Polymer-related off-target effects in non-viral siRNA delivery. *Biomaterials* 32, 2388-2398.

Merkel, O. M., Beyerle, A., Librizzi, D., Pfestroff, A., Behr, T. M., Sproat, B., Barth, P. J., and Kissel, T. (2009). Nonviral siRNA delivery to the lung: investigation of PEG-PEI polyplexes and their in vivo performance. *Mol Pharm* 6, 1246-1260.

Meyerhoff, A. (1999). U.S. Food and Drug Administration approval of AmBisome (liposomal amphotericin B) for treatment of visceral leishmaniasis. *Clin Infect Dis* 28, 42-48; discussion 49-51.

Miyawaki-Shimizu, K., Predescu, D., Shimizu, J., Broman, M., Predescu, S., and Malik, A. B. (2006). siRNA-induced caveolin-1 knockdown in mice increases lung vascular permeability via the junctional pathway. *Am J Physiol Lung Cell Mol Physiol* 290, L405-413.

Moghimi, S. M., and Szebeni, J. (2003). Stealth liposomes and long circulating nanoparticles: critical issues in pharmacokinetics, opsonization and protein-binding properties. *Prog Lipid Res* 42, 463-478.

Morrissey, D. V., Lockridge, J. A., Shaw, L., Blanchard, K., Jensen, K., Breen, W., Hartsough, K., Machemer, L., Radka, S., Jadhav, V., Vaish, N., Zinnen, S., Vargeese, C., Bowman, K., Shaffer, C. S., Jeffs, L. B., Judge, A., MacLachlan, I., and Polisky, B. (2005). Potent and persistent in vivo anti-HBV activity of chemically modified siRNAs. *Nat Biotechnol* 23, 1002-1007.

Nel, A. E., Madler, L., Velegol, D., Xia, T., Hoek, E. M., Somasundaran, P., Klaessig, F., Castranova, V., and Thompson, M. (2009). Understanding biophysicochemical interactions at the nano-bio interface. *Nat Mater* 8, 543-557.

Neu, M., Fischer, D., and Kissel, T. (2005). Recent advances in rational gene transfer vector design based on poly(ethylene imine) and its derivatives. *J Gene Med* 7, 992-1009.

Novina, C. D., and Sharp, P. A. (2004). The RNAi revolution. *Nature* 430, 161-164.

Ogris, M., Brunner, S., Schuller, S., Kircheis, R., and Wagner, E. (1999). PEGylated DNA/transferrin-PEI complexes: reduced interaction with blood components, extended circulation in blood and potential for systemic gene delivery. *Gene Ther* 6, 595-605.

Omidi, Y., Barar, J., and Akhtar, S. (2005). Toxicogenomics of cationic lipid-based vectors for gene therapy: impact of microarray technology. *Curr Drug Deliv* 2, 429-441.

Omidi, Y., Barar, J., Heidari, H. R., Ahmadian, S., Yazdi, H. A., and Akhtar, S. (2008). Microarray analysis of the toxicogenomics and the genotoxic potential of a cationic lipid-based gene delivery nanosystem in human alveolar epithelial a549 cells. *Toxicol Mech Methods* 18, 369-378.

Omidi, Y., Hollins, A. J., Benboubetra, M., Drayton, R., Benter, I. F., and Akhtar, S. (2003). Toxicogenomics of non-viral vectors for gene therapy: a microarray study of lipofectin- and oligofectamine-induced gene expression changes in human epithelial cells. *J Drug Target* 11, 311-323.

Oupicky, D., Ogris, M., Howard, K. A., Dash, P. R., Ulbrich, K., and Seymour, L. W. (2002). Importance of lateral and steric stabilization of polyelectrolyte gene delivery vectors for extended systemic circulation. *Mol Ther* 5, 463-472.

Pal, A., Ahmad, A., Khan, S., Sakabe, I., Zhang, C., Kasid, U. N., and Ahmad, I. (2005). Systemic delivery of RafsiRNA using cationic cardiolipin liposomes silences Raf-1 expression and inhibits tumor growth in xenograft model of human prostate cancer. *Int J Oncol* 26, 1087-1091.

Palliser, D., Chowdhury, D., Wang, Q. Y., Lee, S. J., Bronson, R. T., Knipe, D. M., and Lieberman, J. (2006). An siRNA-based microbicide protects mice from lethal herpes simplex virus 2 infection. *Nature* 439, 89-94.

Panyam, J., and Labhasetwar, V. (2003). Biodegradable nanoparticles for drug and gene delivery to cells and tissue. *Adv Drug Deliv Rev* 55, 329-347.

Petersen, H., Fechner, P. M., Fischer, D., and Kissel*, T. (2002a). Synthesis, Characterization, and Biocompatibility of
Polyethylenimine-graft-poly(ethylene glycol) Block Copolymers. *Macromolecules* 35, 6867-6874.

Petersen, H., Fechner, P. M., Martin, A. L., Kunath, K., Stolnik, S., Roberts, C. J., Fischer, D., Davies, M. C., and Kissel, T. (2002b). Polyethylenimine-graft-poly(ethylene glycol) copolymers: influence of copolymer block structure on DNA complexation and biological activities as gene delivery system. *Bioconjug Chem* 13, 845-854.

Pison, U., Welte, T., Giersig, M., and Groneberg, D. A. (2006). Nanomedicine for respiratory diseases. *Eur J Pharmacol* 533, 341-350.

Ren, X. L., Xu, Y. M., Bao, W., Fu, H. J., Wu, C. G., Zhao, Y., Li, Z. K., Zhang, J., Li, S. Q., Chen, W. Q., Wang, T., Zhang, R., Zhang, L. H., Qian, G. S., Chen, S. Y., Jia, L. T., and Yang, A. G. (2009). Inhibition of non-small cell lung cancer cell proliferation and tumor growth by vector-based small interfering RNAs targeting HER2/neu. *Cancer Lett* 281, 134-143.

Robbins, M., Judge, A., Ambegia, E., Choi, C., Yaworski, E., Palmer, L., McClintock, K., and MacLachlan, I. (2008). Misinterpreting the therapeutic effects of small interfering RNA caused by immune stimulation. *Hum Gene Ther* 19, 991-999.

Robbins, M., Judge, A., and MacLachlan, I. (2009). siRNA and innate immunity. *Oligonucleotides* 19, 89-102.

Santel, A., Aleku, M., Keil, O., Endruschat, J., Esche, V., Fisch, G., Dames, S., Loffler, K., Fechtner, M., Arnold, W., Giese, K., Klippel, A., and Kaufmann, J. (2006). A novel siRNA-lipoplex technology for RNA interference in the mouse vascular endothelium. *Gene Ther* 13, 1222-1234.

Schatzlein, A. G. (2006). Delivering cancer stem cell therapies - a role for nanomedicines? *Eur J Cancer* 42, 1309-1315.

Schlee, M., Hornung, V., and Hartmann, G. (2006). siRNA and isRNA: two edges of one sword. *Mol Ther* 14, 463-470.

Seguin, R. M., and Ferrari, N. (2009). Emerging oligonucleotide therapies for asthma and chronic obstructive pulmonary disease. *Expert Opin Investig Drugs* 18, 1505-1517.

Sitterberg, J., Ozcetin, A., Ehrhardt, C., and Bakowsky, U. (2010). Utilising atomic force microscopy for the characterisation of nanoscale drug delivery systems. *Eur J Pharm Biopharm* 74, 2-13.

Somia, N., and Verma, I. M. (2000). Gene therapy: trials and tribulations. *Nat Rev Genet* 1, 91-99.

Soutschek, J., Akinc, A., Bramlage, B., Charisse, K., Constien, R., Donoghue, M., Elbashir, S., Geick, A., Hadwiger, P., Harborth, J., John, M., Kesavan, V., Lavine, G., Pandey, R. K., Racie, T., Rajeev, K. G., Rohl, I., Toudjarska, I., Wang, G., Wuschko, S., Bumcrot, D., Koteliansky, V., Limmer, S., Manoharan, M., and Vornlocher, H. P. (2004). Therapeutic silencing of an endogenous gene by systemic administration of modified siRNAs. *Nature* 432, 173-178.

Spagnou, S., Miller, A. D., and Keller, M. (2004). Lipidic carriers of siRNA: differences in the formulation, cellular uptake, and delivery with plasmid DNA. *Biochemistry* 43, 13348-13356.

Tagami, T., Barichello, J. M., Kikuchi, H., Ishida, T., and Kiwada, H. (2007). The gene-silencing effect of siRNA in cationic lipoplexes is enhanced by incorporating pDNA in the complex. *Int J Pharm* 333, 62-69.

Tagami, T., Hirose, K., Barichello, J. M., Ishida, T., and Kiwada, H. (2008). Global gene expression profiling in cultured cells is strongly influenced by treatment with siRNA-cationic liposome complexes. *Pharm Res* 25, 2497-2504.

Tan, Y., and Huang, L. (2002). Overcoming the inflammatory toxicity of cationic gene vectors. *J Drug Target* 10, 153-160.

Thomas, M., Lu, J. J., Ge, Q., Zhang, C., Chen, J., and Klibanov, A. M. (2005). Full deacylation of polyethylenimine dramatically boosts its gene delivery efficiency and specificity to mouse lung. *Proc Natl Acad Sci U S A* 102, 5679-5684.

Tong, A. W. (2006). Small RNAs and non-small cell lung cancer. *Curr Mol Med* 6, 339-349.

Tuschl, T., Zamore, P. D., Lehmann, R., Bartel, D. P., and Sharp, P. A. (1999). Targeted mRNA degradation by double-stranded RNA in vitro. *Genes Dev* 13, 3191-3197.

Urban-Klein, B., Werth, S., Abuharbeid, S., Czubayko, F., and Aigner, A. (2005). RNAi-mediated gene-targeting through systemic application of polyethylenimine (PEI)-complexed siRNA in vivo. *Gene Ther* 12, 461-466.

Verma, U. N., Surabhi, R. M., Schmaltieg, A., Becerra, C., and Gaynor, R. B. (2003). Small interfering RNAs directed against beta-catenin inhibit the in vitro and in vivo growth of colon cancer cells. *Clin Cancer Res* 9, 1291-1300.

Werth, S., Urban-Klein, B., Dai L., Höbel S., Grzelinski M., Bakowsky U., Czubayko F., Aigner A. (2006). A low molecular weight fraction of polyethylenimine (PEI) displays increased trasnfection efficiency of DNA and siRNA in fresh or lyophilized complexes. *J Control Rel* 112, 257-270.

Williams, J. H., Sirsi, S. R., Latta, D. R., and Lutz, G. J. (2006). Induction of dystrophin expression by exon skipping in mdx mice following intramuscular injection of antisense oligonucleotides complexed with PEG-PEI copolymers. *Mol Ther* 14, 88-96.

Zamora-Avila, D. E., Zapata-Benavides, P., Franco-Molina, M. A., Saavedra-Alonso, S., Trejo-Avila, L. M., Resendez-Perez, D., Mendez-Vazquez, J. L., Isaias-Badillo, J., and Rodriguez-Padilla, C. (2009). WT1 gene silencing by aerosol delivery of PEI-RNAi complexes inhibits B16-F10 lung metastases growth. *Cancer Gene Ther* 16, 892-899.

Zimmermann, T. S., Lee, A. C., Akinc, A., Bramlage, B., Bumcrot, D., Fedoruk, M. N., Harborth, J., Heyes, J. A., Jeffs, L. B., John, M., Judge, A. D., Lam, K., McClintock, K., Nechev, L. V., Palmer, L. R., Racie, T., Rohl, I., Seiffert, S., Shanmugam, S., Sood, V., Soutschek, J., Toudjarska, I., Wheat, A. J., Yaworski, E., Zedalis, W., Koteliansky, V., Manoharan, M., Vornlocher, H. P., and MacLachlan, I. (2006). RNAi-mediated gene silencing in non-human primates. *Nature* 441, 111-114.

Zintchenko, A., Philipp, A., Dehshahri, A., and Wagner, E. (2008). Simple modifications of branched PEI lead to highly efficient siRNA carriers with low toxicity. *Bioconjug Chem* 19, 1448-1455.
Zuhorn, I. S., Engberts, J. B., and Hoekstra, D. (2007). Gene delivery by cationic lipid vectors: overcoming cellular barriers. *Eur Biophys J* 36, 349-362.

6

Toxicogenomics of Nonviral Cationic Gene Delivery Nanosystems

Yadollah Omidi, Vala Kafil and Jaleh Barar
Research Center for Pharmaceutical Nanotechnology
Faculty of Pharmacy, Tabriz University of Medical Sciences, Tabriz
Iran

1. Introduction

To date, both viral and nonviral vectors have been exploited for delivery of gene-based therapies to target cells/tissues. Despite high efficiency of the viral vectors (e.g., retroviruses and adenoviruses), these vectors appear to be immunogenic and potentially harmful when used in clinical gene therapy protocols (Ferber, 2001b). Besides, the preparation and purification of the viral vectors appear to be laborious, cost-prohibitive and not amenable to industrial-scale manufacture. Nonviral vectors such as cationic lipids (CLs) and cationic polymers (CPs) have been categorized as advanced materials and their low immunogenicity, lack of pathogenicity, and ease of pharmacologic production continue to make them attractive alternatives to viral vectors (Medina-Kauwe et al., 2005). However, these vectors may also suffer from relatively low levels of gene transfer compared to viruses. Thus, the drive to advance these vectors continues resulting in considerable progresses in improved transfection efficiency. Nonviral vectors (in particular cationic gene delivery systems) are able to bind and enter the target cells, however they yield low gene expression. No substantial information is available on interactions of these vectors with cellular biomolecules. Since these medicaments tend to act at genomic levels, thus understanding the genomic impacts of the nonviral vectors may help develop more efficient gene delivery systems. Nonetheless, this needs recruitment of high throughput screening methodologies.

To date, exploitation of the "omics" concepts (e.g., genomics, proteomics and metabolomics) is going to change the face of pharmacotherapy towards significantly more advanced and efficient pharmaceuticals (e.g., gene based nanomedicines) with minimal adverse consequences (Aardema & MacGregor, 2002). Enormous efforts have also been devoted for application of the global gene expression profiling in pharmacologic and toxicological investigations. The gene expression profiling technology has been primarily exploited for identification of underlying mechanisms for toxicity of pharmaceuticals and their genomic signatures, by which the safety liabilities can be determined and manifestations of undesired genotoxicity can be prohibited (Suter et al., 2004; Yang et al., 2004).

This methodology can be successfully used for the discovery and development of any chemicals and pharmaceuticals including gene delivery nanosystems. The main focus of the current book chapter is to provide some useful information about "genocompatibility" and "toxicogenomics" of the nonviral vectors using global gene expression profiling techniques i.e. DNA microarray.

2. Gene therapy challenges and dilemmas

The principle of gene therapy possesses undeniable therapeutic advantages over the conventional therapeutic modalities that are basically dependent upon exploitation of small molecules or biological pharmaceuticals. These advantages are: 1) specific or selective treatment of diseased cells/tissue, 2) minimal adverse consequences, 3) correction of the genetic cause of a disease, and 4) long-term treatment after single application (Rubanyi, 2001). Basically, to silence/suppress a target gene or to correct a genetic defect, the gene-based therapeutics such as oligodeoxynuleutides (ODNs), plasmid DNA, ribozymes, DNAzymes or short interfering RNA (siRNA) need to be shuttled to the target site. Delivery of gene-based therapeutics has been also advanced by development and implementation of various strategies, including: biological (e.g., viral vectors), physical (e.g., microinjection and electroporation, gene gun, ultrasound, and hydrodynamic delivery), and chemical (e.g., non-viral vectors) approaches. However, gene transfer into various target cells still faces major obstacles including poor delivery efficiency, cellular toxicity, immunogenicity and oncogenicity, as well as short-term transgenic expression and poor expression levels.

The first clinical test of gene therapy was accomplished a decade ago with the transfer of the missing "adenosine deaminase" gene into lymphocytes isolated from patients with severe combined immune-deficiency syndrome (i.e., as ex-vivo gene therapy approach). However, despite the early promising prophecy on the high effectiveness of gene therapy, the existing clinical experience indicate insufficient therapeutic efficacy coupled with increasing safety concerns and ethical issues (Verma & Somia, 1997). In some cases, aptamer-based genomedicines (e.g., Pegaptanib sodium, Macugen™) have been successfully utilized for treatment of the age related macular degeneration (Barar et al., 2008). Gendicine™ is an adenoviral p53-based gene medicine that was approved by the Chinese FDA in 2003 for treatment of head and neck cancer, while Advexin™ (a similar gene therapy approach from Introgen) was turned down by the US FDA in 2008. In fact, the death of Jesse Gelsinger in a gene therapy experiment in 1999 imposed a significant setback to gene therapy research in the United States, however many scientists aimed to resolve problems associated with the gene therapy strategies. In 2006, an international group of scientists announced the successful use of gene therapy to treat two adult patients for a disease affecting myeloid cells (Ott et al., 2006). Also in 2007, the world's first gene therapy trial for inherited retinal disease was announced for treatment of Leber's congenital amaurosis which is a inherited blinding disease caused by mutations in the RPE65 gene (Maguire et al., 2008). It should be evoked that the performance and pathogenicity of viral vectors (e.g., retroviruses, lentiviruses, adenoviruses, and adeno-associated viruses) and nonviral vectors have been evaluated in animal models. Promising results form the basis for clinical trials to treat genetic disorders and acquired diseases, however vector development/advancement remains a seminal concern for improved gene therapy technologies (Verma & Weitzman, 2005). Fundamentally, an ideal gene delivery method should protect the transgene against degradation, transport the transgene into the cytoplasm and then nucleus of target cells with little undesired detrimental effects (Gao et al., 2007).

Results obtained from *in vitro* studies have revealed that treatment of cells with antisense oligonucleotides (As-ODNs) for a period of only a few hours can bestow the desired effects of As-ODNs, while animal experiments demand repeated administration through multiple injections for prolonged exposure to As-ODNs. Despite promising results of some in vivo studies with free As-ODNs, improved delivery systems are essential to increase the efficacy of As-ODNs and to reduce its amount and frequency of administration (Hughes et al., 2001). Successful delivery of desired genes are important for both *ex vivo*, where cells undergo gene therapy in culture prior to implantation into the patient, or *in vivo* gene therapy where nucleic acids are administered directly to the patient to attain the desired gene change. Preferably, in either approach, only the therapy-intended gene expression changes should occur. However, this is not always the case, for example viral vectors are known to be efficient delivery systems for nucleic acids but can also induce immunogenic responses (Audouy et al., 2002; Ferber, 2001a; Ferber, 2001b). Hence, several nonviral gene delivery nanosystems such as cationic polymer- or lipid-based formulations have been developed for nucleic acid delivery. These cationic nanostructures can readily condense DNA into complexes and form polyplexes/lipoplexes to be used for *ex vivo* and *in vivo* gene therapy.

Although the CPs/CLs can principally enhance the delivery and improve the biological end-point of genomic-therapeutics, they often exert cytotoxicity depending on delivery system and target cell/tissue (Pedroso de Lima et al., 2001). Thus, both transfection efficiency evaluation and safety assessment are essential for gene transfer with these gene therapy vectors. A number of factors may affect the efficacy and safety of nonviral vector-mediated gene transfer; in particular their structural properties and type of target cells and tissue. It should be noticed that as various target cells may display different responses, the transfection efficacy and safety of vectors should be carefully optimized upon types of target cells and target organs. Once transfection accomplished, specific attention should be given to the genotoxicity potentials of gene-based medicines. Surprisingly, no substantial information is available about the genomic signature of the cationic delivery systems. We have previously investigated the potential of the commercially available nonviral vectors (e.g., Polyamidoamine (PAMAM) dendrimers such as Polyfect™ (PF) and Superfect™ (SF)) and lipids (e.g., Lipofectin™ (LF) and Oligofectamine™ (OF)) on global gene expression within human epithelial A431 and A549 cells by exploiting the cDNA microarray technology (Barar et al., 2009; Omidi et al., 2003; Omidi et al., 2005a; Omidi et al., 2005b; Omidi et al., 2008). These investigations revealed occurrence of inadvertent nonspecific gene expression changes within target cells upon treatments with these cationic gene delivery nanosystems. These findings led us to screen series of lipid- or polymer-based non-viral vectors for their toxicogenomic and genomic toxicity potentials in target cells.

Fig. 1 represents schematic illustrations of polymer/lipid based micro/nano systems used for delivery of genes/drugs.

3. Cellular trafficking and toxicity of polycationic nanostructures

For achievement of an efficient systemic delivery of gene-based nanomedicines, various factors appear to play crucial role, including: 1) the physicochemical characteristics of the gene-based therapies, 2) the effects of biological environment, 3) the functionality of membranes and barriers, and 4) the biological impacts of cellular microenvironment.

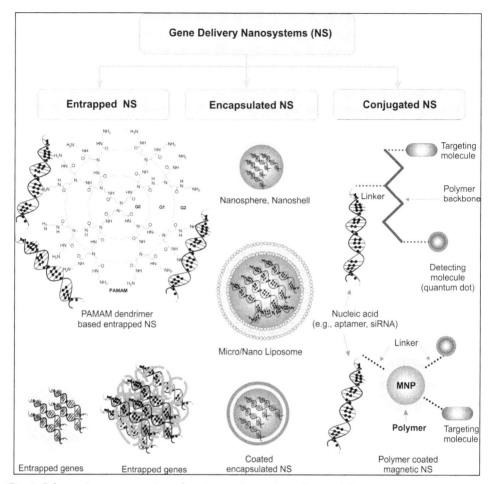

Fig. 1. Schematic representation of various polymer based gene delivery nanosystems. To prepare gene medicine nanosystems (NS) nucleic acids (e.g., antisense, siRNA, and aptamer) are generally entrapped, encapsulated or conjugated with polymers. Genes can be conjugated to magnetic nanoparticles (MNP) and quantum dots for concurrent detection and therapy.

Within the circulation system, blood cells, proteins, enzymes and serum components may bind to the genomedicines and cause instability and lowered transfection efficiency (Konopka et al., 2005). In addition, the circulating gene therapies must circumvent the immune system clearance and cross the capillary endothelial cells to reach the target cells/tissue. Once inside the target cells (normally via receptor-mediated endocytosis pathway), the genomedicine must overcome the subcellular and/or biomolecular impacts. In fact, the amphipathic sheet like lipid bilayer architecture of the biological membranes along with the integrated proteins separate cells from their environment and form the boundaries of different organelles inside the cells, at which exchange of materials among the different parts of a cell is controlled (Omidi & Gumbleton, 2005). Nonviral vectors may bind to cells by means of one or both of two types of cell binding interaction machineries, i.e. receptor and non-receptor mediated bindings (Medina-Kauwe et al., 2005). At cellular level, trafficking of the gene-based nanomedicines is basically performed through vesicular transportation pathways, in which they may engineer their own escape from demise in the lysosome. Endocytosis of macromolecular nanomedicines occurs through various cellular pathways, including clathrin coated pits, caveolae membranes and lipid rafts (Conner & Schmid, 2003; Spang, 2008). More likely, these complexes enter cells through nonspecific exploitation of these endocytic machineries, presumably mainly involving clathrin-mediated endocytic pathway. This route initiates and stabilizes membrane curvature formation, in which the adaptor proteins bind to clathrin pits and augment the inward pull of the membrane towards the cytoplasm leading to vesicle formation (Young, 2007).

It has been evidenced that the N-1(-(2,3-dioleoyloxy)propyl)-N,N,N-trimethylammoniummethylsulphate (DOTAP) lipoplexes are internalized by cells solely via clathrin-mediated endocytosis, however PEI polyplexes were shown to be internalized both by clathrin-mediated and caveolae-mediated endocytosis (Rejman et al., 2005). Once inside the cytoplasm, DNA is released from vesicular compartment upon physicochemical properties of the genomedicine. The endosomal escape of DNA at an early stage of endocytosis is deemed to be critical for cytosolic DNA delivery and determination of overall transfection efficiency. Among CPs and CLs, fusogenic lipid dioleoylphosphatidylethanolamine (DOPE) as a helper lipid for liposome-based DNA delivery were reported to induce membrane fusion between the endosome and the liposome and result in membrane destabilization and release of DNA into the cytoplasm (Farhood et al., 1995). Such destabilization of the vesicular membrane further highlights the interaction of cationic lipids with cellular compartments. This inadvertent nonspecific interaction may be exacerbated for *in vivo* systemic gene, which requires high and potentially toxic doses of nonviral vectors. Utilization of the cell-specific ligands or antibodies were reported to lower the cytotoxicity, while facilitating tissue targeting (Rawat et al., 2007), in which the ligand choice is largely dictated by whether or not the target receptor undergoes vesicular trafficking and the endocytic pathway used by the vector is dependent upon the targeting ligand as well as cell type. The structural architecture of the gene delivery nanosystems was shown to be important from gene expression changes viewpoints (Omidi et al., 2005b), which is also largely dependent upon cell type, in particular the membrane lipid composition and membrane phase state (Kabanov, 2006). Adsorption of polycations such as poly(N -ethyl-4-vinylpyridinium) salts (PEVP) in liposomic biomembranes was shown to induce flip-flop of negatively charged lipids (e.g., cardiolipin, phosphatidylserine, and phosphatidic acid) from the inner to the outer leaflet of the liquid liposomal membrane, but not in solid membranes (Yaroslavov et al., 1994; Yaroslavov et al., 2006). Among polycations, starburst PAMAM dendrimers and PEI appeared to elicit the most dramatic increase in membrane permeability by interacting the membranous biomolecules and forming holes in lipid membranes (Hong et al., 2006; Leroueil et al., 2007). Such structures could function as gates, through which the lipid molecules can be transported across the biomembranes (Kabanov, 2006). Fig. 2 represents cytotoxicity of linear and branched PEI in A431 cells (Kafil & Omidi, 2011).

Upon differences in cell types, the polyions can bind to the cellular compartments and accordingly induce compartmentalization within certain areas of the membranes and inadvertently trigger various signaling paths. Furthermore, nanoscaled defects were shown to be induced by PAMAM dendrimers through removing lipid from the fluid domains at a significantly greater rate than for the gel domains (Erickson et al., 2008). This reinforces a possibility of compartmentalization of synthetic polymers within different membrane domains as well as a differential effect of polymers on functional systems in the membranes that consecutively provoke inadvertent cytoplasmic/nucleic consequences directly and indirectly via secondary messengers such as G proteins.

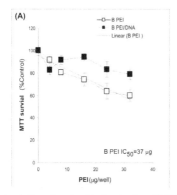 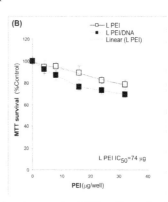

Fig. 2. Cytotoxicity of polyethylenimine (25 kDa) polymers in A431 cells evaluated by MTT assay. A) Cytotoxicity of B PEI with IC_{50}=37 µg. B) Cytotoxicity of LPEI with IC_{50}=74 µg. BPEI: Branched polyethylenimine; LPEI: linear polyethylenimine; adapted with permission from (Kafil & Omidi, 2011).

Fischer et al. (2003) monitored cytotoxicity of various polycationic gene delivery systems in L929 mouse fibroblasts using MTT assay and the release of the cytosolic enzyme lactate dehydrogenase (LDH). They showed a pattern for cellular toxicity as follow, poly(ethylenimine)=poly(L-lysine)>poly(diallyl-dimethyl-ammonium chloride)>diethylaminoethyl-dextran>poly(vinyl pyridinium bromide)>Starburst dendrimer>cationized albumin>native albumin. These researchers, interestingly, confirmed the molecular weight and the cationic charge density of the polycations as key parameters for the interaction with the cell membranes and accordingly the cell damage (Fischer et al., 2003). Besides, interaction of dendrimers with erythrocyte membrane proteins was shown to trigger echinocytosis (Domanski et al., 2004), while the cationic liposomes are less cytotoxic than dendrimers. The toxicity by CLs appeared to be dependent upon the type of cationic lipid macromolecule, concentration, molecular weight and the presence of DNA, where complexation of the polycations with DNA resulted in reduced tissue damage. However, Gebhart et al. (2001) showed increased cytotoxicity in the cos-7 cells upon complexation of various polymers with DNA (Gebhart & Kabanov, 2001).

Filion et al. (1997) have performed an important body of work by evaluating the toxicity of liposomes, formulated with various cationic lipids, towards murine macrophages and T lymphocytes and the human monocyte-like U937 cell line. They reported occurrence of pronounced toxicity by cationic liposomes formulated from DOPE and cationic lipids based on diacyltrimethylammonium propane (dioleoyl-, dimyristoyl-, dipalmitoyl-, disteroyl-: DOTAP, DMTAP, DPTAP, DSTAP) or dimethyldioctadecylammonium bromide (DDAB) in the phagocytic cells (macrophages and U937 cells), but not within non-phagocytic T lymphocytes. They also showed the rank order of toxicity as follows: DOPE/DDAB > DOPE/DOTAP > DOPE/DMTAP > DOPE/DPTAP > DOPE/DSTAP.

Once complexed with nucleic acid (e.g., antisense oligonucleotide or plasmid vector), lipoplexes revealed marginally reduced toxicity towards macrophages (Filion & Phillips, 1997b). Furthermore, since cationic lipids display intrinsic anti-inflammatory activity, they should be cautiously utilized as a gene delivery system to transfer nucleic acids for gene therapy *in vivo*.

DNA microarray technology has advanced and accelerated the identification process for mechanistic toxicology to illuminate genomic aspects of toxicology that could consequently postulate early effect within targets cells/tissues upon exposure to the toxicants (de et al., 2004). Recently, an interesting study was performed to compare different commercially available cationic liposome–DNA lipoplexes (Masotti et al., 2009), and it was reported that the lipoplex size and cationic lipid to DNA ratio are the two main parameters affecting the transfection efficiency of lipoplexes. The lipofection efficiency was determined mainly by lipoplex size, but not by the extent of lipoplex–cell interactions including binding, uptake or fusion. In the presence or absence of serum, lipoplex size was found to be a major factor determining lipofection efficiency. These researchers concluded that, by controlling lipoplex size, an efficient lipid delivery system may be achieved for *in vitro* and *in vivo* gene therapy.

Florea et al. (2002) evaluated PEIs with different molecular weights for their efficiency in transfecting undifferentiated COS-1 and well-differentiated human submucosal airway epithelial Calu-3 cells and showed that transfection efficiency was dependent upon the cell types, but not molecular weights. These researchers reported that gene transfer by PEI was 3 orders of magnitude more effective in COS-1 than in Calu-3 cells, perhaps because of secretion of mucins by Calu-3 cells (Florea et al., 2002). However, the larger molecular weights of PEI were also shown to yield the highest transfection efficiency in EA.hy 926 cell line derived from a fusion of the human A549 cell line with human umbilical vein endothelial cells, HUVEC (Godbey et al., 2001). Two types of cytotoxicities in process of PEI -mediated cell transfection have been reported: 1) an immediate toxicity associated with free PEI, 2) a delayed toxicity associated with cellular processing of PEI/DNA complexes (Godbey et al., 1999; Godbey et al., 2001). The immediate toxicity seems to occur upon interaction of the free PEIs with negatively charged serum proteins (e.g., albumin) and red blood cells (cytotoxic effects), while the delayed toxicity by PEI/DNA complex appeared to be closely related to the release of DNA (genomic effects). In cell culture, free PEI interacts with cellular components and inhibits normal cellular process. It causes several changes to cells, which include cell shrinking, reduced number of mitoses and vacuolization of the cytoplasm. We have observed significant genotoxicity impacts induced by PEI in A431 cells (Kafil & Omidi, 2011) and xenografted mice (our unpublished data).

Toxicity impacts of nanostructured materials have been recently reviewed (Nel et al., 2006), while many aspects of this issue (in particular at genomics/protemics levels) still remains unresolved. As a result, necessity of analysis of toxicogenomics of the nanoscaled advanced biomaterials is very clear. It will direct us towards development of safe pharmaceutical formulations with maximal efficiency and wide therapeutic index yet displaying minimal toxicity profiles since the conventional assessment of toxicity solely provide preliminary information with little devotion to the global genomic/proteomic impacts (Hollins et al., 2007; Kabanov et al., 2005; Kabanov, 2006; Omidi et al., 2005a). If this is the case, then the gene and drug delivery paradigms are going to stumble upon new era to deal with "functionalized excipients".

4. Genocompatibility and toxicogenomics of polycationic nanostructures

To pursue the genomic impacts of any gene based medicine, it is necessary to exploit high throughput screening methodologies (e.g., DNA microarray) for evaluation of global gene changes induced by the gene medicine or any other chemicals/compounds. Such genome based impact could be termed as "genotoxicity" or "toxicogenomics".

The DNA microarray technology combines standard molecular techniques with high-throughput screening to monitor the expression of up to ~40000 genes, which may provide a means for toxicity prediction prior to classical toxicological endpoints such as histopathology or clinical chemistry (Goldsmith & Dhanasekaran, 2004). In gene silencing experiments, such approach may allow a genomic characterization of delivery systems leading to identification of possible incompatibilities with intended target genes or biological effects of the gene based medicine. This may allow screening of compatible or useful delivery systems early in drug development that could subsequently save time and money in pre-clinical and clinical studies (Fielden & Kolaja, 2006; Lettieri, 2006).

Cytotoxicity and genotoxicity potentials of CPs and CLs are going to be well acknowledged, and accordingly these cationic nanosystems should undergo a rigorous genocompatibility evaluation prior to *in vitro* and *in vivo* exploitation (Kabanov, 2006; Omidi et al., 2005a). These systems alone or in combination with biologically active molecules (e.g., siRNA, antisense, aptamer) are able to alter cell signaling and biological responses in cells and organisms, emerging a cluster of genomic and post genomic consequences. In general, toxic responses to these kinds of nanomaterials are deemed to be very profound, in which various signaling pathways such as oxidative stress, immune responses and apoptosis pathways may be involved in response to generation of reactive oxygen species in the membranes (Kabanov, 2006). Cationic liposomes, irrespective of complexation with DNA, can downregulate the synthesis of pro-inflammatory mediators such as nitric oxide (NO) and tumor necrosis factor-alpha (TNF-alpha) in lipopolysaccharide (LPS)/interferon-gamma (IFN-gamma)-activated macrophages (Filion & Phillips, 1997a; Filion & Phillips, 1997b). Under the oxidative stress, cells may undergo the Nrf-2 signaling or the pro-inflammatory signaling cascades such as mitogen-activated protein kinase (MAPK) and nuclear factor kB (NFkB) cascades and eventually a programmed cell death may occur (Kabanov, 2006). Certain proteins such as protein kinase C (PKC) may also be affected detrimentally by cationic amphiphiles (Aberle et al., 1998), which function as PKC inhibitors and may inevitably result in inadvertent toxicity. It seems that the cationic amphiphiles with steroid backbones can exert more potent inhibitors of PKC than their straight-chain analogues, resulting in greater toxic impacts (Bottega & Epand, 1992). Polycations such as PEI formulated with plasmid DNA and administered to mouse lungs was reported to activate the p38 pathway involved in endocytosis, phagocytosis and hydrogen peroxide production. The observed *in vitro* and *in vivo* toxicity of such PEI polyplex formulations appeared to link to a general stress reaction, inflammatory responses, cell cycle regulation and DNA damage repair (Regnstrom et al., 2006). To obtain a complete image, it is essential to recruit high throughput screening methods such as DNA microarray.

5. DNA microarray technology

Practically, in the exploring stage, the expression of ~40,000 gene spots and replicates can be simultaneously analyzed on a couple of glass array in a single experiment by means of microarray technology. However, for accomplishment of a significant correlation between the gene expression profiles and their functionality expression, it is important to implement substantial complementary investigations to verify the results at the molecular level and as a result extend our understanding of gene expression patterns and molecular pathways.

Microarray technology can be exploited to attain a wealth of data that can be used to develop a more complete understanding of gene expression, which can be used for transcriptional regulation and interactions as well as functional genomics. Despite its successful *in vitro* cell-based implementation, application of this technology for *in vivo* investigations is deemed to be more sophisticated because of complexity of cytotoxicity and genotoxicity studies, which can be confounded by a number of variables such as type of target organ, effect of pharmacokinetics and/or pharmacodynamics parameters (Lobenhofer et al., 2001). Since its advent and application in life sciences, microarray has been widely applied for molecular/biological studies. In fact, a large number of indexed articles in various data banks (e.g., MEDLINE/PubMed) highlight the importance of microarray technology in post-genomics era.

Fig. 3 shows a schematic illustration of step-wise processes of the DNA microarray technology.

Technically, DNA microarray can be generated in two different types including printing pre-synthesized cDNAs (500–2000 bp) or synthesizing short oligonucleotides (20–50 bases) onto glass microscope slides, in which gene spots include either fully sequenced genes of known function or collections of partially sequenced cDNA derived from expressed sequence tags (ESTs) corresponding to the messenger RNAs of unknown genes. For example in practice, one may compare two different cells/tissues from untreated (UT) versus treated (T). For gene expression profiling, normally total RNA is extracted from the untreated and treated samples. Using an indirect labeling methodology, they are converted to labeled cDNA (e.g., with aminoallyle-dUTP). The aminoallyle-dUTP-cDNA is then labeled with cyanine dye (e.g., Cy3 or Cy5). The Cy3 and Cy5 labeled aminoallyle-dUTP-cDNA from UT and T samples are hybridized on a single glass array, which is subjected to several washing steps, scanning with an appropriate scanner (e.g., using RS Reloaded™, TECAN, Switzerland) and data mining (e.g., using GeneMath™ software; Applied Maths, Sint-Martens-Lathem, Belgium); for detailed information reader is directed to see (Hegde et al., 2000; Omidi et al., 2005b; Omidi et al., 2008).

For microarray analysis, significantly upregulated and/or downregulated genes can be identified using traditional method (gene expression changes with a fixed cutoff threshold usually in 2 fold) to infer significance differences (i.e., the so called "fold change method"). The resultant data are normally presented as scatter plots of treated (T) versus untreated (UT) control. To reach this stage, data need to undergo a number of processes called as "transformation" and "normalization" to minimize the experimental erroneousness (i.e., the so called "data mining"). Since a scatter plot of T versus UT genes would cluster along a straight line, normalization of this type of data is equivalent to calculating the best-fit slope using regression techniques and adjusting the intensities so that the calculated slope is one. In many experiments, the intensities are nonlinear, and local regression techniques are more suitable, such as Locally WEighted Scatterplot Smoothing (LOWESS) regression (Berger et al., 2001; Chen et al., 2003).

In our studies, we have successfully exploited both approaches to study the impacts of the nonviral vectors (CPs and CLs based formulation) on global gene expression experiments. To get the significant alterations in gene expression, we rejected the arrays showing non-

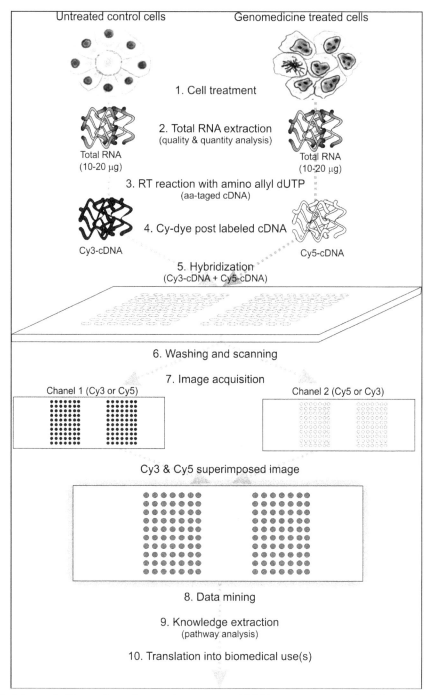

Fig. 3. Schematic illustration of step-wise process of DNA microarray methodology.

equal intensity or variable intensity of control gene spots in replicates on the same slide or between slides in dye-flipping experiments (Hollins et al., 2007; Omidi et al., 2003; Omidi et al., 2005b; Omidi et al., 2008). Data for each gene were typically reported as an "expression ratio" or as the base 2 logarithm ($\log_2$) of the expression ratio of T to UT control. Genes were assumed to be up regulated or downregulated if they revealed an expression ratio of >2 and <0.5 (or >1 and <-1 for $\log_2$ transformed data), respectively.

Based on our findings, the starburst PAMAM dendrimer alone or as complexed with DNA can elicit inadvertent gene expression changes. We also found that the linear and branched PEI (25 kDa) are able to induce gene expression changes in A431 cells, as shown in Fig. 4 (our unpublished data).

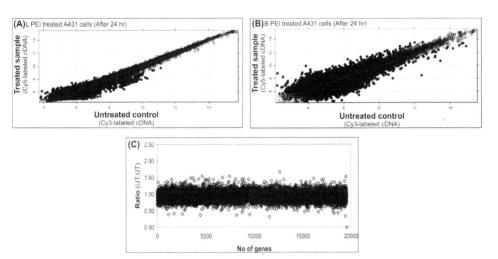

Fig. 4. Scatter plots of gene expression changes induced by cationic linear (A) and branched (B) PEI (25 kDa) in A431 cells. Data represent Log2 transformed gene expression values for large arrays housing 20000 genes. Above 2-fold change in expression of treated to untreated is indicated by bold circles and unchanged genes by unfilled circles. Panel C represents gene expression changes ratio between untreated A431 cells from different experiment. BPEI: branched polyethylenimine; LPEI: linear polyethylenimine (our unpublished data produced by Omidi et al.).

In the case of arrays with thousands of spots, one needs to employ the "feature reduction" or "dimension reduction" to find the minimum number of the features (i.e., genes or maybe even the conditions) that can best describe the data and the classification using statistical methods such as principal component analysis (PCA), correspondence analysis (CA), multi-dimensional scaling (MDS), and cluster analysis, reader is directed to see the following citation (Hegde et al., 2000; Quackenbush, 2001; Quackenbush, 2002). Of the dimension reduction methods, PCA is the most widely used method as a tool in exploratory data analysis, which involves a mathematical procedure that transforms a number of possibly correlated variables into a smaller number of uncorrelated variables called principal components. PCA ignores the dimensions in which data do not vary significantly and it is closely related to factor analysis.

6. Pathway analysis for functional genomics and gene ontology

To understand the functions of the genomic changes, one needs to implement appropriate methods on knowledge extraction from DNA microarray data. Such aim can be performed by means of "pathway analysis" (PA), which should be towards functional enrichment for establishing networks between genes. In fact, understanding the expression dynamics of gene networks helps us infer innate complexities and phenomenological networks among genes. Likewise, studying the regulation patterns of genes in groups, using clustering and classification methods may help us understand different pathways in the cell, their functions, regulations and the way one component in the system affects the other one. For pathway analysis, one of the most widely used methods is comparing the gene list to a pathway which gives a p value as a result. Basically, such scoring enrichment methods compare a list of the genes to that of a pathway and count the hits, so that the greater the number of the hits, the greater the score and the enrichment (Curtis et al., 2005). GenMAPP is an open source package that allows users to visualize microarray and proteomics data in the context of biological pathways (freely available at http://www.genmapp.org/). It represents biological pathways in a special file format called 'MAPPs' which are independent of the gene expression data. It is used to group genes by any organizing principle (e.g., apoptosis pathways). In addition, the gene set enrichment analysis (GSEA) is a novel method that uses all the data on the microarray in the order of expression, determining whether a priori defined set of genes shows statistically significant, concordant differences between two biological states such as phenotypes (Subramanian et al., 2005). In 2003, Hosack et al. developed a powerful software named, "the Expression Analysis Systematic Explorer" (EASE), which is customizable software for rapid biological interpretation of gene lists resulted by "omics" technology such as toxicogenomics, proteomics, or other high-throughput genomic data, in particular DNA microarray gene expression profiles. In fact, the biological themes returned by EASE recapitulate manually determined themes in previously published gene lists and are robust to varying methods of normalization, intensity calculation and statistical selection of genes (Hosack et al., 2003). We have largely exploited EASE to rapidly searching the Genbank in order to find the functional 'themes' in our microarray experiments. We have found various functional themes for the upregulated or downregulated genes induced by CLs in human epithelial cells, mainly: signal transducer activity, catalytic activity, response to external stimulus, cell growth and/or maintenance, cell cycle, response to biotic stimulus, regulation of programmed cell death, humoral immune response, cellular defense response, positive regulation of biosynthesis, negative regulation of cell proliferation, regulation of interferon-gamma biosynthesis, transcription factor binding, DNA repair, regulation of nucleocytoplasmic transport, apoptosis, apoptosis inhibitor activity, positive regulation of apoptosis, nuclease activity, transcriptional elongation regulator activity, regulation of caspase activation, response to oxidative stress, DNA damage response, and cell-mediated immune response (Omidi et al., 2005a).

As a secondary goal of array experiments it necessitates to look for groups of genes that behave similarly across a series of treatments (i.e. clustering analysis). There are a number of methodologies for clustering that can be employed upon experimental and statistical objectives; for clustering methods see citations (Azuaje, 2003; Sturn et al., 2002; Yang et al., 2001). In our studies on toxicogenomics of gene delivery systems, we have used softwares such as GeneSight™ or GeneMath™gene expression to present data as a single linkage

Hierarchical clustering plot. The algorithm used subjects the expression intensity ratio of treated versus untreated samples to single-linkage Hierarchical clustering (by means of Euclidean distance metric) analyses in order to arrange each gene with its related group members exhibiting a similar ratio of change in expression. We have shown that some overexpressed - or underexpressed genes display not only a similar pattern of expression but also a related cellular functionality and themes (e.g. apoptotic related genes) (Omidi et al., 2003; Omidi et al., 2005a). Such Hierarchical clustering maybe considered as a "genomic signature" of any chemical.

Taken all these facts together, surprisingly, still little information is available upon specific genomic effects elicited by chemicals within various cells/tissues despite implementing the "omics" technology for discovery of intrinsic genomic signature of chemicals/compounds in various targets. As a result, extensive investigations are yet to be performed to get sufficient information on genetic-signature of chemical and pharmaceuticals in target cells/tissues. Accordingly, many individuals and some organizations have attempted to accomplish such aim. For example, the Comparative Toxicogenomics Database (CTD) is a useful platform providing insights into complex chemical–gene and protein interaction networks (http://ctd.mdibl.org/about) that can be used for successfully advancement of novel pharmaceuticals.

7. Genomic impacts of cationic lipids

To date, cationic lipids have been the most widely used delivery system for delivery of nucleic acids both *in vitro* and *in vivo*. For example, Lipofectin™ is the 1:1 mixture of DOTMA and DOPE. It is the first cationic lipid formulation that was received widespread attention. We found that cationic liposomes such as LF and OF, at concentrations routinely used to obtain efficient delivery of gene based medicines, were able to induce gene expression changes in human epithelial A431 cells (Table 1). Such alterations in gene expressions appeared to be largely dependent upon the physicochemical characteristics of the lipid, wherein OF elicited greater gene expression than LF, i.e., up to 16% of the genes studied (Omidi et al., 2003). We speculate that the surface charge may play a key role in terms of such genotoxicity. In these cells, we witnessed that the affected genes were functionally involved in various cellular processes such as cell proliferation, differentiation and apoptosis. The upregulated or downregulated genes include some important genes such as bcl-2-related protein a1 (BCL2A1), caspase 8 isoform c (CASP8), heat shock protein 70 (HSP70) and 60 (HSP60), annexin a2 (ANXA2), and tubulin beta 5 (TUBB5) (Omidi et al., 2003). Up regulation of caspase-8 clearly impart activation of procaspases and caspases that may provoke activity of a series of apoptotic signaling cascades such as electron carrier protein cytochrome C, adaptor protein Apaf-1, Bcl-2 family, p53 and various transcription factors (Kanduc et al., 2002). Given that the heat shock protein 70 acts as an inhibitor of apoptosis (Li et al., 2000), it's upregulation by OF in A431 cells is deemed to be a cellular compensatory or defense response. We assume that cells recognize the xenobiotics upon their biological properties. To examine such concept, we compared OF genotoxicities within two epithelial cell lines (i.e., A431 and A549 cells).

In A549 cells, the genomic impacts were intriguingly dissimilar compared to that of A431 cells (Table 1). Further, we observed some commonalities in gene expression modulation between two different cell lines (Omidi et al., 2008). Upon EASE analyses, the changes in gene expression fell into a number of various functional genomic ontologies. For example, the upregulated genes by OF nanoliposomes included the genes involved in apoptosis, oxidative stress and external/biotic stimulus (e.g., IL9R, DUSP1, CSK, CSE1L); while the downregulated genes were related to the cell growth and/or cell maintenance, cell proliferation and apoptosis (e.g., SEP6, PSMA4).

Gene ID (Accession No.)	Gene description	LF-A431	OF-A431	OF-A549
NM_004417	Dual specificity phosphatase 1; DUSP1	−	+	+
NM_033356	Caspase 8, isoform c; CASP8	NC	+	NC
NM_002467	V-mycmyelocytomatosis viral oncogene homolog (avian); MYC	NC	+	NC
NM_004049	Bcl2-related protein a1; BCL2A1	NC	+	NC
NM_003195	Transcription elongation factor a (sii), 2; TCEA2	NC	+	NC
NM_001983	Excision repair cross-complementing rodent repair deficiency, complementation group 1 (includes overlapping antisense sequence); ERCC1	NC	+	NC
NM_004094	Eukaryotic translation initiation factor 2, subunit 1 (alpha, 35kd); EIF2S1	NC	+	NC
NM_000994	Rbosomal protein l32; RPL32	NC	+	NC
NM_001274	Chk1 checkpoint homolog (s. pombe); CHEK1	NC	+	NC
NM_002849	Protein tyrosine phosphatase, receptor type, r; PTPRR	NC	+	NC
NM_002156	Heat shock 60kd protein 1 (chaperonin); HSPD1	NC	+	+
NM_002957	Retinoid x receptor, alpha; RXRA	NC	+	NC
NM_001242	Cd27 antigen; TNFRSF7	NC	+	NC
NM_006083	Red protein; IK	NC	+	NC
L12723	Heat shock protein 70; HSP70	NC	+	+
NM_004383	C-src tyrosine kinase; CSK	NC	+	+
NM_004635	Mitogen-activated protein kinase-activated protein kinase 3; MAPKAPK3	NC	+	NC
NM_005546	Il2-inducible t-cell kinase; ITK	NC	+	NC
NM_006235	Pou domain, class 2, associating factor 1; POU2AF1	NC	+	NC
NM_002623	Prefoldin 4; PFDN4	NC	NC	NC
NM_001316	Cse1 chromosome segregation 1-like (yeast); CSE1L	NC	NC	+
NM_002953	Ribosomal protein s6 kinase, 90kd, polypeptide 1; RPS6KA1	NC	NC	NC
NM_000660	Transforming growth factor, beta 1; TGFB1	NC	NC	NC
NM_000043	Apoptosis (apo-1) antigen 1; TNFRSF6	NC	NC	NC
NM_001961	Eukaryotic translation elongation factor 2; EEF2	NC	NC	NC
NM_001786	Cell division cycle 2 protein, isoform 1; CDC2	NC	NC	NC
NM_021103	Thymosin beta, TMSB10	NC	NC	NC
NM_004315	N-acylsphingosineamidohydrolase (acidceramidase);	−	NC	NC

Gene ID (Accession No.)	Gene description	LF-A431	OF-A431	OF-A549
	ASAH			
NM_002026	Fibronectin 1, isoform 1 preproprotein; FN1	—	NC	NC
NM_001238	Cyclin e1, isoform 1; CCNE1	NC	NC	NC
NM_002186	Interleukin 9 receptor; IL9R	NC	NC	+
NM_002945	Replicationprotein a1 (70kd); RPA1	NC	NC	NC
NM_003875	Guanine monophosphate synthetase; GMPS	—	NC	NC
NM_000887	Integrinalpha x precursor; ITGAX	NC	NC	+
NM_000075	Cyclin-dependent kinase 4, isoform 1; CDK4	NC	NC	—
NM_032959	Dna directed rna polymerase ii polypeptide j, isoform b; POLR2J	NC	NC	+
NM_000970	Ribosomal protein l6; RPL6	—	NC	NC
NM_005319	H1 histone family, member 2; H1F2	NC	NC	NC
NM_002592	Proliferating cell nuclear antigen; PCNA	—	NC	NC
NM_020300	Microsomal glutathione s-transferase 1; MGST1	NC	NC	NC
NM_021065	H2a histone family, member g; H2AFG	NC	—	NC
NM_004832	Glutathione-s-transferase like; GSTTLP28	NC	—	NC
NM_006087	Tubulin, beta, 5; TUBB5	NC	—	NC
NM_002789	Proteasome (prosome, macropain) subunit, alpha type, 4; PSMA4	NC	—	—
NM_005566	Ldha	NC	—	NC
NM_015129	Septin 6; SEP6	NC	—	—
NM_004039	Annexin a2; ANXA2	NC	—	NC

Table 1. Gene expression changes induced by cationic liposomes in A431 and A549 cells. LF: Lipofectin™ ; OF: Oligofectamine™; NC: no changes; +: upregulation; —: downregulation; adapted with permission (Barar et al., 2009).

For example, among the genes upregulated by OF in A549 cells (but not A431 cells), the IL9R gene encodes IL9 receptor protein which is a cytokine receptor that specifically mediates the biological effects of IL9. The ligand binding of this receptor leads to the activation of various JAK kinases and STAT proteins, which connect to different biologic responses, in particular some genetic studies, suggested an association of this gene with the development of asthma (Gaga et al., 2007).

The heat shock proteins 60 and 70 as well as c-src tyrosine kinase (CSK) were observed to be upregulated in both cell lines (Table 1). Of these, the heat shock proteins family of molecular chaperones appears to act in protein folding, translocation, and assembly into complexes; while CSK is mainly involved in protein-tyrosine kinase activity as well as protein metabolism and modifications. Once looked at the overlapped activities of these genes, we found that they are cooperating mostly to activate the binding activity - we speculate that these genes somehow are collaborating perhaps in terms of protein folding and binding.

Since liposomal formulations are being explored for pulmonary drug/gene delivery, and thus their ability to activate IL9R should be assessed when used clinically for lung gene therapy. The CSK along with some other genes were upregulated in A549 cells treated with cationic lipids similar to what we observed previously in A431 cells (Omidi et al., 2003) and is mainly involved in cell growth and/or cell maintenance. The SEP6 and PSMA4 were downregulated genes by OF in both cell lines. The SEP6 gene is a member of the septin family of GTPases. Members of this family are required for cytokinesis. One version of pediatric acute myeloid leukemia is the result of a reciprocal translocation between chromosomes 11 and X, with the breakpoint associated with the genes encoding the mixed-lineage leukemia and septin 2 proteins. This gene encodes four transcript variants encoding three distinct isoforms. An additional transcript variant has been identified, but its biological validity has not been determined. The PSMA4 is a multicatalytic proteinase complex with a highly ordered ring-shaped 20S core structure. They are distributed throughout eukaryotic cells at a high concentration and cleave peptides in an ATP/ubiquitin-dependent process in a non-lysosomal pathway.

Because of the gene expression commonalities and distinctions between the two cell lines, we conceptualized that these cells may respond to the cationic lipid "OF" differently upon their cellular characteristics. These cells appeared to undergo somewhat adaptation upon exposure to xenobiotics, as a result of which they could dynamically respond as expressing/activating related cellular elements for recognition and internalization of the cationic lipid. Of interest, we found that the genotoxicity elicited by the cationic lipid nanosystems were largely dependent upon the structural architecture and/or physicochemical properties of the cationic lipid since no extensive overlap was observed in the gene expression profile induced by either LF or OF in A431 cells. Besides, the responsiveness of the target cells to the lipids could be different since the transfection efficiency is significantly depended upon the target cells and lipids used. Likewise, Filion and Phillips (1997) reported high toxicity rate elicited by some cationic lipids in phagocytic cells such as macrophages and U937 cells, but not in non-phagocytic T lymphocytes.

Taken all these findings together, it seems that for attaining detailed characterization of the toxicogenomics of these lipid delivery systems (based on their molecular structure), the gene expression patterns/profiles need to be determined in different cell types perhaps with known cell surface architecture.

8. Genomic impacts of cationic polymers

Despite plethora of investigations on application of polymers in drug/gene delivery, surprisingly, little attention has been devoted about possible biofunction of polymer per se in particular genomic effects. Many researchers have now consensus upon functionalities of polymers, and accordingly new domains of polymer science such as "polymer genomics", "polymer genocompatibly" and "polymer genotoxicity" have been arisen. To examine the polymer genocompatibly concept, we have previously reported that starburst PAMAM dendrimers (i.e., PF and SF) as well as polypropylene imine (PPI) dendrimers (e.g., DAB8 and DAB16) can inadvertently induce alterations in gene expression (Hollins et al., 2007; Omidi et al., 2005b). These dendrimers have been successfully exploited for delivery of gene based medicines. Of these dendrimers, we have previously shown dramatic alteration in gene expression induced by DAB16 dendrimer in A431 and A549 cells (Omidi et al., 2005b).

Table 2 represents the gene expression changes by DAB polymers in A431 and A549 cells. Of the altered genes in A431 cells, some are related to cell defense and response to stress (e.g., ALOX5, TNFRSF7) and apoptosis (e.g., TNFRSF7). In A549 cells, some of the altered genes

Gene ID (Accession No.)	Description	A431 cells		A549 cells	
		DAB8	DAB16	DAB16	DAB16:DNA
NM_006716	Activator of s phase kinase; ASK	NC	−	NC	NC
NM_000034	Aldolase a; ALDOα	NC	NC	NC	NC
NM_004039	Annexin a2; ANXα2	NC	+	NC	NC
NM_000698	Arachidonate 5-lipoxygenase; ALOX5	NC	−	NC	NC
NM_004049	Bcl2-related protein a1; BCL2α1	NC	NC	NC	+
NM_000591	Cd14 antigen precursor; CD14	NC	NC	+	NC
NM_001242	Cd27 antigen; TNFRSF7	NC	−	NC	NC
NM_001786	Cell division cycle 2 protein, isoform 1; CDC2	NC	NC	−	NC
NM_003467	Chemokine (c-x-c motif), receptor 4 (fusin); CXCR4	NC	NC	NC	−
NM_001274	Chk1 checkpoint homolog (s. pombe); CHEK1	NC	NC	NC	−
NM_004383	C-src tyrosine kinase; CSK	NC	NC	NC	−
NM_003914	Cyclin a1; CCNα1	NC	NC	+	NC
NM_001239	Cyclin h; CCNH	NC	NC	−	NC
NM_000075	Cyclin-dependent kinase 4, isoform 1; CDK4	NC	+	NC	NC
NM_001801	Cysteine dioxygenase, type i; CDO1	NC	NC	NC	−
NM_004417	Dual specificity phosphatase 1; DUSP1	NC	−	NC	+
NM_003875	Guanine monophosphate synthetase; GMPS	NC	−	NC	+
NM_021065	H2a histone family, member g; H2AFG	NC	+	NC	NC
NM_002156	Heat shock 60kd protein 1 (chaperonin); HSPD1	NC	−	NC	NC
NM_000879	Interleukin 5 (colony-stimulating factor, eosinophil); IL5	NC	NC	NC	−
NM_002186	Interleukin 9 receptor; IL9R	NC	NC	+	NC
NM_002358	Mad2-like 1; MAD2L1	NC	NC	NC	+
NM_002424	Matrix metalloproteinase 8 preproprotein; MMP8	NC	NC	NC	−
NM_000245	Met proto-oncogene precursor; Met	+	NC	−	NC
NM_004315	N-acylsphingosine amidohydrolase (acid ceramidase); ASAH	NC	NC	NC	+
NM_006235	Pou domain, class 2, associating factor 1; POU2AF1	NC	NC	NC	−
NM_000946	Primase, polypeptide 1 (49kd); PRIM1	NC	NC	NC	+
NM_002592	Proliferating cell nuclear antigen; PCNA	NC	NC	−	NC
NM_000532	Propionyl coenzyme a carboxylase, beta polypeptide; PCCβ	NC	−	NC	NC
NM_002789	Proteasome (prosome, macropain)	NC	+	NC	NC

Gene ID (Accession No.)	Description	A431 cells		A549 cells	
		DAB8	DAB16	DAB16	DAB16:DNA
	subunit, alpha type, 4; PSMα4				
NM_002796	Proteasome (prosome, macropain) subunit, beta type, 4; PSMβ4	NC	NC	–	NC
NM_002737	Protein kinase c, alpha; PRKCα	NC	NC	NC	–
NM_006083	Red protein; IK	NC	–	NC	NC
NM_002914	Replication factor c (activator 1) 2 (40kd); RFC2	NC	NC	NC	–
NM_002947	Replicationprotein a3 (14kd); RPα3	NC	–	NC	NC
NM_002957	Retinoid x receptor, alpha; RXRα	NC	NC	+	NC
NM_007209	Ribosomal protein l35; RPL35	NC	NC	NC	+
NM_033301	Ribosomal protein l8; RPL8	NC	–	NC	NC
NM_003139	Signal recognition particle receptor ('docking protein'); SRPR	NC	NC	NC	+
NM_003072	Swi/snf related, matrix associated regulator of chromatin, SMARCA4	NC	–	NC	–
NM_003236	Transforming growth factor, alpha; TGFα	NC	NC	+	NC
NM_000660	Transforming growth factor, beta 1; TGFβ1	NC	NC	NC	+
NM_003292	Translocated promoter region (to activated met oncogene); TPR	NC	NC	+	NC
NM_006087	Tubulin, beta, 5; TUBβ5	NC	+	NC	NC
NM_003299	Tumor rejection antigen (gp96) 1; TRA1	NC	NC	+	NC
NM_006826	Tyrosine 3-monooxygenase/tryptophan 5-monooxygenase activation protein, theta polypeptide; YWHAQ	NC	–	NC	NC

Table 2. Gene expression changes by DAB polymers in A431 and A549 cells. NC: no changes; +/-: up/down regulation; adapted with permission from (Omidi et al., 2005b).

were in association with cell defense, DNA repair/damage and apoptosis (e.g., CCNH; ERCC1; PCNAM, CD14).

With a particular interest on toxicogenomic of the DBA16:DNA nanoparticles in A549 cells, expression changes (upregulation/downregulation) were found for some important genes (i.e., TGFβ1,BCL2α1, IL5, CXCR4 and PCKα). Of these, TGFβ1 is a member of a super-family of multifunctional cytokines that regulate cell proliferation, differentiation, and apoptosis (Chiarugi et al., 1997; Haufel et al., 1999), while the BCL2 protein family is involved in a wide variety of cellular activities that also act as anti- and pro-apoptotic regulators. The protein encoded by BCL2 is able to reduce the release of pro-apoptotic cytochrome c from mitochondria and block caspase activation which is the main apoptosis pathway. Further, this gene is a direct transcription target of NF-KAPPAβ in response to inflammatory mediators, and has been shown to be upregulated by different extracellular signals, such as granulocyte-macrophage colony-stimulating factor (GM-CSF), CD40, phorbol ester and inflammatory cytokine TNF and IL1, which suggests a cyto-protective function that is essential for lymphocyte activation as well as cell survival; reader is directed to see following citations (May et al., 1994; Ruvolo et al., 2001). The upregulation of TGFβ1 and BCL2α conceivably imply incitement of apoptosis in A549 cells upon treatments with DAB16:DNA polyplexes.

It was also found that the altered genes induced by PF, DAB16 and OF in A431 cells shows some commonalities and differences in pattern, presumably due to their positive charge and structural architecture. In A431 cells, treated with either DAB8 or DAB16 resulted in ~13% and ~7% similar and opposite patterns of gene expression changes, respectively. For example, BCL2α1 which acts as anti- and pro-apoptotic regulator was largely affected by DAB16 compared to DAB8. This could be due to higher surface charge and/or interaction capacity of DAB16. Similar pattern was seen for proteasomeα4, but Met proto-oncogene revealed opposite pattern. Once DAB16 was tested in different cell line (i.e., A549 cells), similar and opposite patterns of gene expression changes were ~11% and ~9%, respectively. Intriguingly, upregulation of some important genes (e.g., IL9R, TGFα) was seen solely in A549 cells, but not in A431 cells. It can be speculated that A549 cells can show greater response than A431 cells. Hence, these dendrimers could potentially affect cell growth and immune response of cells by altering the expression of some related genes at doses which did not distinctly modify cell viability (Table 2). It should be also evoked that the identity of the genes whose expression was significantly altered (i.e. the "gene signature" of the delivery system) was markedly different in the two cell lines, despite the similar expression of the majority of the genes (80%) that remained unaffected (Akhtar & Benter, 2007).

Table 3 shows the gene expression of some selected genes induced by branched and linear polyethylenimine (BPEI and LPEI, respectively) in A431 cells. These data solely present the upregulated and downregulated genes, similarly induced by these cationic polymers, while there are a large number of genes showed opposite pattern (data not shown). Based on these results, it was found that the alterations in gene expression by BPEI were significantly greater than LPEI. We contemplate that this could be because of the greater interaction of BPEI with subcellular biomolecules.

To examine the late effect of BPEI in target cells, we evaluated gene expression pattern of caspases genes in A431 cells as a time series approache (i.e., immediately after transfection, 24 h and 48 h after transfection). Fig. 5 represents the gene expression profile of selected caspase pathway genes in A431 cells treated with BPEI, showing significant impacts of BPEI even 48 h after treatment. Of these genes, as previously mentioned, caspase 8 play a key role in apoptosis.

These findings directed us to examine some other cationic polymers such as PAMAM and PEI. Upon our examination on SF and PF, we found that PF induced gene expression changes much greater than SF. This could be due to differences in dendrimers architecture. Significant decrease in gene expression changes were observed upon PF complexation with a DNA at the supplier recommended ratio of 10:1 (w/w) of PF:DNA. Reduced in number, but not in nature and magnitude, of expressed genes were observed upon PF:DNA complexation. In treated A431 cells with cationic dendrimer PF or cationic lipid OF, opposite and similar patterns of gene expression changes were 20% and 16%, respectively (Barar et al., 2009).

Function	Gene ID	T/UT ratio		
		BPEI	LPEI	
gi:407955 - membrane-associated protein hem-1	M58285	4.10	1.95	+
gi:7106883 - HSPC247	AF151081	2.74	1.98	+
gi:13569894 - diaphanous homolog 3; DIAPH3	NM_030932	2.23	2.44	+
gi:14010613 - methylmalonyl-coa epimerase	AF364547	2.13	2.21	+
gi:14248538 - STONIN2	AF255309	2.10	2.13	+
gi:188560 - prepro-mullerian inhibiting substance	K03474	2.10	2.69	+
gi:285915 - epimorphin	D14582	2.07	3.17	+
gi:7109206 - four alpha helix cytokine; ZCYTO10	AF224266	1.99	2.00	+
gi:558098 - protein kinase c-theta; PRKCT	L01087	1.97	1.93	+
gi:9843747 - putative pyroglutamyl-peptidase i; PGPEP1	AJ278828	1.93	2.82	+
gi:22041589 - similar to data source:sptr, source key:q9h4b3, evidence:iss~homolog to mucolipidin~putative; loc255231	XM70908	0.58	0.25	-
gi:14588660 - histidase; hal	AB042217	0.57	0.27	-
gi:10439114 - homo sapiens cdna: flj22644 fis, clone hsi07088; unnamed protein product.	AK026297	0.53	0.26	-
gi:10944321 - myozenin; MYOZ	AF240633	0.53	0.26	-
gi:2613124 - small cell vasopressin subtype 1b receptor	AF030512	0.52	0.26	-
gi:20278870 - delta 4 progesterone receptor; pr	AB084248	0.46	0.26	-
gi:7020101 - cdna clone unnamed protein product	AK000183	0.45	0.27	-
gi:7209599 - melatonin 1b receptor	AB033598	0.44	0.26	-
gi:307425 - nerve terminal protein; SNAP	L19760	0.43	0.25	-
gi:18182679 - nkg2d	AF461811	0.41	0.25	-
gi:347133 - succinate dehydrogenase flavoprotein subunit; SDH	L21936	0.39	0.23	-
gi:2738815 - p2y1 receptor; p2yr1	AF018284	0.28	0.26	-
gi:21928730 - seven transmembrane helix receptor	AB065731	0.26	0.27	-
gi:3088552 - cystatin-related epididymal spermatogenic protein; cres	AF059244	0.24	0.24	-
gi:22048232 - similar to riken cdna 2610027o18; KIAA1393	XM_050793	0.21	0.22	-

Table 3. Gene expression changes of selected genes induced by branched and linear polyethylenimine (BPEI and LPEI, respectively) in A431 cells (our unpublished data produced by Omidi et al.). +/-: up/down regulation

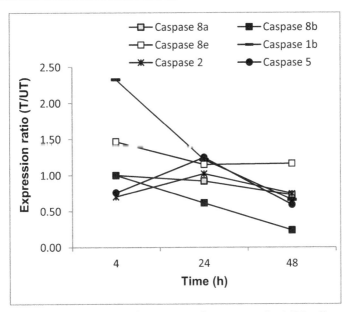

Fig. 5. Gene expression ratio of selected caspase pathway genes in A431 cells treated with BPEI after 4, 24 and 48 h (our unpublished data produced by Omidi et al.).

Likewise, Pluronic® block copolymers were shown to cause various functional alterations in cells through interacting with cellular biomolecules and thus affecting various cellular functions such as mitochondrial respiration, ATP synthesis, activity of drug efflux transporters, apoptotic signal transduction, and transcriptional activation of gene expression both *in vitro* and *in vivo* (Batrakova & Kabanov, 2008). This polymer is able to enhance expression of reporter genes under the control of cytomegalovirus promoter and NF-KB response element in stably and transiently transfected mouse fibroblasts and myoblasts *in vitro*. It has been shown that these block copolymers are able to act as biological response modifying agents through upregulating the transcription of genes via activation of selected signaling pathways such as NF-KB (Sriadibhatla et al., 2006).

Furthermore, Pluronic® P85 (P85) was reported to promote transport of the pDNA to the nucleus in cells transiently transfected with DNA/PEI polyplex (Kabanov, 2006). It has also been successfully exploited for DNA vaccine delivery, however some investigations revealed that P85 simultaneously increase transgene expression and activate immunity, in which P85 alone and P85:DNA complexes were shown to increase the systemic expansion of CD11c+ (DC), and local expansion of CD11c+, CD14+ (macrophages) and CD49b+ (natural killer) cell populations. DNA/P85 polyplex can also increase maturation of local DC (CD11c+ CD86+, CD11c+ CD80 +, and CD11c+ CD40+ (Gaymalov et al., 2009). Thus, the activation of immunogenes in the antigen-presenting cells by P85:DNA complexes can highlight new insights for these kinds of polymers.

In addition, Pluronic® can cause some alterations in HSP60 expression, suggesting that this polymer may affect stress-related pathways or there is a cross-talk between the stress and other pathways activated by the copolymer (Sriadibhatla et al., 2006). These results are in accord with what we have observed for some other cationic polymers or lipids. Pluronic®

(a mixture of Pluronic L61 and F127; also called as SP1017) has been reported to deliver plasmid DNA in skeletal and cardiac muscle, as well as in solid tumors. Unlike other polycations, Pluronic® does not bind and condense the nucleic acids, it does not protect DNA from degradation or facilitate transport of the DNA into the cell and its effects involve transcriptional activation of gene expression (Kabanov, 2006). The effect of Pluronic® was reported to be related to the activation of gene expression by activating the NF-κB and p53 signaling pathways, in which pro-apoptotic AP-1 gene that is frequently regulated by the NF-κB system, was not responsive. This, perhaps, indicates that Pluronic-mediated influence on transcription is selective and it is not a result of a general nonspecific activation of immune defense system such as NO-mediated burst (Kabanov, 2006). Nonetheless, to ensure about this supposition, it is essential to recruit global gene expression screening methods such as microarray technology as we have witnessed dramatic alterations in gene expression *in vitro* and *in vivo* upon treatment with different polymers using microarray technology. Kabanov's group has reported that Pluronic block copolymers interact with biomembranes and induce gene expressions through mechanisms that differ from the delivery of the DNA into the cell. They also questioned whether upregulation of expression of genes delivered into cells can also take place by other nonviral polymer-based gene delivery systems? We have observed that various polymers, in particular polycations, are able to alter gene expressions related to immune response and cell defense (Barar et al., 2009; Hollins et al., 2007; Omidi et al., 2008).

It appears that the cytotoxicity of nonviral vectors is largely dependent upon the cationic nature of the vector, which attains different level to different structural architecture. For cationic lipid, the cytotoxic effects are mainly determined by the structure of its hydrophilic group (Prokop & Davidson, 2008), e.g. the quaternary ammonium amphiphiles are more toxic than their tertiary amine counterparts. Such toxicity (due to positive charge of the head group) can be reduced by importing a heterocyclic ring such as imidazolium or pyridinium.

The biodegradability potential of the advanced nanobiomaterials are also determined their toxicity. For example, poly(lactic-co-glycolic acid) nanoparticles elicit very low level of cytotoxicity and toxicogenomic compared to cationic polymers, but not the modified PLGA-grafted poly(L-lysine) nanosystems (Omidi & Davaran, 2011).

Surprisingly, the effect of hydrophobic chain on toxicity has not been adequately addressed to date even though it is deemed that the hydrophobic moieties may disrupt the integrity of lipid bilayer. Like cationic lipid, cationic polymers with acid-labile linkage can be rapidly degraded and less toxic. It has been reported that the toxicity of polymers (e.g., PEI, PLL or dendrimers) increases with high molecular weight (Bieber & Elsasser, 2001). Polymers synthesized by linking low molecular weight with acid-labile show low toxicity (Li et al., 2004). The creation of amphiphilic cationic polymer based on PEI or PLL, by linking PEG or other groups, reduces toxicity without compromising the gene delivery efficiency (Zhang et al., 2008).

Upon our observations the biodegradable cationic polymers (e.g., polysaccharides) which display high degree of biodegradability possess low toxicity, thus we speculate that they may be extensively used for *in vivo* transfection in the future. Further, high transfection efficiency and low toxicity can be obtained by the addition of co-lipids or co-polymers (PEGylation). Water soluble lipopolymer, to combine the advantages of both cationic polymer and liposome, seems to be our next approach for optimized gene transfer. Besides, adding cell-specific biomolecules (e.g. aptamer, peptide ligands, antibodies or nanobodies) to gene transfer vectors potentially improve the specific problem by permitting lower and safer vector doses while facilitating tissue targeting.

9. Concluding remarks

Synthetic lipids or polymers used for gene delivery may impose selective "phenotypic effects" in cells by affecting cell signaling involved in various biological functions such as cell defense, inflammation, differentiation, proliferation and apoptosis. It is believed that these effects result basically from their interactions with cell membranes, intracellular organelles and subcellular biomolecules, as a result the target cells can respond to these effects phenotypically or genotypically. In some cases, these effects can be relatively benign as they do not induce sever cytotoxic effects, while in the case of nonviral cationic vectors it is not the case since the interaction of the polycationic gene delivery nanosystems with target cells is significantly greater than non-cationic polymers. It is now deemed that one unifying property of polycationic gene delivery nanosystems is their potential to interact with cellular/subcellular biomolecules, upon which profound changes in various cell processes may occur. From this standpoint, it becomes clear that these polycations are able to penetrate into cells and reach different critical subcellular targets and induce inventible biological functions, for which the nanoscaled range of sizes is an important factor. Different cell types as biological targets may response differently, and even modify the activities of such nanomaterials. While the genome-based therapeutics (e.g., oligonucleotides and gene silencing siRNAs) have already been lined up for clinical trials (up to 1700 trials), our knowledge is lacking upon genomic signature of such gene based medicines. As concluding statement, it is suggested that the inadvertent intrinsic genomic signature of nonviral delivery systems should be assessed and taken into consideration for a gene therapy trial since gene silencing/stimulation experiments are to target a specific gene while the gene delivery system may potentially mask or interfere with the desired genotype and/or phenotype end-point of gene therapy. The upregulation or downregulation of genes induced by gene delivery systems or any other drug carriers and excipients appears to instigate a new directionality such as "functional excipients". But, this approach simply represents the gene expression changes which are solely based on intensities of expressed genes for various signaling pathways, while we should look for ways to correlate such gene expression intensities with functional genomics.

10. References

Aardema, M.J. & MacGregor, J.T. (2002). Toxicology and genetic toxicology in the new era of "toxicogenomics": impact of "-omics" technologies. *Mutat.Res.*, Vol.499, No.1, (January 2002), pp. 13-25, ISSN 0027-5107

Aberle, A.M.; Tablin, F.; Zhu, J.; Walker, N.J.; Gruenert, D.C. & Nantz, M.H. (1998). A novel tetraester construct that reduces cationic lipid-associated cytotoxicity. Implications for the onset of cytotoxicity. *Biochemistry*, Vol.37, No.18, (1998), pp. 6533-6540, ISSN 0006-2960

Akhtar, S. & Benter, I. (2007). Toxicogenomics of non-viral drug delivery systems for RNAi: potential impact on siRNA-mediated gene silencing activity and specificity. *Adv.Drug Deliv.Rev.*, Vol.59, No.2-3, (March 2007), pp. 164-182, ISSN 0169-409X

Audouy, S.A.; de Leij, L.F.; Hoekstra, D. & Molema, G. (2002). In vivo characteristics of cationic liposomes as delivery vectors for gene therapy. *Pharm Res*, Vol.19, No.11, (2002), pp. 1599-1605, ISSN 1043-6618

Azuaje, F. (2003). Clustering-based approaches to discovering and visualising microarray data patterns. *Brief.Bioinform.*, Vol.4, No.1, (March 2003), pp. 31-42, ISSN 1467-5463

Barar, J.; Hamzeiy, H.; Mortazavi-Tabatabaei, S.A.; Hashemi-Aghdam, S.E. & Omidi, Y. (2009). Genomic signature and toxicogenomics comparison of polycationic gene delivery nanosystems in human alveolar epithelial A549 cells. *Daru*, Vol.17, No.3, (2009), pp. 139-147, ISSN 1560-8115

Barar, J.; Javadzadeh, A.R. & Omidi, Y. (2008). Ocular novel drug delivery: impacts of membranes and barriers. *Expert.Opin.Drug Deliv.*, Vol.5, No.5, (May 2008), pp. 567-581, ISSN 1742-5247

Batrakova, E.V. & Kabanov, A.V. (2008). Pluronic block copolymers: evolution of drug delivery concept from inert nanocarriers to biological response modifiers. *J.Control Release*, Vol.130, No.2, (September 2008), pp. 98-106, ISSN 0168-3659

Berger, J.A.; Hautaniemi, S.; Jarvinen, A.K.; Edgren, H.; Mitra, S.K. & Astola, J. (December 2004). Optimized LOWESS normalization parameter selection for DNA microarray data. *BMC.Bioinformatics.*, Vol.5, No.1, (December 2004), pp. 194, ISSN 1471-2105

Bieber, T. & Elsasser, H.P. (2001). Preparation of a low molecular weight polyethylenimine for efficient cell transfection. *Biotechniques*, Vol.30, No.1, (2001), pp. 74-77, ISSN 0736-6205

Bottega, R. & Epand, R.M. (1992). Inhibition of protein kinase C by cationic amphiphiles. *Biochemistry*, Vol.31, No.37, (September 1992), pp. 9025-9030, ISSN 0006-2960

Chen, Y.J.; Kodell, R.; Sistare, F.; Thompson, K.L.; Morris, S. & Chen, J.J. (2003). Normalization methods for analysis of microarray gene-expression data. *J.Biopharm.Stat.*, Vol.13, No.1, (February 2003), pp. 57-74, ISSN 1054-3406

Chiarugi, V.; Magnelli, L. & Cinelli, M. (1997). Complex interplay among apoptosis factors: RB, p53, E2F, TGF-beta, cell cycle inhibitors and the bcl2 gene family. *Pharmacol Res*, Vol.35, No.4, (1997), pp. 257-261, ISSN 1043-6618

Conner, S.D. & Schmid, S.L. (2003). Regulated portals of entry into the cell. *Nature*, Vol.422, No.6927, (March 2003), pp. 37-44, ISSN 0028-0836

Curtis, R.K.; Oresic, M. & Vidal-Puig, A. (2005). Pathways to the analysis of microarray data. *Trends Biotechnol.*, Vol.23, No.8, (August 2005), pp. 429-435, ISSN 0167-7799

de, L.F.; Bertholet, V. & Remacle, J. (2004). DNA microarrays as a tool in toxicogenomics. *Comb.Chem.High Throughput.Screen.*, Vol.7, No.3, (May 2004), pp. 207-211, ISSN 1386-2073

Domanski, D.M.; Bryszewska, M. & Salamonczyk, G. (2004). Preliminary evaluation of the behavior of fifth-generation thiophosphate dendrimer in biological systems.

Biomacromolecules., Vol.5, No.5, (September 2004), pp. 2007-2012, ISSN 1525-7797

Erickson, B.; Dimaggio, S.C.; Mullen, D.G.; Kelly, C.V.; Leroueil, P.R.; Berry, S.A.; Baker, J.R., Jr.; Orr, B.G. & Banaszak Holl, M.M. (2008). Interactions of Poly(amidoamine) Dendrimers with Survanta Lung Surfactant: The Importance of Lipid Domains. *Langmuir, Vol.24, No.19, (September 2008), pp. 11003-11008, ISSN 0743-7463*

Farhood, H.; Serbina, N. & Huang, L. (1995). The role of dioleoyl phosphatidylethanolamine in cationic liposome mediated gene transfer. *Biochim.Biophys.Acta*, Vol.1235, No.2, (May 1995), pp. 289-295, ISSN 0006-3002

Ferber, D. (2001). Gene therapy. Repair kits for faulty genes. *Science*, Vol.294, No.5547, (2001), pp. 1639, ISSN 0036-8075

Ferber, D. (2001). Gene therapy. Safer and virus-free? *Science*, Vol.294, No.5547, (2001), pp. 1638-1642, ISSN 0036-8075

Fielden, M.R. & Kolaja, K.L. (2006). The state-of-the-art in predictive toxicogenomics. *Curr.Opin.Drug Discov.Devel.*, Vol.9, No.1, (January 2006), pp. 84-91, ISSN 1367-6733

Filion, M.C. & Phillips, N.C. (1997a). Anti-inflammatory activity of cationic lipids. *Br.J.Pharmacol.*, Vol.122, No.3, (October 1997), pp. 551-557, ISSN 0007-1188

Filion, M.C. & Phillips, N.C. (1997b). Toxicity and immunomodulatory activity of liposomal vectors formulated with cationic lipids toward immune effector cells. *Biochim Biophys Acta*, Vol.1329, No.2, (1997), pp. 345-356, ISSN 0006-3002

Fischer, D.; Li, Y.; Ahlemeyer, B.; Krieglstein, J. & Kissel, T. (2003). In vitro cytotoxicity testing of polycations: influence of polymer structure on cell viability and hemolysis. *Biomaterials*, Vol.24, No.7, (2003), pp. 1121-1131, ISSN 0142-9612

Florea, B.I.; Meaney, C.; Junginger, H.E. & Borchard, G. (2002). Transfection efficiency and toxicity of polyethylenimine in differentiated Calu-3 and nondifferentiated COS-1 cell cultures. *AAPS PharmSci*, Vol.4, No.3, (2002), pp. E12, ISSN 1530-9932

Gaga, M.; Zervas, E.; Grivas, S.; Castro, M. & Chanez, P. (2007). Evaluation and management of severe asthma. *Curr.Med Chem.*, Vol.14, No.9, (2007), pp. 1049-1059, ISSN 0929-8673

Gao, X.; Kim, K.S. & Liu, D. (2007). Nonviral gene delivery: what we know and what is next. *AAPS.J.*, Vol.9, No.1, (2007), pp. E92-104, ISSN 1550-7416

Gaymalov, Z.Z.; Yang, Z.; Pisarev, V.M.; Alakhov, V.Y. & Kabanov, A.V. (2009). The effect of the nonionic block copolymer pluronic P85 on gene expression in mouse muscle and antigen-presenting cells. *Biomaterials*, Vol.30, No.6, (February 2009), pp. 1232-1245,

Gebhart, C.L. & Kabanov, A.V. (2001). Evaluation of polyplexes as gene transfer agents. *J Control Release*, Vol.73, No.2-3, (2001), pp. 401-416, ISSN 0168-3659

Godbey, W.T.; Wu, K.K. & Mikos, A.G. (1999). Poly(ethylenimine) and its role in gene delivery. *J Control Release*, Vol.60, No.2-3, (1999), pp. 149-160, ISSN 0168-3659

Godbey, W.T.; Wu, K.K. & Mikos, A.G. (2001). Poly(ethylenimine)-mediated gene delivery affects endothelial cell function and viability. *Biomaterials*, Vol.22, No.5, (2001), pp. 471-480, ISSN 0142-9612

Goldsmith, Z.G. & Dhanasekaran, N. (2004). The microrevolution: applications and impacts of microarray technology on molecular biology and medicine (review). *Int.J.Mol.Med.*, Vol.13, No.4, (April 2004), pp. 483-495, ISSN 1107-3756

Haufel, T.; Dormann, S.; Hanusch, J.; Schwieger, A. & Bauer, G. (1999). Three distinct roles for TGF-beta during intercellular induction of apoptosis: a review. *Anticancer Res*, Vol.19, No.1A, (1999), pp. 105-111, ISSN 0250-7005

Hegde, P.; Qi, R.; Abernathy, K.; Gay, C.; Dharap, S.; Gaspard, R.; Hughes, J.E.; Snesrud, E.; Lee, N. & Quackenbush, J. (2000). A concise guide to cDNA microarray analysis. *Biotechniques*, Vol.29, No.3, (September 2000), pp. 548-562, ISSN 0736-6205

Hollins, A.J.; Omidi, Y.; Benter, I.F. & Akhtar, S. (2007). Toxicogenomics of drug delivery systems: Exploiting delivery system-induced changes in target gene expression to enhance siRNA activity. *J.Drug Target*, Vol.15, No.1, (January 2007), pp. 83-88, ISSN 1061-186X

Hong, S.; Leroueil, P.R.; Janus, E.K.; Peters, J.L.; Kober, M.M.; Islam, M.T.; Orr, B.G.; Baker, J.R., Jr. & Banaszak Holl, M.M. (2006). Interaction of polycationic polymers with supported lipid bilayers and cells: nanoscale hole formation and enhanced membrane permeability. *Bioconjug.Chem.*, Vol.17, No.3, (May 2006), pp. 728-734, ISSN 1043-1802

Hosack, D.A.; Dennis, G., Jr.; Sherman, B.T.; Lane, H.C. & Lempicki, R.A. (2003). Identifying biological themes within lists of genes with EASE. *Genome Biol*, Vol.4, No.10, (2003), pp. R70, ISSN 1474-760X

Hughes, M.D.; Hussain, M.; Nawaz, Q.; Sayyed, P. & Akhtar, S. (2001). The cellular delivery of antisense oligonucleotides and ribozymes. *Drug Discov Today*, Vol.6, No.6, (2001), pp. 303-315, ISSN 1359-6446

Kabanov, A.V.; Batrakova, E.V.; Sriadibhatla, S.; Yang, Z.; Kelly, D.L. & Alakov, V.Y. (2005). Polymer genomics: shifting the gene and drug delivery paradigms. *J.Control Release*, Vol.101, No.1-3, (January 2005), pp. 259-271, ISSN 0168-3659

Kabanov, V.A. (2006). Polymer Genomics: An Insight into Pharmacology and Toxicology of Nanomedicines. *Adv Drug Deliv Rev*, Vol.58, No.15, (2006), pp. 1597-1621, ISSN 0169-409X

Kafil, V. & Omidi, Y. (2011). Cytotoxic impacts of linear and branched polyethylenimine nanostructures in A431 cells. *BioImpacts*, Vol.1, No.1, (2011), pp. pp. 23-30, ISSN 2228-5652

Kanduc, D.; Mittelman, A.; Serpico, R.; Sinigaglia, E.; Sinha, A.A.; Natale, C.; Santacroce, R.; Di Corcia, M.G.; Lucchese, A.; Dini, L.; Pani, P.; Santacroce, S.; Simone, S.; Bucci, R. & Farber, E. (2002). Cell death: apoptosis versus necrosis (review). *Int J Oncol*, Vol.21, No.1, (2002), pp. 165-170, ISSN 1019-6439

Konopka, K.; Fallah, B.; Monzon-Duller, J.; Overlid, N. & Duzgunes, N. (2005). Serum-resistant gene transfer to oral cancer cells by Metafectene and GeneJammer:

application to HSV-tk/ganciclovir-mediated cytotoxicity. *Cell Mol.Biol.Lett.*, Vol.10, No.3, (2005), pp. 455-470, ISSN 1425-8153

Leroueil, P.R.; Hong, S.; Mecke, A.; Baker, J.R., Jr.; Orr, B.G. & Banaszak Holl, M.M. (2007). Nanoparticle interaction with biological membranes: does nanotechnology present a Janus face? *Acc.Chem.Res.*, Vol.40, No.5, (May 2007), pp. 335-342, ISSN 0001-4842

Lettieri, T. (2006). Recent applications of DNA microarray technology to toxicology and ecotoxicology. *Environ.Health Perspect.*, Vol.114, No.1, (January 2006), pp. 4-9, ISSN 0091-6765

Li, C.Y.; Lee, J.S.; Ko, Y.G.; Kim, J.I. & Seo, J.S. (2000). Heat shock protein 70 inhibits apoptosis downstream of cytochrome c release and upstream of caspase-3 activation. *J Biol Chem*, Vol.275, No.33, (2000), pp. 25665-25671, ISSN 0021-9258

Li, W.; Huang, Z.; Mackay, J.A.; Grube, S. & Szoka, F.C., Jr. (2004). Low-pH-sensitive poly(ethylene glycol) (PEG)-stabilized plasmid nanolipoparticles: effects of PEG chain length, lipid composition and assembly conditions on gene delivery. *J.Gene Med*, Vol.7, No.1, (October 2004), pp. 67-79, ISSN 1099-498X

Lobenhofer, E.K.; Bushel, P.R.; Afshari, C.A. & Hamadeh, H.K. (2001). Progress in the application of DNA microarrays. *Environ.Health Perspect.*, Vol.109, No.9, (September 2001), pp. 881-891, ISSN 0091-6765

Maguire, A.M.; Simonelli, F.; Pierce, E.A.; Pugh, E.N., Jr.; Mingozzi, F.; Bennicelli, J.; Banfi, S.; Marshall, K.A.; Testa, F.; Surace, E.M.; Rossi, S.; Lyubarsky, A.; Arruda, V.R.; Konkle, B.; Stone, E.; Sun, J.; Jacobs, J.; Dell'Osso, L.; Hertle, R.; Ma, J.X.; Redmond, T.M.; Zhu, X.; Hauck, B.; Zelenaia, O.; Shindler, K.S.; Maguire, M.G.; Wright, J.F.; Volpe, N.J.; McDonnell, J.W.; Auricchio, A.; High, K.A. & Bennett, J. (2008). Safety and efficacy of gene transfer for Leber's congenital amaurosis. *N.Engl.J.Med.*, Vol.358, No.21, (May 2008), pp. 2240-2248, ISSN 0028-4793

Masotti, A.; Mossa, G.; Cametti, C.; Ortaggi, G.; Bianco, A.; Grosso, N.D.; Malizia, D. & Esposito, C. (2009). Comparison of different commercially available cationic liposome-DNA lipoplexes: Parameters influencing toxicity and transfection efficiency. *Colloids Surf.B Biointerfaces.*, Vol.68, No.2, (February 2009), pp. 136-144,

May, W.S.; Tyler, P.G.; Ito, T.; Armstrong, D.K.; Qatsha, K.A. & Davidson, N.E. (1994). Interleukin-3 and bryostatin-1 mediate hyperphosphorylation of BCL2 alpha in association with suppression of apoptosis. *J Biol Chem*, Vol.269, No.43, (1994), pp. 26865-26870, ISSN 0021-9258

Medina-Kauwe, L.K.; Xie, J. & Hamm-Alvarez, S. (2005). Intracellular trafficking of nonviral vectors. *Gene Ther.*, Vol.12, No.24, (December 2005), pp. 1734-1751, ISSN 0969-7128

Nel, A.; Xia, T.; Madler, L. & Li, N. (2006). Toxic potential of materials at the nanolevel. *Science*, Vol.311, No.5761, (February 2006), pp. 622-627, ISSN 0036-8075

Omidi, Y.; Barar, J. & Akhtar, S. (2005a). Toxicogenomics of cationic lipid-based vectors for gene therapy: impact of microarray technology. *Curr.Drug Deliv.*, Vol.2, No.4, (October 2005), pp. 429-441, ISSN 1567-2018

Omidi, Y.; Barar, J.; heidari, H.R.; Ahmadian, S.; Ahmadpour Yazdi, H. & Akhtar, S. (2008). Microarray Analysis of the Toxicogenomics and the Genotoxic Potential of a Cationic Lipid-Based Gene Delivery Nanosystem in Human Alveolar Epithelial A549 Cells. *Toxicology Mechanisms and Methods*, Vol.18, No.4, (2008), pp. 369-378, ISSN 1537-6524

Omidi, Y. and Davaran, S. (2011). Impacts of biodegradable polymers: towards biomedical applications, In: *Handbook of Applied Biopolymer Technology: Synthesis, Degradation and Applications*, Sharma, S. and Mudhoo, A., pp. 388-418, Royal Society of Chemistry (RSC), ISBN 978-1-84973-151-5, London

Omidi, Y. and Gumbleton, M. (2005). Biological Membranes and Barriers, In: *Biomaterials for Delivery and Targeting of Proteins Nucleic Acids*, Mahato, R. I., pp. 232-274, CRC Press, ISBN 0849323347, New York

Omidi, Y.; Hollins, A.J.; Benboubetra, M.; Drayton, R.; Benter, I.F. & Akhtar, S. (2003). Toxicogenomics of non-viral vectors for gene therapy: a microarray study of lipofectin- and oligofectamine-induced gene expression changes in human epithelial cells. *J Drug Target*, Vol.11, No.6, (2003), pp. 311-323, ISSN 1061-186X

Omidi, Y.; Hollins, A.J.; Drayton, R.M. & Akhtar, S. (2005b). Polypropylenimine dendrimer-induced gene expression changes: the effect of complexation with DNA, dendrimer generation and cell type. *J.Drug Target*, Vol.13, No.7, (August 2005), pp. 431-443, ISSN 1061-186X

Ott, M.G.; Schmidt, M.; Schwarzwaelder, K.; Stein, S.; Siler, U.; Koehl, U.; Glimm, H.; Kuhlcke, K.; Schilz, A.; Kunkel, H.; Naundorf, S.; Brinkmann, A.; Deichmann, A.; Fischer, M.; Ball, C.; Pilz, I.; Dunbar, C.; Du, Y.; Jenkins, N.A.; Copeland, N.G.; Luthi, U.; Hassan, M.; Thrasher, A.J.; Hoelzer, D.; von, K.C.; Seger, R. & Grez, M. (2006). Correction of X-linked chronic granulomatous disease by gene therapy, augmented by insertional activation of MDS1-EVI1, PRDM16 or SETBP1. *Nat.Med.*, Vol.12, No.4, (April 2006), pp. 401-409, ISSN 1078-8956

Pedroso de Lima, M.C.; Simoes, S.; Pires, P.; Faneca, H. & Duzgunes, N. (2001). Cationic lipid-DNA complexes in gene delivery: from biophysics to biological applications. *Adv Drug Deliv Rev*, Vol.47, No.2-3, (2001), pp. 277-294, ISSN 0169-409X

Prokop, A. & Davidson, J.M. (2008). Nanovehicular intracellular delivery systems. *J.Pharm.Sci.*, Vol.97, No.9, (September 2008), pp. 3518-3590,

Quackenbush, J. (2001). Computational analysis of microarray data. *Nat.Rev.Genet.*, Vol.2, No.6, (June 2001), pp. 418-427, ISSN 1471-0056

Quackenbush, J. (2002). Microarray data normalization and transformation. *Nat Genet*, Vol.32 Suppl (2002), pp. 496-501, ISSN 1061-4036

Rawat, A.; Vaidya, B.; Khatri, K.; Goyal, A.K.; Gupta, P.N.; Mahor, S.; Paliwal, R.; Rai, S. & Vyas, S.P. (2007). Targeted intracellular delivery of therapeutics: an overview. *Pharmazie*, Vol.62, No.9, (September 2007), pp. 643-658, ISSN 0031-7144

Regnstrom, K.; Ragnarsson, E.G.; Fryknas, M.; Koping-Hoggard, M. & Artursson, P. (2006). Gene expression profiles in mouse lung tissue after administration of two cationic polymers used for nonviral gene delivery. *Pharm.Res.*, Vol.23, No.3, (March 2006), pp. 475-482, ISSN 1043-6618

Rejman, J.; Bragonzi, A. & Conese, M. (2005). Role of clathrin- and caveolae-mediated endocytosis in gene transfer mediated by lipo- and polyplexes. *Mol.Ther.*, Vol.12, No.3, (September 2005), pp. 468-474, ISSN 1525-0016

Rubanyi, G.M. (2001). The future of human gene therapy. *Mol Aspects Med*, Vol.22, No.3, (2001), pp. 113-142, ISSN 0098-2997

Ruvolo, P.P.; Deng, X. & May, W.S. (2001). Phosphorylation of Bcl2 and regulation of apoptosis. *Leukemia*, Vol.15, No.4, (2001), pp. 515-522, ISSN 0887-6924

Spang, A. (2008). The life cycle of a transport vesicle. *Cell Mol.Life Sci.* (August 2008), ISSN 1420-682X

Sriadibhatla, S.; Yang, Z.; Gebhart, C.; Alakhov, V.Y. & Kabanov, A. (2006). Transcriptional activation of gene expression by pluronic block copolymers in stably and transiently transfected cells. *Mol.Ther.*, Vol.13, No.4, (April 2006), pp. 804-813, ISSN 1525-0016

Sturn, A.; Quackenbush, J. & Trajanoski, Z. (2002). Genesis: cluster analysis of microarray data. *Bioinformatics.*, Vol.18, No.1, (January 2002), pp. 207-208, ISSN 1367-4803

Subramanian, A.; Tamayo, P.; Mootha, V.K.; Mukherjee, S.; Ebert, B.L.; Gillette, M.A.; Paulovich, A.; Pomeroy, S.L.; Golub, T.R.; Lander, E.S. & Mesirov, J.P. (2005). Gene set enrichment analysis: a knowledge-based approach for interpreting genome-wide expression profiles. *Proc.Natl.Acad.Sci.U.S.A*, Vol.102, No.43, (October 2005), pp. 15545-15550, ISSN 0027-8424

Suter, L.; Babiss, L.E. & Wheeldon, E.B. (2004). Toxicogenomics in predictive toxicology in drug development. *Chem.Biol.*, Vol.11, No.2, (February 2004), pp. 161-171, ISSN 1074-5521

Verma, I.M. & Somia, N. (1997). Gene therapy -- promises, problems and prospects. *Nature*, Vol.389, No.6648, (September 1997), pp. 239-242, ISSN 0028-0836

Verma, I.M. & Weitzman, M.D. (2005). Gene therapy: twenty-first century medicine. *Annu.Rev.Biochem.*, Vol.74 (2005), pp. 711-738, ISSN 0066-4154

Yang, Y.; Blomme, E.A. & Waring, J.F. (2004). Toxicogenomics in drug discovery: from preclinical studies to clinical trials. *Chem.Biol.Interact.*, Vol.150, No.1, (November 2004), pp. 71-85, ISSN 0009-2797

Yang, Y.H.; Buckley, M.J. & Speed, T.P. (2001). Analysis of cDNA microarray images. *Brief.Bioinform.*, Vol.2, No.4, (December 2001), pp. 341-349, ISSN 1467-5463

Yaroslavov, A.A.; Kul'kov, V.E.; Polinsky, A.S.; Baibakov, B.A. & Kabanov, V.A. (1994). A polycation causes migration of negatively charged phospholipids from the inner to outer leaflet of the liposomal membrane. *FEBS Lett.*, Vol.340, No.1-2, (1994), pp. 121-123, ISSN 0014-5793

Yaroslavov, A.A.; Melik-Nubarov, N.S. & Menger, F.M. (2006). Polymer-induced flip-flop in biomembranes. *Acc.Chem.Res.*, Vol.39, No.10, (October 2006), pp. 702-710, ISSN 0001-4842

Young, A. (2007). Structural insights into the clathrin coat. *Semin.Cell Dev.Biol.*, Vol.18, No.4, (August 2007), pp. 448-458, ISSN 1084-9521

Zhang, X.; Pan, S.R.; Hu, H.M.; Wu, G.F.; Feng, M.; Zhang, W. & Luo, X. (2008). Poly(ethylene glycol)-block-polyethylenimine copolymers as carriers for gene delivery: effects of PEG molecular weight and PEGylation degree. *J.Biomed.Mater.Res.A*, Vol.84, No.3, (March 2008), pp. 795-804, ISSN 1549-3296

7

Modular Multifunctional Protein Vectors for Gene Therapy

Hugo Peluffo

Department of Histology and Embryology, Faculty of Medicine, University of the Republic (UDELAR) and Neurodegeneration Laboratory, Institut Pasteur de Montevideo
Uruguay

1. Introduction

The introduction of genes into the organism or the regulation of the expression of endogenous genes has emerged in the last decade as a very potent strategy for correcting monogenic inherited diseases, treating acute disorders, and slowing down the progression of diseases without known cure. In addition it constitutes an important tool for research, which has been widely used and has contributed to show the mechanisms behind several physiological processes and pathologies.

Adequate carriers able to transfer DNA or RNA into target cells have been largely explored. However, this is an area under continuous expansion as there is no ideal vector suitable for all applications. In fact, no individual vector will meet all the characteristics for a perfect or ideal vector, as many of the needs are different and even contradictory. For example, immunogenicity is in most cases an undesirable side effect, while it is a valuable property when treating tumours as it contributes to their clearance. Another example of contradictory needs of one single vector would be the capacity of a vector to determine the overexpression of the transgenic protein for life. This would be an essential property for the treatment of inherited diseases produced by the lack of a particular protein, however for the treatment of acute injuries the lifelong expression of a therapeutic protein will probably be deleterious. Moreover, some vectors do not transduce post-mitotic cells like neurons or muscle fibres, which is a drawback for targeting these cell types but may be an advantage for the targeting of cancer cells. Thus, there is a need for diverse type of vectors for diverse therapeutic or experimental paradigms, and in particular versatile tuneable vectors would be very interesting. Moreover, several basic problems with the known vectors persist, like toxicity, oncogenicity, immunogenicity, low transfection efficiency, or poor bioavailability, which need further consideration and efforts.

Due to their natural efficiency, viruses have been modified to act as vectors, and they have shown a good degree of success. Non-viral vectors have also been developed by combining several properties necessary for transfection: nucleic acid attachment and condensation, cell attachment, cell entry, endosomal escape, intracellular trafficking, nuclear entry, and nucleic acid release. Some of these vectors are quite simple, as the ones formed by the combination of nucleic acids and lipid components or other carriers like polyethylene glycol (PEG). Others include the previous components but have in addition attached targeting molecules like antibodies, enabling these vectors to preferentially transfect a given tissue. In fact even magnetic fields have been used to concentrate suitable engineered vectors to a given area (Corchero and Villaverde 2009).

An interesting type of non-viral vectors is the one based on multifunctional proteins (Aris and Villaverde 2004; Mastrobattista *et al.* 2006). The combination of functional domains in a single polypeptide is a simple yet powerful approach for the development of vectors suitable for gene therapy. In fact, this approach has generated the first prototypes of modular protein gene therapy vectors. Three general methods have been used for the engineering of these molecules: i) production of a recombinant protein by the direct fusion of the functional domains; ii) production of a recombinant protein by combining a known scaffold protein and several functional domains inserted into exposed regions of the scaffold protein; and iii) chemical conjugation of functional domains and proteins. Many of these vectors can be produced recombinantly, generating reproducible and stable stocks appropriate for the formulation of clinically usable drugs. Moreover, the modular nature of these versatile vectors enables the combination of different domains to fulfil the changing requirements of pathological end experimental situations.

2. Functional domains available

2.1 Nucleic acid attachment and condensation

Trans-membrane transport of DNA is an inefficient process, and thus the successful introduction of a transgene into a target cell must include two important steps regarding the plasmid or oligonucleotid DNA that is included in the vector. First, the extended DNA needs to be condensed into an ordered compact nano-particle, and second, once inside the nucleus, the DNA must be de-condensed and thus accessible to transcription. Basic peptides or polycations have been exploited for the interaction with the DNA backbone due to their electrostatic interactions (Bloomfield 1996; Saccardo *et al.* 2009)(see Table 1). When DNA is mixed with these condensing agents, smaller molecules of different shapes are formed mainly depending on DNA size (Vijayanathan *et al.* 2002). For instance, in the absence of DNA, the HNRK modular vector that uses poly-lysine for DNA condensation, self-organize as amorphous, polydisperse particulate entities ranging from a few nanometres up to around one micron. However, in the presence of DNA, protein-DNA complexes appear as tight and rather monodisperse spherical-like nanoparticles of around 80 nm in diameter (Domingo-Espín *et al.* 2011). The most widely used condensing agent is a poly-lysine chain (Saccardo *et al.* 2009). Poly-lysine polymers containing at least 6 lysines will efficiently condense DNA, however, additional 4 to 9 lysines are needed to fully condensate the DNA into smaller particles of 50-100nm, increasing in this way many folds the transfection capacity (Wadhwa *et al.* 1997). Other basic peptides used are the poly-arginine peptides, which not only induce DNA condensation, but also show membrane translocation potential (Futaki *et al.* 2001) and nuclear translocation capacity, determining in this way transgene expression (Kim *et al.* 2003; Vazquez *et al.*).

The condensed DNA by these peptides is partially protected from cellular acid nucleases of the lysosomal compartment (Krishnamoorthy *et al.* 2003; Ross *et al.* 1998; Wolfert and Seymour 1998) and serum nucleases, inducing an extended half-life in serum (Kumar *et al.* 2007) and in the circulation, making tissue targeting possible (Kawabata *et al.* 1995; Nishikawa *et al.* 2000a). For example, the addition of the acid nuclease inhibitor DMI-2 induced a 10-fold increase in receptor-mediated transfection in cultured cells exposed to a

Surfactant Protein A-poly-lysine modular vector or a transferrin-poly-lysine modular vector (Ross *et al.* 1998). Naturally DNA condensing proteins have also been used for the construction of modular vectors. For instance, Histones condense plasmid DNA and protects it from endonucleases, being the lysine-rich H1 Histone the most effective one (Pyhtila *et al.* 1976). Moreover, some nuclear localization signals like the NLS peptide from SV40 virus large T-antigen are lysine-rich peptides that when used as a tetramer can efficiently condense DNA without loosing its nuclear localization properties (Ritter *et al.* 2003).

2.2 Cell attachment and cell targeting

When a viral or non-viral gene therapy vector is injected intravenously, most of the vectors will localize mainly in the liver but also in the kidneys, lungs and spleen. While this is normally a problem to circumvent for most gene therapy applications, it constitutes an advantage for the expression of molecules in the liver. There are many fetal metabolic diseases resulting from a defect or a deficiency of hepatocyte-derived proteins. Moreover, the liver can be considered as a platform to produce various proteins secreted into the blood. Therefore, many pioneer studies focused on the development of more efficient gene delivery systems for the introduction of therapeutic genes selectively into hepatocytes (Wu and Wu 1988). Intravenously injected plasmids are cleared from the circulation by the liver non-parenchymal cells by a scavenging receptor mediated mechanism (Kawabata *et al.* 1995). When Nishikawa and colleagues administered naked ^{32}PDNA into the tail vein of mice, about 40% and 10% of the radioactivity rapidly accumulated in the liver and kidneys, respectively (Nishikawa *et al.* 2000b). Again, the main cell-types targeted were the liver non-parenchymal cells: Kupffer cells and endothelial cells. When they injected a vector composed of ^{32}PDNA/polyornithine, little effect on the distribution of the DNA was observed. However, the injection of the ^{32}PDNA/Gal-pOrn galactose-mediated hepatocyte-targeting vector induced a 60% hepatic accumulation of radioactivity, but more interestingly, most of the targeted cells were now hepatocytes instead of Kupffer or endothelial cells. The same effect was observed at the level of luciferase transgene expression, indicating that the DNA/Gal-pOrn vector was not only able to adhere and enter preferentially into hepatocytes, but it could also transfect them.

Many different domains of known proteins and sugars have been used for cell targeting of modular vectors, like galactose (Wu and Wu 1987), transferrin (Wagner *et al.* 1990), foot-and-mouth disease virus integrin interacting peptide (Aris *et al.* 2000; Aris and Villaverde 2003; Domingo-Espín *et al.* 2011), nerve growth factor (Ma *et al.* 2004; Zeng *et al.* 2004), surfactant protein A (Ross *et al.* 1995), rabies virus glycoprotein (Kumar *et al.* 2007), tetanus toxin fragment Hc (Box *et al.* 2003; Knight *et al.* 1999), cholera toxin b chain (Barrett *et al.* 2004), and neurotensin (Navarro-Quiroga *et al.* 2002). In an interesting study, Arango-Rodríguez and colleagues showed that they could target only substantia nigra neurotensin high affinity receptor positive neurons by means of a modular vector that displayed neurotensin, while no other neurons were transfected (Arango-Rodriguez *et al.* 2006). *In vivo*, many of these targeting systems have shown success (see Table 1). An additional interesting targeting strategy is the use of antibodies (Berhanu and Kush 2008; Buschle *et al.* 1995; Thurnher *et al.* 1994). For instance, the use of the 1E3 antibody against the Tn antigen expressed on many carcinomas coupled to polylysine induced an important increase in the transfection of a cancer cell line (Thurnher *et al.* 1994). Another vector, named fkAbp75-ipr, possess several

Name	Functional Domains	Production Method	Particle Size with nucleic acid (nm)	Gene	Target cells	Administration route	Time of transgene expression	Functional effect	Toxicity	Authors
ASOR-PL	Asialoorosomucoid glycoprotein, Poly-Lys	Chemical conjugation	ND	Human serum albumin	Asialoglyco-protein receptor+ Hepatocytes	i.v.	At least 4 weeks	Partial correction of analbuminemia and hypercholesterolemia	ND	(Wilson et al. 1992; Wu et al. 1991; Wu and Wu 1987)
F105-P	αHIV-gp160 Fab fragment, protamine	Expressed in COS cells	ND	c-myc, MDM2, VEGF siRNA	HIV-gp160 overexpressing cancer cells	i.v.	ND	Partial inhibition of tumour growth	No interferon response detected	(Song et al. 2005)
Gal-PL	Galactose, Poly-Lys	Chemical conjugation	10-12	Human Factor IX	Asialoglyco-protein receptor+ Hepatocytes	i.v.	At least 140 days	No, but increased blood human Facto IX	ND	(Perales et al. 1994)
Man-PL	Mannose, Poly-Lys	Chemical conjugation	220	Chloramphenicol acetyltransferase	Mannose receptor+ hepatic Kupffer cells	i.v.	At least 2 days	ND	ND	(Nishikawa et al. 2000a)
PEI600/DNA/NL4-10K	PEI600, NGF loop4, Poly-Lys	Chemical synthesis and charge interaction assembly	180.4± 5.5	Luciferase	DRG neurons	i.t.	At least 2 days	ND	No	(Zeng et al. 2007)
MC192-P-L-I	MAB MC192 αp75NTR, Poly-Lys	Chemical conjugation	ND	GDNF	p75NTR+ cells	Gel foam at nerve transection site	At least 8 weeks	Neuroprotection of motor neurons after peripheral nerve transection	ND	(Barati et al. 2006)
fkAbp75-ipr	MAB MC192 αp75NTR, HA2, Poly-Lys, SV40-NLS	Chemical conjugation	ND	TrkA siRNA	p75NTR+ cells	i.c.v. Osmotic pump	20 days	Impaired spatial memory after TrkA downregulation	ND	(Berhanu and Rush 2008)
249AL	β-Galactosidase scaffold, integrin binding FMDV RGD, Poly-Lys	Bacterial recombinant	20-40x100-200 filaments	GFP	αvβ3 and other αv integrin+ cells	i.c.	3 days	ND	No	(Aris et al. 2000; Peluffo et al. 2003)
NLSCt	β-Galactosidase scaffold, integrin binding FMDV RGD, Poly-Lys, SV40-NLS	Bacterial recombinant	ND but probably similar to 249AL	Cu/Zn SOD	αvβ3 and other αv integrin+ cells	i.c.	3 days	Neuroprotection from excitotoxic brain lesion after Cu/Zn SOD overexpression	No, in fact neuroprotective per se	(Aris and Villaverde 2003; Peluffo et al. 2006)

Name	Functional Domains	Production Method	Particle Size with nucleic acid (nm)	Gene	Target cells	Administration route	Time of transgene expression	Functional effect	Toxicity	Authors
LDL-DNA	Several domains of the Apo B100 protein of LDL	Isolated from human and rat plasma	ND	GFP and luciferase	Apoprotein B100 receptor+ cells	i.v.	2 days	ND	ND	(Guevara et al.)
RV-G+9R	Rabies virus glycoprotein (29aa), Poly-Arg	Chemical synthesis	ND	GFP siRNA, Cu/ZnSOD siRNA, and FvEJ siRNA	Acetylcholine receptor+ cells	i.v.	2-3 days	Downregulation of genes, protection from mortal viral encephalitis	No inflammation nor specific antibodies produced	(Kumar et al. 2007)
Gal-pOrn-mHA2	Galactose, Poly-Orn, mHA2	Chemical synthesis	130.9 ± 22.6	Luciferase	Asialoglyco-protein receptor+ Hepatocytes	i.v.	2 days	ND	ND	(Nishikawa et al. 2000b)
Fusogenic-karyophilic-NT-polyplex	Neurotensin, HA2, Poly-Lys, SV40-NLS	Charge interaction assembly and chemical conjugation	<200	GFP, GDNF	High affinity Neurotensin receptor+ cells	i.c.	2 months	Neuroprotection and functional recovery in a model of Parkinsons Disease	ND	(Arango-Rodriguez et al. 2006; Gonzalez-Barrios et al. 2006; Navarro-Quiroga et al. 2002)
SPKR/L1-2/PEI600	SPKR, NGF loops 1 and 2, poly-His	Recombinant and charge interaction assembly	100-200	Luciferase	TrkA and p75NTR+ cells	i.t.	3 days	ND	ND	(Ma et al. 2004)
DNA/TfPEI/PEG	Transferrin, PEI, PEG	Charge interaction assembly and chemical conjugation	200-400	Luciferase	Transferrin receptor+ cells	i.v.	2 days	Preferential tumour targeting	ND	(Ogris et al. 1999)
Tat-PTD-DRBD	Tat-PTD, DRBD, poly-His	Recombinant	ND	Luciferase siRNA	Non-selective	i.n.	3-4 days	No, but downregulation of luciferase	ND	(Eguchi et al. 2009)
Tf-HSV-TK	Biotinylated-DNA, streptavidin, biotinylated-transferrin	Chemical conjugation	ND	herpes simplex virus thymidine kinase	Transferrin receptor+ cells	i.v.	At least 7 days	Decreased metastasis and increased survival	ND	(Sato et al. 2000)

Abbreviations: RGD: Arg-Gly-Asp; NGF: Nerve growth factor; i.v.: intravenous; i.c.: intracerebral; i.t.: intrathecal; i.c.v.: intracerebroventricular; i.n.: intranasal; LDL: low-density lipoprotein; HA2: peptide from influenza virus hemagglutinin subunit HA-2; i.t. intrathecal; SPKR: DNA binding motif derived from Histone H1; MDV: foot-and-mouth disease virus; PEG: poly (ethylene glycol); PEI: polyethyleneimine; Tat-PTD: Tat peptide transduction domain; DRBD: (ds)RNA-binding domain; GDNF: Glial derived neurotrophic factor; TK: thymidine kinase.

Table 1. Modular protein vectors effective in vivo

functional domains (see Table 1), being one of them the monoclonal antibody MC192 against p75NTR, the low affinity neurotrophin receptor (Berhanu and Rush 2008). By injecting it intracerebroventricularly coupled to siRNA against TrkA, one of the high affinity neurotrophin receptors, Berhanu and Rush were able to down-regulate TrkA expression in p75NTR expressing cells and correlate this with functional alterations like impaired spatial memory.

2.3 Endosomal escape

A limiting step for receptor-mediated gene delivery is the escape from endosomes, as the vector needs to gain access to the cytosol to enter the nuclei. Fusogenic peptides are reported to strongly enhance *in vitro* gene transfer after being incorporated into carrier systems by chemical linkage (Box *et al.* 2003; Fisher and Wilson 1997; Navarro-Quiroga *et al.* 2002; Nishikawa *et al.* 2000b; Ogris *et al.* 2001; Wagner *et al.* 1992) or by ionic interaction (Gottschalk *et al.* 1996; Plank *et al.* 1994), but co-treatment of the cells with the vector and the fusogenic peptide may also be effective (Read *et al.* 2005). The most widely used method for endosome escape is based on the amino-terminal motif of influenza virus hemagglutinin subunit HA2 (Plank *et al.* 1994; Wagner *et al.* 1992). For example, Nishikawa and colleagues showed that when an acid-sensitive fusogenic peptide derived from HA2 was incubated with mouse erythrocytes at pH 5.0, it induced hemolysis while it did not show any significant hemolytic activity at pH 7.4 (Nishikawa *et al.* 2000b). Interestingly, the same study showed that the *in vivo* liver transgene expression obtained after intravenous injection of the vector DNA/Gal-pOrn-mHA2 was 300 fold higher than that obtained with the same vector lacking the HA2 domain (Nishikawa *et al.* 2000b).

Other domains used for DNA condensation or vector purification as polylysine or polyhistidine have shown endosome disrupting activities (Read *et al.* 2005; Zauner *et al.* 1997). The most effective ones were histidine rich polyplexes formed by the condensation of approximately 50 monomers of Cys-His$_6$-Lys$_3$-His$_6$-Cys and DNA (Read *et al.* 2005). In this study, the endosomolytic agent chloroquine, which normally enhance the transfection capacity of most non-viral vectors, did not enhance the transfection with the histidine rich polyplexes while it enhanced transfection with other non-viral vectors, suggesting that the poly-his domains are in fact endosomolytic. Though polycations like polylysine may be toxic to cells, especially if they have membrane-disrupting activity, this polyhistidine vector showed no toxicity. Histidine becomes positively charged when the pH decrease to less than 7 and thus becomes useful for the permeabilization of the endosomal membrane induced by acidification of endosomes, increasing cell transfection (Midoux *et al.* 1998). *In vivo*, many of these endosomal escape systems have shown success (see Table 1). For an extensive review on different strategies and domains used for endosomal escape please refer to Ferrer-Miralles et al. (Ferrer-Miralles *et al.* 2008).

For the introduction of siRNA and DNA into cells, several cationic peptide transduction domains or also called cell-penetrating domains have been used. TAT, 8xArg, Hph-1or Antp domains can deliver a wide variety of cargo into primary cells, to most tissues, and are in addition being evaluated in clinical trials (Gump and Dowdy 2007). For instance, when the Tat-domain was combined with a poly-His domain and the (ds)RNA-binding domain DRBD, the vector coupled to siRNA could successfully down-regulate Luciferase expression in the nasal and tracheal passages for 4 days after intranasal administration (Eguchi *et al.* 2009). An important characteristic of these systems using cell-penetrating peptides is that they are not cell-specific, and thus should be used for general non-selective transfection. A careful evaluation of the toxicity of this cell penetrating domains in *in vivo* settings has to be performed as toxicity of Tat protein has been reported (Cardozo *et al.* 2007), specially for the CNS (Bonavia *et al.* 2001; Nath *et al.* 1996). In addition, toxicity of the Antp domain has also been reported for many cell types (Cardozo *et al.* 2007).

2.4 Nuclear translocation

The transgene expression levels obtained after plasmid DNA injection into the cytoplasm or the nucleus showed that de nuclear double membrane and its pores are important barriers for naked DNA (Liu *et al.* 2003; Pollard *et al.* 1998). The selection of macromolecules that will be actively imported into the nucleus occurs at the nuclear pore complex, which is composed of more than 50 different proteins. The pore complex will recognise importin proteins bound to short (normally 4-8 amino acids) nuclear localization signals which can be located almost anywhere in the amino acid sequence of the protein, and which are rich in the positively charged amino acids lysine and arginine and usually contains proline (Pouton 1998). This mechanism has been exploited for the design of modular protein vectors, introducing nuclear localization sequences like the SV40 NLS peptide from the T antigen (Aris and Villaverde 2003; Fritz *et al.* 1996). For instance, Aris and co-workers introduced this nuclear localization sequence into the 249AL modular vector (see Table 1) and they observed an enhanced transgene expression with the resulting vector termed NLSCt (Aris and Villaverde 2003). However, studies performed in cells in culture show that even in the presence of nuclear localizations sequences, complexes of more than 60nm seem to be excluded (Chan *et al.* 2000). This data are in contrast to the high transfection efficiency obtained, even *in vivo*, with different modular protein vectors that exceeds this size, reaching 200nm (see Table 1). One can speculate that in fact some molecules of up to 200nm can be imported into the nucleus by being flexible, or that during the interaction of the vector with the nuclear import machinery the vector is disassembled and only the DNA is imported.

Another important step for efficient transgene expression may be the release of the nucleic acid from the vector once in the nucleus. Several studies have addressed the possible enhancement of the release of the DNA by the cellular reducing conditions. For example, histidine rich polyplexes were able to release the complexed DNA when exposed to the reducing agent Dithiothreitol (DTT), suggesting that in cells a similar mechanism would occur (Read *et al.* 2005). In fact, the increase in the cellular antioxidant and reducing agent glutathione, induced an important 200 fold increase in the transfection observed with the histidine rich polyplexes, but only a 3fold increase was observed with the PEI/DNA vector, another non-viral vector with no reduction-dependent release of DNA. Though this is an interesting phenomenon, it is difficult to understand why the cytosol reducing conditions do not disassemble the vector too early, determining that the DNA is released into the cytosol instead of inside the nucleus, not favouring the transfection process.

2.5 Trophic vectors/functional vectors

An attractive possibility is the combination of the effects mediated by the overexpression of a transgene and the direct effects of the vector per se. In fact, as modular vectors normally take advantage of a cell attaching motif for receptor mediated endocytosis, they tend to display intrinsic activities. More importantly, the use of trophic factors or toxin domains for cell attachment and internalization is ideal, as their natural mechanism of action includes the attachment to high affinity cell surface receptors, the endocytosis to early endosomes, and even being transported to the cell soma in the case of neurons (Lalli and Schiavo 2002). An interesting modular vector was produced combining a polylysine tail with the loop 4 of the nerve growth factor (NGF) (Zeng *et al.* 2004; Zeng and Wang 2005). This "trophic vector" maintained the trophic effects of NGF, was able to condensate DNA, and when combined with polyethylenimine (PEI600), transfected cells in culture that expressed NGF receptors but not cells without these receptors. Interestingly, the DNA-PEI600 showed a size of 445nm and an zeta potential of 6,2mV, but the addition of the NGF loop4 poly-lysine peptide to the complex induced the formation of smaller 180nm particles with a zeta potential of 23,2mV (Zeng *et al.* 2007). This shows that the addition of targeting peptides to non-specific DNA/condensing products complexes may in fact contribute to enhance not only the targeted delivery but also to decrease the particle size and charge of the resulting vector. A somehow more complex trophic vector including NGF loops was also produced. It combined the loops 1 and 2 of NGF and the SPKR4 domain derived from histone H1 DNA binding motif, linked together by a α-helical linker (Ma *et al.* 2004). Both NGF-loop derived vectors could even transfer a transgene *in vivo* preferentially to dorsal root ganglia neurons (which express NGF receptors) after intrathecal spinal cord injection (Ma *et al.* 2004; Zeng *et al.* 2007). Several toxins have been used as cell attachment motifs (Andreu *et al.* 2008; Box *et al.* 2003; Knight *et al.* 1999), and some motifs of these toxins can in fact display trophic effects (Chaib-Oukadour *et al.* 2004), and have thus been used to design trophic vectors.

An important consideration regarding many acute injuries is that the therapeutic time window is short. In those cases, a direct trophic or functional effect of the vector per se could extend the therapeutic window, giving time for the transgene to be expressed and mediate its own effects. For example, the neuroprotection observed after an acute brain injury using the vector termed NLSCt was partially mediated by the transgene overexpressed, but also partially mediated by the RGD integrin-interacting motif of the vector itself (Peluffo *et al.* 2006; Peluffo *et al.* 2007). In this experimental setting the direct injection of the vector into the lesioned brain area was performed 4 hours after the lesion. The CNS is a tissue that tolerates injures very badly due to its high dependence on blood flow and oxygen consumption, and its poor regeneration capacity. This determines that the therapeutic window for the treatment of acute injuries is very short. Interestingly, even in this experimental paradigm, the modular recombinant NLSCt vector overexpressing the anti-oxidant enzyme Cu/Zn superoxide dismutase (SOD) could mediate neuroprotection (Peluffo *et al.* 2006). These studies shows the wide possibilities of combining the vectors themselves with active protein domains like trophic factors, which will exert rapid direct effects, which in turn may increase the therapeutic window or the potency of the effect of the transgene used.

3. Immunogenicity and inflammation

The introduction of modular protein vectors into the organism may be accompanied by a humoral or cell-mediated immune response against the inserted motifs, which in many cases are derived from viral molecules. However, when injected intravenously, the Rabies virus glycoprotein (29aa)-Poly-Arg vector (RVG-9R) (see Table 1) did not induce an antibody response or an increase in several pro-inflammatory cytokines evaluated (Kumar *et al.* 2007). In another example, when the recombinant 249AL vector (see Table 1) was injected into the normal postnatal brain, no changes were observed in glial activation, demyelination, recruitment of cytotoxic CD8 lymphocytes, or expression of IL1β. Interestingly, when a very similar vector termed NLSCt (see Table 1) was injected into the postnatal brain after an excitotoxic injury, an increase in macrophage/microglia number and in the levels of IL1β and Cox2 enzyme were observed in the lesion (Gonzalez *et al.* 2011). Most interesting, the same set of studies discovered that this vector, with or without accomplished control DNA, besides inducing an inflammatory response, also induced a decrease in the brain lesion volume and in the number of degenerating neurons (Peluffo *et al.* 2006; Peluffo *et al.* 2007), an effect that was mediated by the prototypic RGD-integrin interacting motif of the vector (Peluffo *et al.* 2007). These data may suggest that the modulation of the inflammation by the vector may be beneficial under some circumstances. Another vector termed Tat-PTD-DRBD (see Table 1) did not induce interferon (IFN)-α or tumour necrosis factor (TNF)-α responses when incubated with primary human peripheral blood mononuclear cells (Eguchi *et al.* 2009). Thus, the overall data suggests that these types of vectors are less immunogenic and pro-inflammatory than most viral and other non-viral vectors.

4. Administration routes and transgene expression

If these types of vectors are useful for gene therapy applications is still an open question, and adequate testing of these vectors in preclinical and actual clinical studies need to be performed. In fact, it has been well established that there is no ideal vector for all gene therapy applications, being the characteristics of each vector critical for each pathological paradigm. The use of modular protein vectors is limited to pathologies accepting an acute treatment, but would be ineffective for chronic ones as the transgene expression that they determine is normally short lived. The time of transgene expression varies from a few days to more than two months, depending on the doses and the method of administration. For instance, multifunctional recombinant vectors can induce the *in vivo* brain expression of a reporter gene after direct injection into the bran in a model of acute brain injury, lasting the transgenic protein in the brain for 3 days (Peluffo *et al.* 2003), but another vector was able to determine expression in normal brain for two months after intracerebral injection (Navarro-Quiroga *et al.* 2002). In the case of other administration routes and pathologies, as for example the intravenous administration of these vectors, the time for transgenic protein expression in the liver may range from a few days to more that 4 months (Perales *et al.* 1994). In another study, the liver-selective and transient overexpression of the therapeutic protein human coagulation factor IX could be achieved using a synthetic modular glycoprotein vector, and secreted factor IX into the serum could be detected for 30 days (Ferkol *et al.* 1993). This same paradigm could be used for vaccination, overexpressing transiently the desired immunogenic protein (Chen and Huang 2005). Even the use of modular vectors coupled to plasmids producing shRNA show potent downregulation of an endogenous gene during 20 days when infused with osmotic pumps into the nervous system (Berhanu and Rush 2008). In all this approaches, the transient expression of a protein by means of multifunctional vectors would be desirable when compared to viral vector inoculation, which present higher risks of oncogenic and inflammatory complications, may produce very high levels of transgenic protein, and will produce the transgenic protein for life or for extended periods.

5. Pharmacokinetics and biodistribution

Various approaches have been undertaken to overcome the interaction of vectors with blood components to avoid aggregation as well as embolisms. Moreover for most strategies, the phagocytic clearing system of the organism must be eluded. Pharmacokinetic analysis has shown that physicochemical properties of the vectors such as molecular weight, electrical charge and immunogenicity (or pre-existing antibodies in the organism) are important determinants for the *in vivo* success of the treatment. In addition, the volume and shape of the final vector is also important as it determines if the complex will be internalized into the cell and the cell nucleus. P^{32}plasmid DNA is rapidly eliminated from the circulation after intra-venous injection in mice (Kawabata *et al.* 1995), mainly by a scavenger receptor mechanism-mediated uptake by hepatic phagocytes (Kawabata *et al.* 1995; Takakura *et al.* 1999). Thus, the *in vivo* plasmid delivery needs to modify its physicochemical properties by condensing carriers. One interesting example is the Mannose-Poly-Lysine vector (Man-PL), which was designed to accommodate plasmid DNA for the mannose receptor-mediated transfection of liver endothelial cells and Kuppfer phagocytes. After intravenous injection, the Man-PL-P32DNA vector disappeared from the plasma with a half-life of 1 minute, being 80% of the radioactivity recovered from the liver at 10 minutes (mainly in the mannose receptor+ target cells) and less than 1% at lungs or kidneys at 1 hour after (Nishikawa *et al.* 2000a). This vector had a size of 220nm and a zeta potential of 12,1mV, while the DNA alone had a size of 200nm and a zeta potential of -36,4. This type of study clearly shows the importance of the condensation of plasmid DNA into small less charged particles. In accordance, it has been described that positively charged DNA complexes can activate the alternative complement pathway (Plank *et al.* 1996). The conjugation of vectors with hydrophilic polymers has been shown to decrease their interaction with plasmatic proteins and blood cells, increasing their half-life in circulation. One of the most used polymers is poly (ethylene glycol) (PEG). In an interesting study, Ogris and colleagues compared the blood stability of DNA/transferrin/PEI vectors with or without covalently linked PEG. The non-PEGylated vectors aggregated in plasma, bound several plasmatic proteins like IgM, fibrinogen, fibronectin, and complement C3, and also induced erythrocyte aggregation (Ogris *et al.* 1999). Interestingly, the PEGylated vector showed stable complex size, reduced surface charge, reduced binding of plasmatic proteins and erythrocyte aggregation, and most important, increased *in vivo* circulation half-life combined with enhanced transfection selectivity towards tumours.

An interesting vector for improving pharmacokinetics could be the use of natural circulating molecules, like the low-density lipoprotein (LDL). In fact it has been shown that LDL can act as a vector when mixed with plasmid DNA and injected intravenously, reaching several organs including the brain, heart, kidneys and spleen (Guevara *et al.*). The LDL molecule is composed of a highly hydrophobic core, surrounded by a shell of phospholipids and unesterified cholesterol, as well as a single copy of Apo B100 protein (Segrest *et al.* 2001). The B100 protein contains several motifs that explain the vector profile of the LDL: i) a motif that enable nucleic acid binding, ii) a motif that mediate cellular uptake, and iii) a motif that is apparently involved in transferring DNA into the cell nucleus (Guevara *et al.*). Interestingly, low-density particles composed of lipid, Apo B100, RNA, and core protein of hepatitis C virus were reported in the plasmas of individuals infected with this virus (Andre *et al.* 2002). This and other studies suggested that virus might utilize the potential of the LDL particle to act as a vector as a mechanism for persistent chronic infection.

6. Preclinical studies

Many interesting preclinical studies have been performed with modular multifunctional protein vectors (see Table 1). The first studies showing *in vivo* functional effects using modular protein vectors were made by Wu and colleagues. By injecting intravenously the asialoorosomucoid glycoprotein-polylysine vector (ASOR-PL, see Table 1), they targeted hepatocytes and were able to partially and temporary correct analbuminemia and hypercholesterolemia by overexpressing human serum albumin or functional LDL receptor respectively (Wilson *et al.* 1992; Wu *et al.* 1991; Wu and Wu 1987). In another study, neuroprotection from an acute brain injury was achieved after direct intracerebral injection of the NLSCt vector overexpressing the antioxidant enzyme Cu/ZnSOD (see Table 1). In this experimental setting the overexpression of the therapeutic protein could not only induce reduced infarct volume but also functional improvement of the animals (Peluffo *et al.* 2006). Here, the vector was injected directly into the lesioned brain by a tightly controlled microinjector, using a similar protocol reported for the injection of cells into the human Parkinsonian brain (Brundin *et al.*), or for the intracerebral injection of adeno-associated viral vectors for the treatment of infantile lysosomal storage disease (Worgall *et al.* 2008). Thus, this direct intracerebral injection approach could show some benefits in clinical cases of focal traumatic or ischemic injuries, were a delimited area is lesioned and were in some cases even a decompressing craniectomy is needed leaving a direct entrance to the brain parenchyma. Modular protein vectors have also been used for neuroprotection after acute peripheral nerve transection. For example, Barati and colleagues (Barati *et al.* 2006) delivered a polylysine-based polyplex targeting p75[NTR] positive cells accomplishing the plasmid encoding for GDNF after a peripheral nerve transection (see Table 1). They showed an almost complete reversal in neuronal death caused by GDNF transgene expression. Though this is a very interesting study, the authors performed a subtle pre-lesion to the nerve one week before the nerve transection injury to upregulate p75[NTR] receptor, and thus the same experiment should be repeated but under more clinically relevant conditions. In another preclinical setting, the intravenous injection (once a day during 3 consecutive days) of the RVG-9R vector accomplished to the antiviral siRNA siFvEJ (see Table 1) was able to induce 80% survival of animals 30 days after their inoculation with a fatal flavivirus (Kumar *et al.* 2007). Thought many modular vectors have been shown to mediate over-expression or down-regulation of reporter genes, they need to be tested *in vivo* in clinically relevant models for the establishment of their real potential.

7. Conclusion

More complex modular protein vectors including all the important domains for efficient nucleic acid delivery need to be engineered. They should include domains for DNA attachment and condensation, cell attachment and endocytosis, endosomal escape, cytosol trafficking towards the nucleus, nuclear import, and DNA release. HNRK (Domingo-Espín *et al.* 2011), fkAbp75-ipr (Berhanu and Rush 2008), and the fusogenic-karyophilic-NT-polyplex (Navarro-Quiroga *et al.* 2002) (see Table 1) are three prototypes of this increasingly complex vectors, but additional domains have to be inserted. In addition, an interesting strategy could be the exploitation of several domains that have dual functions, like poly-his with DNA attachment and endosomal escape properties, like melittin with endosomal escape properties and nuclear import potential, or histones with DNA attachment and nuclear import potential. Considering the fact that for example several cellular nuclear proteins have several nuclear localization domains, the introduction of several domains with the same function in the same vector may further increase their efficiency. In fact, dual targeting of cancer cell lines using both transferrin and RGD domains showed synergistic effects (Nie *et al.*). Furthermore, the combination of engineered modular protein vectors with engineered plasmids for long term-regulated expression *in vivo* will be essential. For instance, the pEPI DNA vector was the first prototype of episomal vector whose function relies exclusively on chromosomal elements, replicating autonomously in low copy numbers in all cells tested (Piechaczek *et al.* 1999). This vector was further engineered to show regulated expression and to be removed from transduced cells when transgene expression is no longer needed (Rupprecht *et al.*). Finally, vectors have to be tested *in vivo*, but evaluating biological effects and not only reporter gene expression, and the comparison of different vectors in a same *in vivo* experimental setting will also contribute to the selection of the best prototypes.

8. Acknowledgments

This work was supported by the Comisión Sectorial de Investigación Cienctífica (CSIC) of the Universidad de la República (UDELAR) and by the Agencia Nacional de Investigación e Innovación (ANII) of the Ministerio de Cultura, Uruguay.

9. References

Andre, P., F. Komurian-Pradel, S. Deforges, M. Perret, J.L. Berland, M. Sodoyer, S. Pol, C. Brechot, G. Paranhos-Baccala and V. Lotteau. 2002. Characterization of low- and very-low-density hepatitis c virus rna-containing particles. J Virol 76, no. 14: 6919-28.

Andreu, A., N. Fairweather and A.D. Miller. 2008. Clostridium neurotoxin fragments as potential targeting moieties for liposomal gene delivery to the cns. Chembiochem 9, no. 2: 219-31.

Arango-Rodriguez, M.L., I. Navarro-Quiroga, J.A. Gonzalez-Barrios, D.B. Martinez-Arguelles, M.J. Bannon, J. Kouri, P. Forgez, W. Rostene, R. Garcia-Villegas, I. Jimenez and D. Martinez-Fong. 2006. Biophysical characteristics of neurotensin polyplex for *in vitro* and in vivo gene transfection. Biochim Biophys Acta 1760, no. 7: 1009-20.

Aris, A., J.X. Feliu, A. Knight, C. Coutelle and A. Villaverde. 2000. Exploiting viral cell-targeting abilities in a single polypeptide, non-infectious, recombinant vehicle for integrin-mediated DNA delivery and gene expression. Biotechnol Bioeng 68, no. 6: 689-96.

Aris, A. and A. Villaverde. 2003. Engineering nuclear localization signals in modular protein vehicles for gene therapy. Biochem Biophys Res Commun 304, no. 4: 625-31.

Aris, A. and A. Villaverde. 2004. Modular protein engineering for non-viral gene therapy. Trends Biotechnol 22, no. 7: 371-7.

Barati, S., P.R. Hurtado, S.H. Zhang, R. Tinsley, I.A. Ferguson and R.A. Rush. 2006. Gdnf gene delivery via the p75(ntr) receptor rescues injured motor neurons. Exp Neurol 202, no. 1: 179-88.

Barrett, L.B., M. Berry, W.B. Ying, M.N. Hodgkin, L.W. Seymour, A.M. Gonzalez, M.L. Read, A. Baird and A. Logan. 2004. Ctb targeted non-viral cdna delivery enhances transgene expression in neurons. J Gene Med 6, no. 4: 429-38.

Berhanu, D.A. and R.A. Rush. 2008. Targeted silencing of trka expression in rat forebrain neurons via the p75 receptor. Neuroscience 153, no. 4: 1115-25.

Bloomfield, V.A. 1996. DNA condensation. Curr Opin Struct Biol 6, no. 3: 334-41.

Bonavia, R., A. Bajetto, S. Barbero, A. Albini, D.M. Noonan and G. Schettini. 2001. Hiv-1 tat causes apoptotic death and calcium homeostasis alterations in rat neurons. Biochem Biophys Res Commun 288, no. 2: 301-8.

Box, M., D.A. Parks, A. Knight, C. Hale, P.S. Fishman and N.F. Fairweather. 2003. A multi-domain protein system based on the hc fragment of tetanus toxin for targeting DNA to neuronal cells. J Drug Target 11, no. 6: 333-43.

Brundin, P., R.A. Barker and M. Parmar. Neural grafting in parkinson's disease problems and possibilities. Prog Brain Res 184: 265-94.

Buschle, M., M. Cotten, H. Kirlappos, K. Mechtler, G. Schaffner, W. Zauner, M.L. Birnstiel and E. Wagner. 1995. Receptor-mediated gene transfer into human t lymphocytes via binding of DNA/cd3 antibody particles to the cd3 t cell receptor complex. Hum Gene Ther 6, no. 6: 753-61.

Cardozo, A.K., V. Buchillier, M. Mathieu, J. Chen, F. Ortis, L. Ladriere, N. Allaman-Pillet, O. Poirot, S. Kellenberger, J.S. Beckmann, D.L. Eizirik, C. Bonny and F. Maurer. 2007. Cell-permeable peptides induce dose- and length-dependent cytotoxic effects. Biochim Biophys Acta 1768, no. 9: 2222-34.

Chaib-Oukadour, I., C. Gil and J. Aguilera. 2004. The c-terminal domain of the heavy chain of tetanus toxin rescues cerebellar granule neurones from apoptotic death: Involvement of phosphatidylinositol 3-kinase and mitogen-activated protein kinase pathways. J Neurochem 90, no. 5: 1227-36.

Chan, C.K., T. Senden and D.A. Jans. 2000. Supramolecular structure and nuclear targeting efficiency determine the enhancement of transfection by modified polylysines. Gene Ther 7, no. 19: 1690-7.

Chen, W.C. and L. Huang. 2005. Non-viral vector as vaccine carrier. Adv Genet 54: 315-37.

Corchero, J.L. and A. Villaverde. 2009. Biomedical applications of distally controlled magnetic nanoparticles. Trends Biotechnol 27, no. 8: 468-76.

Domingo-Espín, J., E. Vazquez, J. Ganz, O. Conchillo, E. García-Fruitós, J. Cedano, U. Unzueta, V. Petegnief, N. Gonzalez-Montalbán, A.M. Planas, X. Daura, H. Peluffo, N. Ferrer-Miralles and A. Villaverde. 2011. The nanoparticulate architecture of protein-based artificial viruses is supported by protein-DNA interactions. Nanomedicine In Press.

Eguchi, A., B.R. Meade, Y.C. Chang, C.T. Fredrickson, K. Willert, N. Puri and S.F. Dowdy. 2009. Efficient sirna delivery into primary cells by a peptide transduction domain-dsrna binding domain fusion protein. Nat Biotechnol 27, no. 6: 567-71.

Ferkol, T., G.L. Lindberg, J. Chen, J.C. Perales, D.R. Crawford, O.D. Ratnoff and R.W. Hanson. 1993. Regulation of the phosphoenolpyruvate carboxykinase/human factor ix gene introduced into the livers of adult rats by receptor-mediated gene transfer. Faseb J 7, no. 11: 1081-91.

Ferrer-Miralles, N., E. Vazquez and A. Villaverde. 2008. Membrane-active peptides for non-viral gene therapy: Making the safest easier. Trends Biotechnol 26, no. 5: 267-75.

Fisher, K.J. and J.M. Wilson. 1997. The transmembrane domain of diphtheria toxin improves molecular conjugate gene transfer. Biochem J 321 (Pt 1): 49-58.

Fritz, J.D., H. Herweijer, G. Zhang and J.A. Wolff. 1996. Gene transfer into mammalian cells using histone-condensed plasmid DNA. Hum Gene Ther 7, no. 12. 1395-404.

Futaki, S., T. Suzuki, W. Ohashi, T. Yagami, S. Tanaka, K. Ueda and Y. Sugiura. 2001. Arginine-rich peptides. An abundant source of membrane-permeable peptides having potential as carriers for intracellular protein delivery. J Biol Chem 276, no. 8: 5836-40.

Gonzalez, P., H. Peluffo, L. Acarin, A. Villaverde, B. Gonzalez and B. Castellano. 2011. Il-10 overexpression does not synergize with the neuroprotective action of rgd-containing vectors after postnatal brain excitotoxicity, but modulates the main inflammatory cell responses. . Under second revision in the Journal of Neuroscience Research.

Gonzalez-Barrios, J.A., M. Lindahl, M.J. Bannon, V. Anaya-Martinez, G. Flores, I. Navarro-Quiroga, L.E. Trudeau, J. Aceves, D.B. Martinez-Arguelles, R. Garcia-Villegas, I. Jimenez, J. Segovia and D. Martinez-Fong. 2006. Neurotensin polyplex as an efficient carrier for delivering the human gdnf gene into nigral dopamine neurons of hemiparkinsonian rats. Mol Ther 14, no. 6: 857-65.

Gottschalk, S., J.T. Sparrow, J. Hauer, M.P. Mims, F.E. Leland, S.L. Woo and L.C. Smith. 1996. A novel DNA-peptide complex for efficient gene transfer and expression in mammalian cells. Gene Ther 3, no. 5: 448-57.

Guevara, J., Jr., N. Prashad, B. Ermolinsky, J.W. Gaubatz, D. Kang, A.E. Schwarzbach, D.S. Loose and N.V. Guevara. 2010. Apo b100 similarities to viral proteins suggest basis for ldl-DNA binding and transfection capacity. J Lipid Res 51, no. 7: 1704-18.

Gump, J.M. and S.F. Dowdy. 2007. Tat transduction: The molecular mechanism and therapeutic prospects. Trends Mol Med 13, no. 10: 443-8.

Kawabata, K., Y. Takakura and M. Hashida. 1995. The fate of plasmid DNA after intravenous injection in mice: Involvement of scavenger receptors in its hepatic uptake. Pharm Res 12, no. 6: 825-30.

Kim, H.H., W.S. Lee, J.M. Yang and S. Shin. 2003. Basic peptide system for efficient delivery of foreign genes. Biochim Biophys Acta 1640, no. 2-3: 129-36.

Knight, A., J. Carvajal, H. Schneider, C. Coutelle, S. Chamberlain and N. Fairweather. 1999. Non-viral neuronal gene delivery mediated by the hc fragment of tetanus toxin. Eur J Biochem 259, no. 3: 762-9.

Krishnamoorthy, G., B. Roques, J.L. Darlix and Y. Mely. 2003. DNA condensation by the nucleocapsid protein of hiv-1: A mechanism ensuring DNA protection. Nucleic Acids Res 31, no. 18: 5425-32.

Kumar, P., H. Wu, J.L. Mcbride, K.E. Jung, M.H. Kim, B.L. Davidson, S.K. Lee, P. Shankar and N. Manjunath. 2007. Transvascular delivery of small interfering rna to the central nervous system. Nature 448, no. 7149: 39-43.

Lalli, G. and G. Schiavo. 2002. Analysis of retrograde transport in motor neurons reveals common endocytic carriers for tetanus toxin and neurotrophin receptor p75ntr. J Cell Biol 156, no. 2: 233-9.

Liu, G., D. Li, M.K. Pasumarthy, T.H. Kowalczyk, C.R. Gedeon, S.L. Hyatt, J.M. Payne, T.J. Miller, P. Brunovskis, T.L. Fink, O. Muhammad, R.C. Moen, R.W. Hanson and M.J. Cooper. 2003. Nanoparticles of compacted DNA transfect postmitotic cells. J Biol Chem 278, no. 35: 32578-86.

Ma, N., S.S. Wu, Y.X. Ma, X. Wang, J. Zeng, G. Tong, Y. Huang and S. Wang. 2004. Nerve growth factor receptor-mediated gene transfer. Mol Ther 9, no. 2: 270-81.

Mastrobattista, E., M.A. Van Der Aa, W.E. Hennink and D.J. Crommelin. 2006. Artificial viruses: A nanotechnological approach to gene delivery. Nat Rev Drug Discov 5, no. 2: 115-21.

Midoux, P., A. Kichler, V. Boutin, J.C. Maurizot and M. Monsigny. 1998. Membrane permeabilization and efficient gene transfer by a peptide containing several histidines. Bioconjug Chem 9, no. 2: 260-7.

Nath, A., K. Psooy, C. Martin, B. Knudsen, D.S. Magnuson, N. Haughey and J.D. Geiger. 1996. Identification of a human immunodeficiency virus type 1 tat epitope that is neuroexcitatory and neurotoxic. J Virol 70, no. 3: 1475-80.

Navarro-Quiroga, I., J. Antonio Gonzalez-Barrios, F. Barron-Moreno, V. Gonzalez-Bernal, D.B. Martinez-Arguelles and D. Martinez-Fong. 2002. Improved neurotensin-vector-mediated gene transfer by the coupling of hemagglutinin ha2 fusogenic peptide and vp1 sv40 nuclear localization signal. Brain Res Mol Brain Res 105, no. 1-2: 86-97.

Nie, Y., D. Schaffert, W. Rodl, M. Ogris, E. Wagner and M. Gunther. Dual-targeted polyplexes: One step towards a synthetic virus for cancer gene therapy. J Control Release.

Nishikawa, M., S. Takemura, F. Yamashita, Y. Takakura, D.K. Meijer, M. Hashida and P.J. Swart. 2000a. Pharmacokinetics and in vivo gene transfer of plasmid DNA complexed with mannosylated poly(l-lysine) in mice. J Drug Target 8, no. 1: 29-38.

Nishikawa, M., M. Yamauchi, K. Morimoto, E. Ishida, Y. Takakura and M. Hashida. 2000b. Hepatocyte-targeted in vivo gene expression by intravenous injection of plasmid DNA complexed with synthetic multi-functional gene delivery system. Gene Ther 7, no. 7: 548-55.

Ogris, M., S. Brunner, S. Schuller, R. Kircheis and E. Wagner. 1999. Pegylated DNA/transferrin-pei complexes: Reduced interaction with blood components, extended circulation in blood and potential for systemic gene delivery. Gene Ther 6, no. 4: 595-605.

Ogris, M., R.C. Carlisle, T. Bettinger and L.W. Seymour. 2001. Melittin enables efficient vesicular escape and enhanced nuclear access of nonviral gene delivery vectors. J Biol Chem 276, no. 50: 47550-5.

Peluffo, H., L. Acarin, A. Aris, P. Gonzalez, A. Villaverde, B. Castellano and B. Gonzalez. 2006. Neuroprotection from nmda excitotoxic lesion by cu/zn superoxide dismutase gene delivery to the postnatal rat brain by a modular protein vector. BMC Neurosci 7: 35.

Peluffo, H., A. Aris, L. Acarin, B. Gonzalez, A. Villaverde and B. Castellano. 2003. Nonviral gene delivery to the central nervous system based on a novel integrin-targeting multifunctional protein. Hum Gene Ther 14, no. 13: 1215-23.

Peluffo, H., P. González, A. Arís, L. Acarin, A. Villaverde, B. Castellano and B. González. 2007. Rgd domains neuroprotect the immature brain by a glial dependent mechanism. Ann Neurol 62: 251-56.

Perales, J.C., T. Ferkol, H. Beegen, O.D. Ratnoff and R.W. Hanson. 1994. Gene transfer in vivo: Sustained expression and regulation of genes introduced into the liver by receptor-targeted uptake. Proc Natl Acad Sci U S A 91, no. 9: 4086-90.

Piechaczek, C., C. Fetzer, A. Baiker, J. Bode and H.J. Lipps. 1999. A vector based on the sv40 origin of replication and chromosomal s/mars replicates episomally in cho cells. Nucleic Acids Res 27, no. 2: 426-8.

Plank, C., K. Mechtler, F.C. Szoka, Jr. and E. Wagner. 1996. Activation of the complement system by synthetic DNA complexes: A potential barrier for intravenous gene delivery. Hum Gene Ther 7, no. 12: 1437-46.

Plank, C., B. Oberhauser, K. Mechtler, C. Koch and E. Wagner. 1994. The influence of endosome-disruptive peptides on gene transfer using synthetic virus-like gene transfer systems. J Biol Chem 269, no. 17: 12918-24.

Pollard, H., J.S. Remy, G. Loussouarn, S. Demolombe, J.P. Behr and D. Escande. 1998. Polyethylenimine but not cationic lipids promotes transgene delivery to the nucleus in mammalian cells. J Biol Chem 273, no. 13: 7507-11.

Pouton, C.W. 1998. Nuclear import of polypeptides, polynucleotides and supramolecular complexes. Adv Drug Deliv Rev 34, no. 1: 51-64.

Pyhtila, M.J., I. Miettola, T. Kurkela and A. Hoyhtya. 1976. Protection of deoxyribonucleic acid from nuclease action by histones. Acta Chem Scand B 30, no. 8: 797-8.

Read, M.L., S. Singh, Z. Ahmed, M. Stevenson, S.S. Briggs, D. Oupicky, L.B. Barrett, R. Spice, M. Kendall, M. Berry, J.A. Preece, A. Logan and L.W. Seymour. 2005. A versatile reducible polycation-based system for efficient delivery of a broad range of nucleic acids. Nucleic Acids Res 33, no. 9: e86.

Ritter, W., C. Plank, J. Lausier, C. Rudolph, D. Zink, D. Reinhardt and J. Rosenecker. 2003. A novel transfecting peptide comprising a tetrameric nuclear localization sequence. J Mol Med 81, no. 11: 708-17.

Ross, G.F., M.D. Bruno, M. Uyeda, K. Suzuki, K. Nagao, J.A. Whitsett and T.R. Korfhagen. 1998. Enhanced reporter gene expression in cells transfected in the presence of dmi-2, an acid nuclease inhibitor. Gene Ther 5, no. 9: 1244-50.

Ross, G.F., R.E. Morris, G. Ciraolo, K. Huelsman, M. Bruno, J.A. Whitsett, J.E. Baatz and T.R. Korfhagen. 1995. Surfactant protein a-polylysine conjugates for delivery of DNA to airway cells in culture. Hum Gene Ther 6, no. 1: 31-40.

Rupprecht, S., C. Hagedorn, D. Seruggia, T. Magnusson, E. Wagner, M. Ogris and H.J. Lipps. Controlled removal of a nonviral episomal vector from transfected cells. Gene 466, no. 1-2: 36-42.

Saccardo, P., A. Villaverde and N. Gonzalez-Montalban. 2009. Peptide-mediated DNA condensation for non-viral gene therapy. Biotechnol Adv 27, no. 4: 432-8.

Sato, Y., N. Yamauchi, M. Takahashi, K. Sasaki, J. Fukaura, H. Neda, S. Fujii, M. Hirayama, Y. Itoh, Y. Koshita, K. Kogawa, J. Kato, S. Sakamaki and Y. Niitsu. 2000. *In vivo* gene delivery to tumor cells by transferrin-streptavidin-DNA conjugate. Faseb J 14, no. 13: 2108-18.

Segrest, J.P., M.K. Jones, H. De Loof and N. Dashti. 2001. Structure of apolipoprotein b-100 in low density lipoproteins. J Lipid Res 42, no. 9: 1346-67.

Song, E., P. Zhu, S.K. Lee, D. Chowdhury, S. Kussman, D.M. Dykxhoorn, Y. Feng, D. Palliser, D.B. Weiner, P. Shankar, W.A. Marasco and J. Lieberman. 2005. Antibody mediated *in vivo* delivery of small interfering rnas via cell-surface receptors. Nat Biotechnol 23, no. 6: 709-17.

Takakura, Y., T. Takagi, M. Hashiguchi, M. Nishikawa, F. Yamashita, T. Doi, T. Imanishi, H. Suzuki, T. Kodama and M. Hashida. 1999. Characterization of plasmid DNA binding and uptake by peritoneal macrophages from class a scavenger receptor knockout mice. Pharm Res 16, no. 4: 503-8.

Thurnher, M., E. Wagner, H. Clausen, K. Mechtler, S. Rusconi, A. Dinter, M.L. Birnstiel, E.G. Berger and M. Cotten. 1994. Carbohydrate receptor-mediated gene transfer to human t leukaemic cells. Glycobiology 4, no. 4: 429-35.

Vazquez, E., M. Roldan, C. Diez-Gil, U. Unzueta, J. Domingo-Espin, J. Cedano, O. Conchillo, I. Ratera, J. Veciana, X. Daura, N. Ferrer-Miralles and A. Villaverde. Protein nanodisk assembling and intracellular trafficking powered by an arginine-rich (r9) peptide. Nanomedicine (Lond) 5, no. 2: 259-68.

Vijayanathan, V., T. Thomas and T.J. Thomas. 2002. DNA nanoparticles and development of DNA delivery vehicles for gene therapy. Biochemistry 41, no. 48: 14085-94.

Wadhwa, M.S., W.T. Collard, R.C. Adami, D.L. Mckenzie and K.G. Rice. 1997. Peptide-mediated gene delivery: Influence of peptide structure on gene expression. Bioconjug Chem 8, no. 1: 81-8.

Wagner, E., C. Plank, K. Zatloukal, M. Cotten and M.L. Birnstiel. 1992. Influenza virus hemagglutinin ha-2 n-terminal fusogenic peptides augment gene transfer by transferrin-polylysine-DNA complexes: Toward a synthetic virus-like gene-transfer vehicle. Proc Natl Acad Sci U S A 89, no. 17: 7934-8.

Wagner, E., M. Zenke, M. Cotten, H. Beug and M.L. Birnstiel. 1990. Transferrin-polycation conjugates as carriers for DNA uptake into cells. Proc Natl Acad Sci U S A 87, no. 9: 3410-4.

Wilson, J.M., M. Grossman, C.H. Wu, N.R. Chowdhury, G.Y. Wu and J.R. Chowdhury. 1992. Hepatocyte-directed gene transfer in vivo leads to transient improvement of hypercholesterolemia in low density lipoprotein receptor-deficient rabbits. J Biol Chem 267, no. 2: 963-7.

Wolfert, M.A. and L.W. Seymour. 1998. Chloroquine and amphipathic peptide helices show synergistic transfection in vitro. Gene Ther 5, no. 3: 409-14.

Worgall, S., D. Sondhi, N.R. Hackett, B. Kosofsky, M.V. Kekatpure, N. Neyzi, J.P. Dyke, D. Ballon, L. Heier, B.M. Greenwald, P. Christos, M. Mazumdar, M.M. Souweidane, M.G. Kaplitt and R.G. Crystal. 2008. Treatment of late infantile neuronal ceroid lipofuscinosis by cns administration of a serotype 2 adeno-associated virus expressing cln2 cdna. Hum Gene Ther 19, no. 5: 463-74.

Wu, G.Y., J.M. Wilson, F. Shalaby, M. Grossman, D.A. Shafritz and C.H. Wu. 1991. Receptor-mediated gene delivery in vivo. Partial correction of genetic analbuminemia in nagase rats. J Biol Chem 266, no. 22: 14338-42.

Wu, G.Y. and C.H. Wu. 1987. Receptor-mediated in vitro gene transformation by a soluble DNA carrier system. J Biol Chem 262, no. 10: 4429-32.

Wu, G.Y. and C.H. Wu. 1988. Receptor-mediated gene delivery and expression in vivo. J Biol Chem 263, no. 29: 14621-4.

Zauner, W., A. Kichler, W. Schmidt, K. Mechtler and E. Wagner. 1997. Glycerol and polylysine synergize in their ability to rupture vesicular membranes: A mechanism for increased transferrin-polylysine-mediated gene transfer. Exp Cell Res 232, no. 1: 137-45.

Zeng, J., H.P. Too, Y. Ma, E.S. Luo and S. Wang. 2004. A synthetic peptide containing loop 4 of nerve growth factor for targeted gene delivery. J Gene Med 6, no. 11: 1247-56.

Zeng, J. and S. Wang. 2005. Enhanced gene delivery to pc12 cells by a cationic polypeptide. Biomaterials 26, no. 6: 679-86.

Zeng, J., X. Wang and S. Wang. 2007. Self-assembled ternary complexes of plasmid DNA, low molecular weight polyethylenimine and targeting peptide for nonviral gene delivery into neurons. Biomaterials 28, no. 7: 1443-51.

8

Peptides as Promising Non-Viral Vectors for Gene Therapy

Wei Yang Seow and Andrew JT George
Imperial College London, England
United Kingdom

1. Introduction

In its most simplistic sense, gene therapy involves the delivery and expression of DNA by target cells so as to produce a therapeutic protein. In the case of RNA interference (RNAi), it is to shut off or silence the expression of a particular target protein. In order to exert its effects, the nucleic acid must first reach its intended site of action. DNA molecules (frequently as plasmids, which are circularised DNA) have to gain nuclear entry to access the transcription machinery. Conversely, RNAi molecules such as small interfering RNA (siRNA), short hairpin RNA (shRNA) and micro RNA (miRNA) will need to accumulate within the cytoplasm, although shRNA-encoding plasmids will require prior nuclear access before transcription into shRNA. However, if administered alone, a great majority of the nucleic acids will be degraded en route, leading to a lost of therapeutic potential. This then necessitates the development of vectors that protect and deliver nucleic acids to their target site. Arguably, it is the lack of safe and efficient delivery systems, rather than suitable therapeutic molecules that is limiting the success of gene therapy.

In this chapter, we start by examining how issues at the cellular level have shaped the design of modern, multifunctional vectors. We then briefly review the various types of gene delivery system, focusing on peptides as a promising class of non-viral vector. We will concentrate on the delivery of plasmids since the phenomenon of RNAi is relatively recent (Fire et al., 1998). As such, many strategies for RNAi delivery are adapted from DNA delivery technology.

2. Intracellular barriers in gene therapy: Problems and potential solutions

Ensuring the arrival of a plasmid at its site of action in a transcriptional state is the entire aim of gene delivery systems. However, plasmids face a constant threat of being degraded. The challenge begins as soon as they are introduced into the extracellular milieu (Figure 1). In most experimental setups, cells/tissues are maintained at 37°C in serum-supplemented medium where serum nucleases can extensively damage a naked plasmid. The plasmid therefore needs protection. Next, the plasmid needs to be internalised. However, both DNA (phosphate groups within the backbone) and plasma membrane (glycoproteins with their sialic acid groups, glycerophosphates with their phosphate groups and proteoglycans which contain sulphate groups) are negatively charged. Electrostatic repulsion then ensures that there is little chance of the plasmid being naturally taken up by a cell.

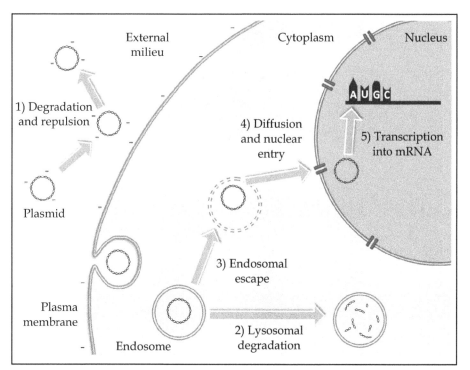

Fig. 1. Chronological sequence of events and challenges that a plasmid faces during its treacherous journey towards the nucleus. 1) A naked plasmid is susceptible to degradation by nucleases and is likely to be repelled from the plasma membrane. 2) Assuming successful endocytosis, the plasmid has to avoid trafficking into lysosomes where it will be degraded. 3) The plasmid has to escape into the cytoplasm. 4) It now has to diffuse through the viscous cytoplasm towards the nucleus while avoiding degradation and penetrate the nuclear membrane. 5) Transcription into mRNA can then occur if the plasmid is still intact.

For these reasons, gene delivery systems are frequently designed to be cationic in character and this fulfils several functions. First, the carrier can use its positive charges to mask the negative charges on the plasmid and package itself as a carrier/DNA complex with an overall positive charge. As expected, positively charged particles are internalised much more readily, as confirmed by an elegant study using PRINT (Particle Replication In Non-wetting Templates) technology to fabricate particles with exquisite control over their size, shape and surface charge (Gratton et al., 2008b). By keeping size and shape constant, positively charged particles were found in 84% of cells after an hour of incubation compared to the <5% uptake of negatively charged particles, proving that surface charge alone can influence uptake dramatically. Second, due to a charge screening effect, the macromolecular plasmid is collapsed (or condensed) into a compact structure more amendable for cellular uptake. This condensing process was clearly demonstrated using transmission electron microscopy which showed an elongated plasmid (long-axis diameter of ~470 nm) being compacted into tight, 80-100 nm toroid-shaped complexes by polylysine carriers (Wagner et al., 1991). Third, the carrier protects its cargo against degradation by nucleases, presumably by steric obstruction. This was shown by first exposing the complexes to DNase and then using gel electrophoresis to validate the physical integrity of the plasmid upon its release from the carrier. Control plasmids that were unprotected gave no bands in the subsequent gel electrophoresis experiment.

A problem with cationic carriers is that negatively charged serum protein can be non-specifically bound. As a result, targeting signals on the carrier can become blocked or complexes can start to aggregate. Reducing or removing serum from the media during *in vitro* transfection can mitigate such effects and improve transfection (Moore et al., 2009; Moulton et al., 2004). However, this strategy fails during *in vivo* experiments where serum proteins are unavoidably present. Another approach is to mix DNA and carrier in precise stoichiometric ratio so as to result in electro-neutral complexes (Funhoff et al., 2005). Along similar lines, zwitterionic (McManus et al., 2004) or anionic (Liang et al., 2005) lipids have been proposed in which binding between carrier and plasmid is dependant on hydrophobic forces and the presence of divalent cations such as Ca^{2+}, Zn^{2+} and Mg^{2+} to screen the disruptive repulsion between like charges. Neutral water-soluble polymers such as polyvinyl alcohol (PVA) and polyvinyl pyrolidone (PVP) similarly exploit non-electrostatic forces such as hydrogen bonding and van der Waal's attraction to condense plasmids (Park et al., 2006). These particles are however less popular because the lack of positive charge is expected to adversely impact cellular uptake. The PEGylation of carriers is another option. PEGylation refers to the surface decoration of carriers with flexible chains of polyethylene glycol (PEG), which is a highly hydrophilic polymer capable of making a surface less susceptible to protein adsorption (Duncan, 2006). Having said that, a major concern is that PEGylation obstructs the positive charges, resulting in carriers which are less efficient in DNA binding and transfection (Lin et al., 2008; Meyer et al., 2008). Moreover, while PEGylated drug formulations are already in clinical use, PEG is non-biodegradable and its chronic use may be a concern (Urakami & Guan, 2008).

The positive charges on cationic carriers have also been implicated in the formation of pores on the membrane, leading to cytotoxicity (Rimann et al., 2008). The observation that carrier/DNA complexes are less toxic to the cells compared to the carrier alone can be interpreted as partial evidence that charge compensation on the carrier may be a reason, albeit a non-exclusive one, for the reduced toxicity (Niidome et al., 1997). However, the exact mechanism is not totally clear. It may be due to the high rate of uptake of cationic carriers – and not the positive charges *per se* – that is to blame for pore formation. Herein lies a dilemma of the gene therapist: a high rate of internalisation can increase transfection efficiency but is also frequently paralleled by toxicity (Gabrielson & Pack, 2006; Pouton & Seymour, 2001). Fortunately, cells do have membrane repair mechanisms. One example is the membrane repair response (MRR) where the influx of Ca^{2+} ions directs lysosomes to donate their vesicular membrane in a concerted effort to plug the hole (Palm-Apergi et al., 2009). As always, the challenge is to strike a fine balance between two counter-acting events.

Assume the plasmid has been successfully taken up by a cell via endocytosis and now resides within an endosome. Another degradative fate awaits as endosomes eventually acidify into lysosomes and activate a broth of acid hydrolases capable of degrading nucleic acids. For this reason, a high rate of uptake may not necessarily translate into high transfection efficiency if, for example, most of the plasmids are degraded in lysosomes (Lundin et al., 2008). To avoid degradation, the plasmid/carrier complex will need to escape from the confines of the endosome into the cytosol. A popularly cited mechanism by which cationic carriers can achieve this is the proton-sponge hypothesis, so called because it relies on the buffering capability of the carrier to absorb H^+ ions and thus function as a proton sink. This model assumes that as the H^+-ATPase endosomal membrane pump injects protons into the vesicle during acidification, a build-up of positive charges will result due to the ability of the carrier to protonate and absorb the protons. This then triggers a concomitant influx of compensatory negative ions (e.g., Cl^-) and water, leading to the osmotic swelling of the vesicle and its eventual rupture. Consistent with this line of argument, carriers must thus contain chemical groups that are capable of undergoing protonation within the pH range of the endo/lysosomal transition, i.e., a pK_a of 7 to 4. This has motivated investigators to design carriers with a large buffering capacity. The polymer polyethylenimine (PEI), for instance, has a combination of protonated amines to bind plasmids at pH 7 and a stockpile of unprotonated amines that can still undergo protonation during the endo/lysosomal transition (Boussif et al., 1995). As such, PEI has a large buffering capacity and this feature is frequently cited as a main reason for PEI's status as one of the most efficient non-viral vector commercially available for *in vitro* transfection (Putnam, 2006).

Another common strategy to promote endosomal escape is to coincubate cells with a lysosomotropic agent such as chloroquine. Traditionally used as an anti-malaria drug, chloroquine is also a weak base capable of buffering the acidification of endosomes. In reality, however, chloroquine is pleiotropic in nature – besides its lysosomotropic property, chloroquine has been reported to be able to aid in the release of plasmid from its carrier and also to inhibit DNase activity (Yang et al., 2009) – and its actual mechanism of action remains controversial. Nevertheless, chloroquine does generally improve the transfecting capability of many carriers (Pouton & Seymour, 2001). A caveat, though, is that chloroquine at the dose normally used (100 µM) is toxic to cells (Wadia et al., 2004; Zauner et al., 1998). Glycerol is another agent reported to augment transfection due to its ability to weaken and make vesicular membrane more susceptible to disruption (Zauner et al., 1997). Interestingly, the more obvious effect of adding glycerol – its osmotic property – was ruled out as the main cause of vesicle escape. Finally, carriers can be functionalised with membrane-disruptive peptides, a strategy which will be reviewed in later sections.

The proton-sponge hypothesis is the most commonly cited explanation to account for the positive correlation between increased buffering capacity and transfection ability. It is hence easy to overlook that no study has provided any convincing evidence in direct support of its mechanism (Won et al., 2009). In fact, discrediting observations exist. For instance, it was reported that ammonium sulphate, also a weak base and should theoretically be able to provide buffering effects, does not boost transfection (Pouton & Seymour, 2001). Recent calculations have also revealed that the amount of strain that lipid vesicles can withstand before rupture is significantly larger than that which can be induced by endosomal buffering (Won et al., 2009). This suggests that the proton-sponge hypothesis can at best contribute, but cannot be the only cause of endosomal escape. Moreover, increased buffering and endosomal escaping properties do not always produce an accompanying increase in transfection (Akita et al., 2010; Moore et al., 2009). This implies that, while important, cytosolic access is not the only bottleneck of the transfection process. Further, it has to be pointed out that of the multiple pathways which a cell can use for internalisation, only the clathrin-mediated one is widely-accepted to involve vesicle acidification (Won et al., 2009; Zauner et al., 1997). Vesicle acidification is, of course, an inherent requirement of the proton-sponge hypothesis but whether vesicles from other pathways acidify is equivocal. Some researchers believe that macropinocytosis (Akita et al., 2010; Pelkmans & Helenius, 2002) and caveolae-mediated endocytosis (Lundin et al., 2008; Sahay et al., 2010) produce vesicles that do not undergo acidification, while others claim that macropinosomes do acidify (Räägel et al., 2009; Wadia et al., 2004). Furthermore, is it safe to assume that vesicles which do not acidify remain distinct from endo/lysosomes? On this, opinion is also polarised, with some claiming that caveosomes (Pelkmans & Helenius, 2002; Sahay et al., 2010) and macropinosomes (Wadia et al., 2004) remain distinct from endo/lysosomes; and others arguing that vesicles from different pathways can eventually interact (Sahay et al., 2010). Thus, the proton-sponge hypothesis even if true, may not always be relevant and on top of that, definitive trafficking studies of the various modes of uptake are required.

In the cytosol, the plasmid continues its migration towards the nucleus. Current dogma suggests that this proceeds via passive diffusion and that nuclear localisation is a hit-or-miss event. The viscous cytosolic environment makes diffusion extremely inefficient. The diffusion coefficient of bovine serum albumin (BSA) in human fibroblasts, for example, is about 70× lower than in buffer (Wojcieszyn et al., 1981). Protecting the plasmid during migration is also important as cytosolic nucleases restrict the half life of naked DNA to about 90 minutes (Belting et al., 2005).

During migration, another feature of the carrier becomes important – the release of its plasmid cargo. To undergo transcription, the plasmid must first be unpackaged from its carrier and the trick here, is one of timing. A plasmid that gets released too early will risk degradation while one that binds too strongly is not accessible for transcription. For this reason, lower molecular weight chitosan transfects better because their higher molecular weight counterpart interacts too strongly with their plasmid cargo (Koping-Hoggard et al., 2004). Another example involves PEI, where acetylation of its polymeric chains (which removes the amines) reduced both its buffering capacity and binding strength, but improved its transfection (Gabrielson & Pack, 2006). This suggests that vector unpackaging can indeed be a rate-limiting step and a carrier that binds in moderation is ideal. Fluorescence resonance energy transfer (FRET) is a powerful technique to study the process of vector unpackaging. It depends on the excitation of an acceptor dye by a donor dye in close physical proximity, which is the case when the plasmid is being tightly condensed. Using FRET, plasmid-release in the perinuclear region has been observed; alternatively, the plasmid/carrier can enter the nucleus as an associated complex (Seow et al., 2009).

Nuclear entry is believed to be achieved in two ways: either via the ~10 nm wide nuclear pores or during mitosis when the nuclear envelope momentarily disintegrates (Luo & Saltzman, 2000a). The latter appears to be a more efficient method for the large-scale accumulation of complexes. It further provides a possible explanation for why amitotic cells or primary cells which proliferate slower are more difficult to transfect than cancer-derived cell lines. A dilution effect after mitotic cell division also accounts for the transient nature of gene expression mediated by non-integrating vectors. Having said that, mitosis is not a pre-requisite (Won et al., 2009) as amitotic cells have been successfully transfected – it merely provides a convenient window of opportunity for nuclear entry. A proposed method to improve nuclear penetration is to attach a nuclear localisation signal (NLS) to the carrier. The quintessential example of a NLS is the short peptide sequence corresponding to the Simian virus 40 (SV40) T antigen. However, responses regarding the benefits of including a NLS have been mixed, with some investigators (Trentin et al., 2005) more convinced than others (Zauner et al., 1998). A key issue pointed out was that studies involving the use of NLS failed to examine the effect of including a NLS on nuclear import *per se* (Lam & Dean, 2010). Instead, reporter gene expression was frequently used as a proxy and an improved expression was simply accepted to be due to the inclusion of NLS. Given that most NLS are cationic, it is debatable if the observed increase in transfection is strctly the result of improved nuclear import *per se*, or due to other non-specific effects such as enhanced plasmid association and uptake. Moreover, the fact that a NLS can be sterically hindered by plasmids upon binding also contradicts the requirement of NLS to be freely accessible for interaction with importins, the nuclear entry regulating proteins.

In light of the many obstacles that nucleic acids and their carriers have to surmount, it is perhaps understandable that less than 10% of the pool of plasmids that made it into a cell will go on to accumulate in the nucleus (Lam & Dean, 2010). The challenge is to design a multifunctional vector that can address the issues highlighted above and yet, remain safe to use in a human body.

3. Overview and classification of gene delivery systems

3.1 Physical systems

Gene delivery systems can be classified based on their means of achieving transfection (Figure 2). There are systems that utilise physical forces, mostly with the aim of disrupting the plasma membrane, to facilitate nucleic acids delivery. For instance, electroporation and sonoporation (Frenkel, 2008) uses electrical and sonication forces respectively to transiently compromise the plasma membrane. The ballistic gene gun method, on the other hand,

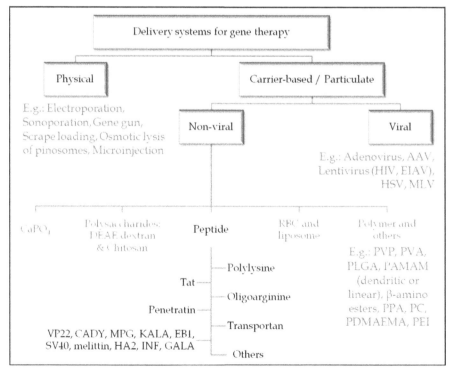

Fig. 2. The different classes and examples of gene delivery systems. This chapter will concentrate on peptide-derived vectors.

directly shoots DNA-coated metal particles (frequently gold) into cells (Merediz et al., 2000). Expectedly, such aggressive methods can irreversibly damage the cell membrane and cause widespread cell death. Scrape loading, first described in 1984, requires the forceful scraping of cells attached to their culture dishes, thereby creating pores on their membranes for plasmid entry (McNeil et al., 1984). This technique, however, is only applicable to adherent cells. The osmotic lysis of pinosomes was proposed in 1982 and requires that cells capable of pinocytosis be initially exposed to a hypertonic medium of sucrose, PEG and the plasmid of interest (Okada & Rechsteiner, 1982). Subsequent exchange to a hypotonic medium then released the pinosomal content. Although cells are constitutively capable of pinocytosis, such wild fluctuations in osmotic conditions can cause cell death. Finally, microinjection refers to the piecemeal injection of plasmids directly into the cell. This technique, while relatively gentle, is extremely laborious. As such, it is prone to failure and the number of cells that can be processed is limited.

3.2 Viral vectors

There are systems that function as particulate carriers by ferrying nucleic acids into or near to their site of action. Such systems can be viral or non-viral in nature. Viral vectors such as adenovirus, adeno-asociated virus (AAV), human immunodeficiency virus (HIV), equine infectious anaemia virus (EIAV), herpes simplex virus (HSV) and murine leukaemia virus (MLV) have been used and comprehensively reviewed elsewhere (Kay et al., 2001). The prime advantage of viral vectors is their transfection efficiency which has benefitted from centuries of selective evolutionary pressure. As a result, viruses are several orders of magnitude more efficient than non-viral vectors (Kircheis et al., 1997) and account for about 70% of all clinical trials involving gene therapy so far (Won et al., 2009). A recent success for viral gene therapy involved the use of lentiviruses to deliver a correct copy of a therapeutic gene to an adult patient suffering from β-thalassaemia (Cavazzana-Calvo et al., 2010). Such patients suffer from defective haemoglobin production and require chronic blood transfusion for survival. Upon reinfusing the patient with his own bone-marrow haematopoietic stem cells that had earlier been transduced *ex vivo*, the patient became transfusion free 1 year after treatment and has been doing well, according to the most recent report at 33 months after treatment. The longer-term outcome, of course, remains to be seen. Having said that, investigators have not abandoned all forms of non-viral research as there are limitations in the use of viral vectors. For example, the technical difficulty of scaling up virus production compliant to good manufacturing practices (GMP) may prevent such therapy from being cheaply accessible (Sheridan, 2011). The size of the construct that can be delivered is also limited. Above all, toxicity and immunogenicity (reviewed by Nayak & Herzog, 2010) provoked by the viral vectors can and have brought clinical trials to premature ends. Repeated administration is also not possible if the body has mounted a systemic immune response. The danger of viral gene therapy was first illustrated about a decade ago by the death of Jesse Gelsinger (Hollon, 2000). Researchers were using experimental adenoviruses to correct his partial ornithine transcarbamylase deficiency affecting the ability of his body to metabolise nitrogen. Unfortunately, the systemic inflammatory response syndrome was triggered and he succumbed, rather rapidly, to multiple organ failure. In another high profile example, stem cells transduced *ex vivo* with MLV were used to treat children suffering from X-linked severe combined immunodeficiency (Hacein-Bey-Abina et al., 2003). However, MLV is an integrating retrovirus and can cause insertional mutagenesis, which is a phenomenon where random viral integration can trigger the activation of an oncogene or disrupt genes with tumor-suppressive properties. Consequently, several patients became leukemic and at least one has died so far (Sheridan, 2011). More recently, retroviruses were also used to treat two patients diagnosed with X-linked chronic granulomatous disease which affected the ability of their phagocytes to clear bacterial infections (Ott et al., 2006). Insertional mutagenesis was again responsible for a clone of cells whose genes responsible for growth were activated, prompting fears that such cells may turn cancerous. Having said that, viral gene therapy is not expected to be perfect and its success should be assessed relative to existing treatments. Nonetheless, researchers have not completely mastered the use of viruses and there is still a need for alternative non-viral vectors with safer profiles.

3.3 Non-viral vectors

Diethylaminoethyl (DEAE)-dextran and calcium phosphate ($CaPO_4$) were two of the earliest systems popular in the 1970s and 80s. DEAE-dextran has a cationic polysaccharide backbone and one of the earliest reports in 1965 used this polymer in a 1:1 mixture with nucleic acids to transfect rhesus monkey kidney cells (Vaheri & Pagano, 1965). Authors of this study also insightfully commented that DEAE-dextran, like histones, could bind and protect nucleic acids from degradation. Although these are now fundamental concepts in modern carrier design, it may not have been obvious in the past. The co-precipitation of $CaPO_4$ with DNA was first described in 1973, when it was observed that Ca^{2+} (not Mg^{2+} or Na^+) and PO_4^{2-} ions, at high enough concentrations, could enhance DNA uptake by cells (Graham & Eb, 1973). This technique was further shown to be sensitive to pH, amount of DNA used and even the level of CO_2 in the incubator (Chen & Okayama, 1987). Using an optimised protocol, $CaPO_4$-mediated transfection achieved up to 50% efficiency with a murine L cell line (Chen & Okayama, 1987).

Chitosan is a polysaccharide obtained by the deacetylation of chitin, an exoskeletal component of crustaceans. Each deacetylation site contains a primary amine (pK_a~6.5) which allows chitosan to bind nucleic acids. The degree of deacetylation also determines its biodegradability and transfection efficiency. Chitosan was first described as a plasmid carrier by Mumper and colleagues in 1995 and is known to be biocompatible, mucoadhesive and virtually non-toxic (MacLaughlin et al., 1998). As such, chitosan has been evaluated in rabbits, although reporter gene expression in that study was low (MacLaughlin et al., 1998). Strong interactions between high molecular chitosan and DNA were blamed for the overly-stable complexes that could not release their plasmid cargos. Using lower molecular weight chitosan, *in vitro* transfection efficiency was improved by up to 24 fold (Koping-Hoggard et al., 2004). Adding histidine (pK_a~6) residues to chitosan further improved buffering capacity and overall transfection efficiency (Chang et al., 2010). Recently, it was also shown that the introduction of thiol groups in N,N,N-trimethylated chitosan improved its efficiency as a siRNA carrier (Varkouhi et al., 2010).

Red blood cells (RBC) were used for the delivery of macromolecules before liposomes became popular. To function as carriers, RBC were first loaded up with the macromolecule under hypotonic conditions to induce mild lysis. A fusogen was then used to cause fusion with target cells. Using this technique, thymidine kinase and BSA were introduced into 3T3-4E mouse cells using Sendai virus as a fusogen (Schlegel & Rechsteiner, 1975). In another study, horseradish peroxidase (HRP) and immunoglobulins (IgG) were delivered into cells expressing hemagglutinin derived from influenza virus by exploiting the fusogenic activity of hemagglutinin under mildly acidic conditions (Doxsey et al., 1985). Fluorescent IgG and

BSA were also delivered into human fibroblast cells using PEG as a fusogen (Wojcieszyn et al., 1981). Dehydration may play a role in PEG-mediated fusion and intriguingly, purification by recrystallisation removed the fusogenic ability of PEG, suggesting that other ingredients in commercial PEG was essential (Wojcieszyn et al., 1983).

Plasmids were initially delivered by synthetic liposomes using concepts adapted from RBC technology. In an early study, plasmids were encapsulated within anionic liposomes and fused with tobacco mesophyll protoplasts using PEG (Deshayes et al., 1985). Since 1987, however, surface binding became popular when liposomes made of N-[1-(2,3,-dioleyloxy)propyl]-N,N,N-trimethylammonium chloride (DOTMA) were synthesised for the first time (Felgner et al., 1987). DOTMA contains cationic quaternary ammonium groups which can be used for DNA binding. Lipofectin®, the prototypical lipid formulation and a workhorse for transfection experiments today, is a 1:1 mixture of DOTMA and the neutral lipid, dioleoyl phosphatidylethanolamine (DOPE). In this formulation, DOPE functions as a fusogen to aid cellular uptake. Several other formulations of liposomes have been reported. Gao and Huang prepared liposomes made out of DOPE and a novel cationic cholesterol derivative, 3β-[N-(N',N'-dimethylamino)ethane-carbamoyl] cholesterol (DC-chol), and used it to transfect several cell lines with high efficiency (Gao & Huang, 1996). A mixture of N',N'-dioctadecyl-N-4,8-diaza-10-aminodecanoylglycine amide (DODAG) and DOPE was also proposed to be a novel liposomal formulation that is good for both DNA and siRNA delivery (Mével et al., 2010). In another study, the cationic lipid 1,2-dilinoleyloxy-3-dimethylaminopropane (DLinDMA) was used as a starting template and systematically modified to yield an optimised construct (Semple et al., 2010). Although toxicity remains one of the chief complaints, liposomes are definitely one of the most successful non-viral vectors around. Already, several sustained-release liposomal drug formulations have been approved for human use and thermosensitive liposomes are being evaluated in clinical trials (Hossann et al., 2010). Lipids also dominate in gene therapy trials aimed at using non-viral vectors to treat cystic fibrosis (Griesenbach & Alton, 2009).

An advantage of polymeric carriers is that they offer so much structural diversity that their potential should, theoretically, be limited only by the imagination of chemists. Two of the more archaic examples including PVP and PVA have been mentioned. Poly(D,L-lactic-co-glycolic acid) (PLGA), a polymer originally developed for controlled drug release, has also been used to encapsulate plasmids for delivery (Wang et al., 1999). Most polymeric carriers, however, are cationic in nature. Dendritic poly(amido amine) (PAMAM) which contained primary amines for DNA binding was further decorated with PEG and sugars (Wood et al., 2005) or peptide (Wood et al., 2008) for targeting purposes. Linear PAMAM was functionalised with disulfide bonds to make the polymer biodegradable and various chemical side-groups were attached to test for its impact on transfection efficiency (Lin et al., 2007). A large library of poly(β-amino ester)s has been synthesised and systematically screened for transfection efficiency (Green et al., 2006). The effects of molecular weight and charge density of polyphosphoramidates (PPA) on DNA binding and buffering capacity have been reported (Ren et al., 2010). A series of novel enzyme-degradable polycarbonates (PC) with various aliphatic side-chains attached were prepared and shown to effectively transfect cells with virtually no toxicity (Seow & Yang, 2009a). Poly(2-(dimethyl-amino)ethylmethacrylate) (PDMAEMA) was also shown to transfect cells with high efficiency (Lin et al., 2008). Indeed, there are so many other classes of polymers being developed that it is impossible to do all justice with this paragraph. Nonetheless, amongst all, the most notable polymer must be PEI. PEI was first developed in 1995 (Boussif et al.,

1995) and is frequently used in its branched, high molecular weight (usually 25 kDa) form. Together with liposomes, they are widely acknowledged to be the best non-viral vectors currently available (Putnam, 2006) and frequently serve as standards to which other novel carriers are referenced. A key feature of PEI is that nitrogen (in a mixture of primary, secondary and tertiary amines) accounts for a third of its molecular weight. Since different classes of amines possess characteristic pK_a, this ensures that not all the nitrogen will be protonated at a given pH. Furthermore, the proximity of the nitrogen atoms also means that a protonated amine can suppress the protonation of its neighbours due to the energetic penalty that gets incurred by situating like charges adjacent to one another (Suh et al., 1994). This blend of protonated and yet-to-be protonated amines is then suggested to endow PEI with its strong DNA binding and buffering abilities. The intracellular trafficking properties of PEI/DNA complexes has been studied (Godbey et al., 1999) and targeting moieties such as mannose (Diebold et al., 1999) and transferrin (Kircheis et al., 1997) were also coupled onto PEI. However, two of the main problems of PEI are its toxicity and non-biodegradability. In response to the latter, PEI was functionalised with reducible disulfide bonds (Lee et al., 2007) or hydrolysable ester bonds (Liu et al., 2008) to facilitate biodegradation and at the same time, to aid its intracellular plasmid release.

4. Peptide-derived vectors for gene therapy

Peptide chains can be fabricated from any of the 20 naturally occurring L-amino acids, which are referred to by their single- or three-lettered code (e.g., R or arg for arginine). Peptides are thus biocompatible and often degradable. Peptide synthesis also does not involve harmful catalysts, which is a concern in the synthesis of some polymeric carriers. Furthermore, synthesis can now be automated, courtesy of advances in solid phase peptide synthesis, which makes the manufacturing process amendable to up-scaling.

Before peptides were seen as proper DNA carriers, studies conducted in the 1960s with histones had already suggested that cationic amino acids such as lysine and arginine can be useful (Akinrimisi et al., 1965). Today, peptide vectors are given fanciful names such as "cell penetrating peptides" (CPP) or "protein transduction domains" (PTD) to celebrate their ability to efficiently penetrate the plasma membrane and mediate the entry of nucleic acids or other macromolecules. Such CPP can be derived from proteins existing in nature (e.g., viral proteins or venom proteins of bees and wasps) or designed *de novo*. There is little in common among CPP and the only unifying theme seems to be the significant presence of cationic residues (mainly lysine and arginine). Amphipathicity has been suggested to be another common feature. However, this is only true for most CPP – oligoarginine being an exception. There are two methods by which peptide vectors carry their cargoes. Nucleic acids are usually non-covalently (electrostatically) attached, while proteins and other macromolecules are typically covalently coupled (chemical cross-linking or by plasmid fusion). The advantages of electrostatic attachment include convenience and the largely unaltered chemical properties of the cargo. However, charge interactions are non-specific and excess peptides are usually needed to completely bind the plasmid. On the other hand, covalent attachment requires chemical modification of the cargo and usually results in stable complexes which, as discussed earlier, may not be desirable. In the following sections, we will review the key classes of peptide vectors and provide non-exhaustive examples of strategies that have been used to improve their efficiency as vectors.

Peptide	Sequence (single letter code)	Short description
Poly-L-lysine	K_n	Frequently, n = 50-400
Tat	YGRK KRRQ RRRP PQ	HIV-derived, sequence 47-60
Oligoarginine	R_n	Frequently, n = 7-9
Penetratin	RQIK IWFQ NRRM KWKK	3rd helix of Antennapedia homeodomain
Tp	GWTL NSAG YLLG KINL KALA ALAK KIL	Galanin + mastoparan (wasp venom)
Tp10	AGYL LGKI NLKA LAAL AKKI L	First 6 residues deleted from Tp
VP22	300-residue long sequence given in (Elliott & O'Hare, 1997)	HSV-1 structural protein
MPG	GALF LGFL GAAG STMG AWSQ PKSK RKV	HIV gp41 + SV40 T-antigen
CADY	GLWR ALWR LLRS LWRL LWRA	Peptide carrier PPTG1-derived
KALA	WEAK LAKA LAKA LAKH LAKA LAKA LKAC EA	Membrane disruptive peptide, also a carrier
GALA	WEAA LAEA LAEA LAEH LAEA LAEA LEAL AA	Membrane disruptive peptide
EB1	LIRL WSHL IHIW FQNR RLKW KKK	Penetratin analogue
HA2	GLFG AIAG FIEN GWEG MIDG	Influenza virus hemagglutinin protein
INF5	(GLFE AIEG FIEN GWEG nIDG)₂K	HA2-derived, lysine-connected dimer. n = norleucine
INF7	GLFE AIEG FIEN GWEG MIDG WYG	HA2-derived, monomer
SV40	PKKK RKV	Simian virus 40 T antigen NLS
Melittin	GIGA VLKV LTTG LPAL ISWI KRKR QQ	Bee venom

Table 1. The amino acid sequences of all the peptides discussed in this chapter.

4.1 Poly-L-lysine (PLL)

The amino acid sequence of PLL and all other peptides subsequently discussed can be found in Table 1. PLL is the first peptide-based vector to be studied intensively. The molecular weight of PLL spans a wide range and depends on the number of repeating units within a chain, or its degree of polymerisation (DP). For the sake of discussion, the molecular weight of PLL is arbitrarily classified as follows: oligolysine (DP<20), low (20≤DP<50), medium (50≤DP≤400) or high (DP>400). Most studies use PLL of medium molecular weight.

PLL has been successfully employed to deliver a host of different cargos. By covalently coupling human serum albumin or HRP to PLL via amide bonds in a 1-ethyl-3-(3-dimethylaminopropyl) carbodiimide (EDC) catalysed reaction, proteins were delivered into L929 mouse fibroblasts for the first time using such a PLL-mediated strategy (Shen & Ryser, 1978). More recently, streptavidin-conjugated quantum dots (QD) were also attached to biotin-tagged PLL and delivered into HeLa cells (Mok et al., 2008). However, PLL is most frequently used to deliver nucleic acids where the electrostatic attachment is preferred. Although polylysine made out of D-amino acids has been suggested to work better – presumably because they are more resistant to enzymatic degradation (Mitchell et al., 2000) – PLL continues to be favoured in transfection studies. Wu and partner provided one of the earliest examples of PLL being used to condense plasmids for receptor-mediated delivery (Wu & Wu, 1987). In that study, asialoorosomucoid (ASOR) was first covalently attached to PLL with N-succinimidyl 3-(2-pyridyldithio) propionate (SPDP) as a linker and then used to bind a reporter plasmid. Complexes then accumulated within HepG2 cells (ASOR receptor positive) but not in SK-Hep1 cells (ASOR receptor negative).

Plasmids dissociated more slowly if bound to a higher molecular weight PLL and this can negatively affect transfection (Schaffer et al., 2000). To facilitate plasmid release, cysteine residues were added to oligolysine, which was then cross-linked using disulfide bonds (McKenzie et al., 2000). The intention was to make use of the intracellular environment – which is much more reductive due to its elevated levels of glutathione (Lee et al., 2007) – to break down the disulfide bonds for polymer disintegration and plasmid release. The number of lysine, cysteine and histidine (for buffering capacity) residues used and the spacing and ordering between the residues were found to influence the final performance of the vector. Upon optimisation, some constructs transfected at levels that were comparable or even higher than LipofectAce, a commercial reagent used as a positive control (McKenzie et al., 2000). Disulfide-linked oligolysine was then further functionalised with triantennary N-glycan signals to target hepatocytes and evaluated *in vivo* (Kwok et al., 2003). However, contrary to results *in vitro*, the particles were not stable enough in the reductive intracellular liver environment and premature plasmid release ultimately limited gene expression.

PLL by itself is generally not considered to be an efficient vector (Meyer et al., 2008) and is frequently coupled with other agents. The imidazole headgroup of histidine ($pK_a{\sim}6$) can provide endosomal buffering and has been added to PLL to boost transfection (Midoux & Monsigny, 1999). Histidine was also added onto a K15-based oligopeptide which was then self assembled for drug and gene co-delivery (Wiradharma et al., 2009). The HA2 subunit of the hemagglutinin glycoprotein present on the surface of influenza virus plays an important role in the endosomal escape of viruses. To do this, HA2 exhibits a pH-dependent membrane fusion activity. HA2 is not normally lytic at neutral pH. However, protonation of its acidic residues during endo/lysosomal transition triggers HA2 to adopt a more α-helical secondary conformation. At the same time, it exposes a highly-conserved hydrophobic sequence which then interacts and destabilises the endosomal membrane (Wagner et al., 1992a). To exploit this membrane-disrupting mechanism, 20 amino acids corresponding to the N-terminus of HA2 were attached to PLL via cysteine-mediated disulfide bonds. The HA2-functionalised PLL was then shown to induce pH-dependent liposomal leakage (Wagner et al., 1992a) and to augment transfection to a greater extent than the use of chloroquine (Midoux et al., 1993). Melittin, a major component of bee venom, is another peptide with fusogenic activity but unlike HA2, melittin is unresponsive to pH. As such, it remains fusogenic at pH 7 and can indiscriminately disrupt plasma membranes (Chen et al., 2006). To confine fusogenic activity within the endosomes, dimethylmaleic anhydride protecting groups were attached to mask the activity of melittin at neutral pH. Upon cleavage of the protecting groups under acidic conditions, the activity of melittin was restored (Meyer et al., 2008). This protected form of melittin was then coupled to PLL via a cysteine-mediated disulfide bond and the entire construct mediated siRNA knockdown more efficiently than PEI. Adenovirus, known to display pH-dependent membrane disruption as part of its infectious cycle (Curiel et al., 1991), has also been coupled to PLL to improve transfection efficiency. Human adenovirus type 5 (dl312) was either biotinylated and coupled to a streptavidinylated PLL (Wagner et al., 1992b), or simply added as free viral particles into the culture medium to be taken up together with the PLL complexes (Curiel et al., 1991). In another study, chicken embryo lethal orphan virus, an adenovirus from chicken, was attached to PLL and augmented transfection as well as human adenovirus (Cotten et al., 1993).

Various signals have also been added onto PLL to improve its uptake or target specificity. For instance, galactose containing an isothiocyanate group was reacted with the amine groups on PLL to form a thiourea bond and used to mediate gene expression in the livers of rats for up to 140 days (Perales et al., 1994). Mannose and lactose were also used to target cell lines that have receptors for the specific sugar (Midoux et al., 1993). ASOR was coupled onto PLL in an EDC catalysed reaction and intravenously injected into rats (Wu et al., 1989). However, reporter gene expression by liver cells disappeared by day four. Transferrin was coupled to PLL via disulfide bonds in a SPDP-mediated reaction to increase its accumulation within cells (Wagner et al., 1991). Insulin was also coupled to PLL in an SPDP-mediated reaction and used with adenovirus (biotin-streptavidin conjugated) to deliver plasmids into pre-implantation mammalian embryos (Ivanova et al., 1999). PEG was grafted onto PLL via amide bonds in an N-hydroxysuccinimide (NHS) catalysed reaction and helped in preventing particle aggregation (Rimann et al., 2008). Stearyl-PLL mixed with a low density lipoprotein was also used to condense plasmids (~600 nm) into ~100 nm complexes, as measured by atomic force microscopy (Kim et al., 1998). Further, the lipoprotein was found to be essential for efficient uptake. Finally, peptides themselves can serve as targeting signals. For example, a short peptide sequence (GACRRETAWACG) suggested to target $\alpha 5\beta 1$ integrins was linked to K_{16} and mixed with Lipofectin® to transfect neuroblastoma cells (Lee et al., 2003). Several groups have also used the RGD motif to target integrins. A recent example involved RGD being linked to K_{16} peptides, which were then used with an intracellularly cleavable PEG-lipid formulation to deliver plasmids into mice bearing subcutaneous tumors (Tagalakis et al., 2011). The integrin-targeting signal was shown to be important. Upon augmentation by the enhanced permeation and retention effect, the complexes were mainly distributed to the tumor.

4.2 Tat

Full length tat has 86 amino acids (sequence 1-86) and it is a regulatory protein encoded by HIV-1 that transactivates viral gene expression. The ability of tat to cross cell membrane was initially observed by two groups independently in 1988 (Frankel & Pabo, 1988; Green & Loewenstein, 1988). In one study, tat was simply added to a culture of HL3T1 cells modified to contain an integrated copy of chloramphenicol acetyltransferase (CAT, a reporter gene) under the control of the HIV-1 LTR (long terminal repeat) promoter and CAT expression was unexpectedly detected (Frankel & Pabo, 1988). Crucially, the amount of CAT expression was dependent on the dosage of tat. Unlike earlier experiments, tat did not require any help from the scrape loading technique to enter cells. Tat 1-86 was further dissected into five regions and region II and III, together spanning roughly residues 38-62, were identified to be essential and sufficient for transactivation activity (Green & Loewenstein, 1988). Region III (roughly residues 49-62), in particular, was interesting and was rich in arginine and lysine. Furthermore, replacing the three arginines at position 55-57 with alanines drastically reduced transactivation activity. Tat was also observed to localise in the nucleus and thought to be a NLS (Green & Loewenstein, 1988).

The region surrounding the arginine- and lysine-rich domain of tat was keenly evaluated as a gene carrier. Today, full length tat is seldom used and among the many truncated versions being studied (Table 2), tat 47-57 and 48-60 are the two most popular sequences. The *in vivo* half life of free tat 47-57 was calculated to be ~3.5 minutes (Grunwald et al., 2009) and tat 48-60 exists as an unstructured random coil in buffer solutions or when bound to lipid vesicles (Caesar et al., 2006). The secondary structure of a carrier has been suggested to affect its membrane translocation ability. However, it remains unclear if it is better for a structure to be rich in α-helices or unordered. On the one hand, structures rich in α-helices have been suggested to be more efficient in inserting themselves and crossing lipid bilayers (Almeida & Pokorny, 2009). This is consistent with the view that α-helical structures are responsible for the membrane disrupting property of fusogenic peptides such as HA2 (Wagner et al., 1992a), melittin (Chen et al., 2006) and GALA (Subbarao et al., 1987). On the other, α-helices has also been negatively correlated with uptake (Ye et al., 2010). Instead, an unordered structure was preferred as it afforded the flexibility needed to adopt the most energetically favourable conformation during membrane translocation (Caesar et al., 2006).

Entry	Sequence	Reference
1	1-86	(Green & Loewenstein, 1988)
2	1-72	(Frankel & Pabo, 1988)
3	37-72	(Fawell et al., 1994)
4	37-57	(Leonetti et al., 2010)
5	43-60	(Eguchi et al., 2001)
6	47-57	(Wang et al., 2010)
7	48-57	(Wadia et al., 2004)
8	48-58	(Fittipaldi et al., 2003)
9	48-59	(Richard et al., 2005)
10	48-60	(Eiriksdottir et al., 2010)
11	49-57	(Saleh et al., 2010)
12	49-60	(Astriab-Fisher et al., 2000)

Table 2. Heterogeneity in tat sequences being reported in the literature. All sequences are with respect to the original sequence 1-86 in the first entry. Only one reference is provided for each entry, although there may be more discussed in text.

Proteins have been delivered by tat and are usually covalently attached. Fawell and colleagues were the first to chemically conjugate several different proteins onto tat 37-72 (Fawell et al., 1994). One of the model proteins used was β-galactosidase (β-gal), which was grafted onto tat using succinimidyl 4-(N-maleimidomethyl)-cyclohexane-1-carboxylate (SMCC) as a heterobifunctional cross-linker. The β-gal/tat conjugate was then intravenously injected into mice and found to accumulate mainly in the heart, liver and spleen. In a separate study, β-gal/tat 47-57 conjugates were generated by plasmid fusion and injected intraperitoneally into mice (Schwarze et al., 1999). The conjugates were then found to be distributed to all tissues, even across the tight blood-brain-barrier. GFP/tat 47-57 fusion protein was also delivered into cells and uptake was discovered to increase if the cells had been pretreated with 10% dimethylsulfoxide (DMSO) for one hour prior to transfection (Wang et al., 2010). Other macromolecules delivered by tat include peptide nucleic acid (PNA), which are artificial nucleic acid-mimicking polymers. PNA was either conjugated to tat 48-59 using 2-aminoethoxy-2-ethoxyacetic acid as a cross-linker (Richard et al., 2003) or linked via a disulfide bond to a cysteine-modified tat 48-60 (Lundin et al., 2008).

Nucleic acids, on the other hand, are mostly electrostatically carried by tat. For instance, tat 48-60 was used to deliver reporter plasmids into HeLa cells and it was shown that its efficiency can be further improved by adding the SV40 NLS and a dendrimer of seven lysine residues (Yang et al., 2009). A short membrane active peptide, LK15 (KLLKLLLKLLLKLLK) was also conjugated onto tat 49-57 and used for plasmid transfection (Saleh et al., 2010). Antisense oligonucleotides were linked via disulfide bonds to cysteine-modified tat 49-60 and delivered into cells to inhibit the expression of P-glycoprotein, a transmembrane pump that is responsible for the multidrug resistance phenotype of tumor cells (Astriab-Fisher et al., 2000). siRNA has also been delivered by tat 47-57 and interestingly, photostimulation promoted the escape of tat complexes into the cytosol (Endoh et al., 2008). Reactive oxygen species produced during laser illumination was postulated to damage the endosomal vesicles for the enhanced cytosolic access. Finally, tat has also played the role of a helper. As an internalisation enhancer, tat 43-60 was displayed on the surfaces of phage particles to augment the delivery of plasmids encapsulated within the phages (Eguchi et al., 2001). In another study, tat 47-57 was used more as a NLS during the transfection of CHO cells (Moore et al., 2009). Unlike many other systems, the presence of serum augmented tat-mediated transfection (Astriab-Fisher et al., 2000; Eguchi et al., 2001).

Although tat can bring nucleic acids and other macromolecules into a cell, the pathway(s) which tat exploits to do so is ambiguous. There is little consensus in the literature, except for the observation that heparan sulphate, an anionic cell membrane glycosaminoglycan, is crucial for uptake (Sandgren et al., 2002; Tyagi et al., 2001). Besides being rapidly internalised via endocytosis (Tyagi et al., 2001), heparan sulphate is probably also involved in the initial binding step before internalisation (Ferrari et al., 2003). It can also act as a co-receptor for endocytosis (Leonetti et al., 2010). Interestingly, other glycosaminoglycans such as chondroitin sulphate and dermatan sulphate have been ruled out in the binding/internalisation of full length tat 1-86 (Tyagi et al., 2001) and tat 37-57 (Leonetti et al., 2010), but not for the shorter tat 48-60 (Sandgren et al., 2002).

Classical endocytosis is an energy- and ATP-dependent mechanism. For the sake of discussion, endocytosis can be further classified into clathrin-mediated endocytosis, caveolae-mediated endocytosis, macropinocytosis and other forms of clathrin- and caveolae-independent endocytosis. Prompted by the observation that tat 48-60 was internalised at 4°C, a temperature normally considered inhibitory for endocytosis, an energy-independent pathway was initially suggested to be responsible (Futaki et al., 2001b). Another group similarly detected low-temperature internalisation of tat 43-60 and reported that uptake was independent of endocytosis but required the presence of caveolae (Eguchi et al., 2001). The ability of free tat 47-57 to enter cells in the presence of sodium azide, which blocks intracellular ATP synthesis, also led the authors to preclude endocytosis as the uptake mechanism (Ignatovich et al., 2003).

Several models of energy-independent uptake have been proposed. A common theme seems to involve the peptide sticking to the cell membrane and creating a local mass imbalance. At the same time, it transforms itself into a more non-polar compound either due to charge neutralisation (Su et al., 2009) or hydrogen bonding (Rothbard et al., 2004) with the anionic membrane proteins. The peptide then partitions into the hydrophobic lipid bilayer (Rothbard et al., 2002) and translocates through the membrane in a process that is driven by the voltage potential across membrane (Rothbard et al., 2004) and/or the need to relieve membrane curvature stress caused by the mass imbalance in the initial step (Su et al., 2009).

In stark contrast, Richard and colleagues reported that the uptake of tat 48-59, in both its free and PNA conjugated forms were sensitive to low temperature and sodium azide, indicative of classical endocytosis (Richard et al., 2003). Endocytosis is also believed to be responsible for the uptake of protein-conjugated tat 37-72 in another study (Fawell et al., 1994). Having agreed that the uptake of tat requires energy, opinions are once again divided regarding which of the specific endocytosis pathways involved. For instance, a study singled out clathrin-mediated endocytosis as the pathway responsible for the uptake of unconjugated tat 48-59 (Richard et al., 2005). In others, caveolae-mediated endocytosis was suggested to be the dominant form of uptake for GFP/tat 48-60 fusion protein (Ferrari et al., 2003), and also for GFP/tat 48-58 and GFP/tat 1-86 fusion proteins (Fittipaldi et al., 2003). To confound matters, macropinocytosis was reported to be mainly responsible for the uptake of PNA-conjugated tat 48-60 (Lundin et al., 2008) and tat 48-57 fusion protein (Wadia et al., 2004). In yet another twist, multiple pathways involving both clathrin-mediated endocytosis and macropinocytosis were proposed for the internalisation of unconjugated tat 48-60 (Räägel et al., 2009).

With this amount of confusion in the literature, is there hope of reconciliation? It seems that the first step is to recognise that there may not be a single mechanism responsible for the uptake of tat or indeed, other CPP that will be discussed. CPP thus cannot be taken in the same light as transferrin (Rejman et al., 2004) or cholera toxin (Torgersen et al., 2001), which are accepted to be internalised exclusively via the clathrin- and caveolae-mediated pathway respectively in a wide variety of cells. The outcome being observed therefore depends on the combination of cell/peptide/detection method chosen for that experiment and heterogeneity in conclusion can be expected due to the following reasons.

Cell: Different cell lines can use different pathways to internalise tat (Ignatovich et al., 2003). The nature of cells (primary versus immortalised or adherent versus suspension) (Eiriksdottir et al., 2010) and culture conditions such as the type of growth medium (Moulton et al., 2004), passage number of cells or even the Young's modulus (Kong et al., 2005) of the substrate were suggested to influence plasmid transfection and uptake.

Peptide: As can be seen from Table 2, there are at least 12 distinct sequences under the same umbrella name of tat – more if one takes into account chain-end modifications. Considering that simply modifying a few residues can drastically affect the property of tat, as discussed earlier, it is understandable why the literature cannot seem to agree. The concentration of peptide used was also shown to be important. For instance, it was reported that below 10 mM, unconjugated tat 47-57 exploited both macropinocytosis and caveolae-mediated endocytosis to gain entry but once above 10 mM, a non-endocytosis mechanism seemed to operate (Duchardt et al., 2007). Perhaps there is a concentration threshold above which there is sufficient amount of surface-bound peptide to cause the mass imbalance and trigger direct transport through the membrane. Finally, the absence or presence and the nature of the cargo can also influence the mechanism of uptake. For example, unconjugated tat 47-57 was reported to enter cells using an energy-independent mechanism but endocytosis was responsible after a plasmid was bound (Ignatovich et al., 2003).

Detection method: The majority of experiments aimed at studying the endocytosis pathways of peptides uses one or both of the following techniques: 1) assaying the effects of drugs that are known to inhibit specific endocytosis pathways at the uptake (by flow cytometry or confocal microscopy) and/or the gene expression level, or 2) using a confocal microscope to trace for any co-localisation with known markers for endocytosis pathways, e.g., transferrin (clathrin), cholera toxin (caveolae) or dextran (macropinocytosis). While both are sensible experiments, one must also be aware of their limitations. Inhibitory drugs are usually pleiotropic and affect more than one pathway concurrently. For instance, dynasore has been used to shut down the clathrin-mediated pathway (Gratton et al., 2008a). However, dynasore is a drug that interferes with the activity of dynamin, an enzyme that is needed in both clathrin- and caveolae-mediated pathway to pinch off vesicles from the cell membrane

(Macia et al., 2006). The same is true for methyl-β-cyclodextrin, which depletes cholesterol from the membrane (Richard et al., 2005) and cytochalasin, which disrupts actin formation (Belting et al., 2005). Both drugs can affect all three forms of endocytosis. Moreover, any drug that interferes with uptake is usually toxic and a safe effective dosage must be established in order not to affect the conclusion. There is also possible redundancy in the uptake mechanisms whereby shutting off one pathway may activate another (Rodal et al., 1999), further complicating interpretation.

Both flow cytometry and confocal microscopy are fluorescent-based techniques and rely on either the carrier or/and its cargo to be labelled with a dye. However, the process of tagging the peptide with a dye can already affect its property. For example, results from isothermal titration calorimetry showed that unlabelled tat 47-57 binds to heparan sulphate much more strongly that tat 47-57 labelled with fluorescein isothiocyanate (FITC), a florescent dye whose hydrophobicity has been implicated in the weakening of binding affinity (Ziegler et al., 2005). In another study, FITC labelling was also observed to alter the trafficking property of an octaarginine conjugate (Puckett & Barton, 2009). Significantly, fixing of cells has been shown to be undesirable and even mild fixing can cause artifactual intracellular accumulation (Richard et al., 2003). As a result of this revelation, the validity of earlier publications has been challenged, especially in studies where cells were fixed and intracellular accumulation could still be observed despite low temperature incubation. Surface-bound peptides are another source of confusion which must be separated from those which have been truly internalised (Richard et al., 2003). A brief trypsin wash is typically enough to digest and remove most of the surface-bound peptides.

Above all, it is fair to say that our understanding of endocytosis is still not perfect. As mentioned earlier, it is still not clear which other pathways, besides the clathrin-mediated one, can produce vesicles that undergo acidification. Whether vesicles from different origin eventually merge is another unresolved issue. Furthermore, both the size (Choi et al., 2006) and shape (Sharma et al., 2010) can affect the uptake of a particle and its *in vivo* distribution (Decuzzi et al., 2010). However, these physical parameters of tat or other CPP complexes are seldom reported. Great care must also be taken when reporting particle sizes based on light scattering as a recent survey has estimated that up to 90% of the published figures can be erroneous due to inappropriate assumptions being made during measurements (Keck & Muller, 2008). With such a plethora of factors that can affect outcome, it seems more realistic to accept that the uptake of tat or its conjugates cannot be ascribed any particular route.

4.3 Oligoarginine (Arg$_n$, usually n = 7 to 9)

The potential of using arginine for gene delivery was firmly established when it was shown that replacing most of the arginine residues in tat 1-86 with alanine drastically reduced internalisation (Tyagi et al., 2001). Replacing the arginine residues within tat 48-60 with lysine had a similar effect and abolished internalisation (Thoren et al., 2004). Clearly, arginine residues are crucial. However, another important (but less obvious) message from these experiments is that arginine is more than just a cationic residue as replacing it with lysine, another cationic residue, is not good enough.

Oligoarginine of various lengths have been evaluated. In one study, oligoarginine with 4, 6, 8, 10, 12 or 16 residues were compared and it was found that both arg$_4$ and arg$_{10}$ were poorly taken up by cells (Futaki et al., 2001b). Instead, arg$_8$ exhibited the highest rate of internalisation both in its free form or when linked via a disulfide bond to a model carbonic anhydrase protein. This demonstrated that cationic charge was not sufficient to afford efficient uptake. Consistent with this, another study showed that arg_7 was internalised much more efficiently into Jurkat cells than lys_7 and his_7 (Mitchell et al., 2000). There was therefore something unique about the chemical structure of arginine that cannot be explained simply by it carrying a cationic charge. Indeed, the guanidine (pK_a~12) sidegroup of arginine was determined to be key as replacing it with a urea (pK_a~0.1) sidegroup removed internalisation. Urea differs from guanidine by only a single nitrogen atom, which in the former is replaced by an oxygen atom. However, this simple modification removed not only the ability of urea to protonate at neutral pH, but also its ability to form hydrogen bonds. This ability to form stable hydrogen bonds with the anionic phosphates and sulphates on cell membrane was then suggested to be the feature that distinguished arginine from lysine and histidine in terms of translocation efficiency (Mitchell et al., 2000).

The spacing between arginine residues can also influence internalisation (Rothbard et al., 2002). To study this, a library of oligoarginines was synthesised, all with seven residues but separated by 1-6 spacers at all the possible permutations. It was argued that the addition of spacers imparted flexibility to the arginine backbone which was important for better membrane translocation.

A length of 7-9 arginines is usually preferred and the chains exist as random coils in buffer solutions and when bound to lipid vesicles (Caesar et al., 2006). Both D- and L-arginines have been explored with some authors preferring D-arginines (Hyun et al., 2010; Puckett & Barton, 2009) and others finding no difference between the stereoisomers (Mitchell et al., 2000; Nakase et al., 2004). Cargoes of different nature have been delivered. Negatively charged QCs were electrostatically bound to arg_8 and delivered into adipose tissue-derived stem cells for imaging purposes (Yukawa et al., 2010). The anti-cancer drug, taxol was covalently bound to arg_8 via disulfide bonds using a novel linker to increase its water solubility and uptake. The drug was also designed to be released intracellularly so as to combat multidrug resistant cell lines which otherwise have limited accumulation of chemotherapeutic drugs (Dubikovskaya et al., 2008). The immunosuppressive drug, cyclosporine A, was coupled with arg_7 using a novel pH-sensitive linker and used for topical delivery in a skin inflammation model (Rothbard et al., 2000). Phosphorodiamidate morpholino oligomers (PMO) are antisense molecules that interfere with mRNA translation but structurally differ from nucleic acids in several aspects. In one study, PMO was electrostatically carried by an arg_9-based carrier, but the efficiency was not as good as covalently linked ones (Moulton et al., 2004). In another study, a short peptide sequence corresponding to the C-terminus of the cystic fibrosis transmembrane regulator was joined to arg_7 during synthesis and laser illumination was used to trigger the release of the conjugate into the cytosol of U2OS cells (Maiolo-III et al., 2004). siRNA was electrostatically carried by an arg_8-based vector and used to transfect mouse bone marrow-derived dendritic cells (Akita et al., 2010). Finally, D-arg_9 with cysteines added on both terminals (i.e., cys-arg_9-cys) was crosslinked via disulfide bonds to form a mesh of reducible poly(oligoarginine) (Hyun et al., 2010). The carrier was then used to deliver plasmids encoding for heme oxygenase-1 (useful for the treatment of ischemia/reperfusion-induced brain stroke) by direct injection into the brain of mice.

Several modifications have been made to oligoarginine to improve its transfection efficiency. For example, arg_8 has been combined with GALA, a pH sensitive fusogenic peptide to enhance its endosomal escaping property (Akita et al., 2010). The addition of a hydrophobic stearyl chain to arg_8 was also shown to greatly increase its transfection ability (Futaki et al., 2001a). This was suggested to be due to a better association between the hydrophobic moieties on the vector and the lipid bilayer (Putnam, 2006). Indeed, a certain degree of hydrophobicity is a common feature of many efficient vectors and this was clearly shown in a recent study where a novel triblock peptide, phobic$_5$-his$_4$-arg$_8$, was developed (Seow & Yang, 2009b; Seow et al., 2009). This design featured a block of five hydrophobic residues (tryptophan, phenylalanine or isoleucine, in order of increasing hydrophobicity) for enhanced uptake, a middle block of four histidines for buffering capacity and a third block of arg$_8$ for DNA binding and membrane penetration. Removing the hydrophobic block drastically reduced the efficiency of the carrier at both the uptake and gene expression level. Transfection efficiency can also be modulated just by changing the hydrophobicity of the hydrophobic block. The buffering capacity of the carriers was also assessed in a series of acid-base titration experiments and shown to vary with the length of the histidine block used. Each block was then systematically studied and an optimised sequence was used to mediate reporter plasmid expression by direct local injection into mice bearing 4T1 tumors. In another study, cholesterol was added as the hydrophobic end of a his5/10-arg10 vector for gene delivery (Guo et al., 2008).

The internalisation of oligoarginine is sharply inhibited by the presence of heparin, which competes with heparan sulphate for binding (Seow et al., 2009). This shows that heparan sulphate is crucial for uptake. Low-temperature internalisation was observed and energy-independence was originally proposed to characterise the uptake of oligoarginine (Futaki et al., 2001b). However, those observation was made with fixed cells. In response to studies that had exposed the flaws of using fixed cells (Richard et al., 2003), authors of the original study re-evaluated the uptake mechanism using live cells. Consequently, they reported macropinocytosis to be a major, but not exclusive pathway for the uptake of oligoarginine (Nakase et al., 2004). Macropinocytosis was also proposed to be the main form of uptake for protein-conjugated (Takayama et al., 2009) and siRNA-bound arg$_8$ (Akita et al., 2010). Nonetheless, an energy-independent form of uptake was still suggested if the concentration of unconjugated arg$_9$ exceeded 10 mM – otherwise, macropinocytosis and caveolae-mediated, but not clathrin-mediated endocytosis seemed to be important (Duchardt et al., 2007). Another study reported that both clathrin-mediated endocytosis and macropinocytosis play a role for the uptake of unconjugated arg$_9$ (Räägel et al., 2009). On the other hand, all three forms of endocytosis (clathrin-mediated, caveolae-mediated and macropinocytosis) were found to be responsible for the uptake of plasmid-bound oligoarginine complexes (Seow et al., 2009). Finally, an energy-dependent but non-endocytosis mechanism was also proposed to be responsible for uptake (Mitchell et al., 2000). Like tat, there is little consensus over the internalisation pathway(s) of oligoarginine, although endocytosis is generally accepted to play a key role in most cases (Richard et al., 2003; Rothbard et al., 2000).

4.4 Penetratin

Homeoproteins are regulatory proteins essential for proper physical development. The DNA binding domain of these proteins is made up of a highly conserved sequence known as the homeobox. The homeobox of the *Drosophila* antennapedia gene (pAntp) is 60-amino acid long (sequence 1-60) and contains three α-helices (Derossi et al., 1994). pAntp was first discovered to effectively translocate into nerve cells and accumulate within their nuclei (Joliot et al., 1991). To demonstrate the usefulness of pAntp as a carrier, a 33-residue peptide cargo corresponding to the C-terminus of rab3, a GTP-binding protein in human, was linked to pAntp via plasmid fusion and shown to translocate into the nuclei of myoblasts and neurons (Perez et al., 1992). A study later revealed that the third helix was actually the domain driving internalisation (Roux et al., 1993). Based on this, penetratin, a 16-residue peptide within the third helix (sequence 43-58 of the original pAntp) was described (Derossi et al., 1994). Penetratin demonstrated membrane penetrating ability but was prone to aggregation. Aggregated particles can enjoy better internalisation due to a sedimentation effect which promotes a more intimate particle-cell contact (Luo & Saltzman, 2000b). While this may have helped the internalisation of penetratin, aggregation alone was excluded as the dominant reason for its efficient internalisation (Derossi et al., 1994).

The secondary structure of penetratin in buffer is unstructured but becomes α-helical when bound to lipid vesicles (Caesar et al., 2006). Raman microscopy on live cells further showed that penetratin within the cytosol was either unstructured or in the β-sheet conformation (Ye et al., 2010). The arginine residues within penetratin are important as replacing them with lysine greatly reduced its translocation ability (Caesar et al., 2006). Various cargoes have been carried by penetratin. Antisense oligonucleotides (Astriab-Fisher et al., 2000), PNA (Lundin et al., 2008) and luciferin protein (Eiriksdottir et al., 2010) have all been coupled onto a cysteine-modified penetratin via disulfide bonds and delivered into cells. siRNA was electrostatically bound to penetratin and although the complexes accumulated favourably within cells, there was limited silencing activity (Lundberg et al., 2007). HA2 was then added to enhance endosomal escape but produced only a modest improvement. Penetratin has been evaluated *in vivo*. In one study, penetratin was directly injected into a rat's brain and the peptide was observed to spread away from the site of injection (Bolton et al., 2000). However, dosage-dependent cell death and inflammatory responses were also provoked.

Penetratin was initially suggested to enter cells using energy-independent mechanisms (Derossi et al., 1994; Perez et al., 1992; Roux et al., 1993), but a caveat is that fixed cells were used in those studies. Nonetheless, an energy-independent mechanism was still suggested to be possible past a concentration threshold of 40 mM, below which all three forms of endocytosis should dominate (Duchardt et al., 2007). Endocytosis was also reported to be responsible for the uptake of siRNA-bound penetratin (Lundberg et al., 2007) while macropinocytosis was suggested to be the main form of uptake for PNA-conjugated penetratin (Lundin et al., 2008).

4.5 Transportan (Tp) and Tp10

Tp uses a lysine residue to join the first 12 N-terminus residues of the neuropeptide, galanin, to the 14 C-terminus residues of the wasp venom, mastoparan. Tp is thus 27 residues long (sequence 1-27) and was first shown to penetrate Bowes' melanoma cells rapidly and efficiently (Pooga et al., 1998). However, Tp at a high concentration was found to inhibit the GTPase activity of cells. To overcome this side effect, a series of Tp analogues was prepared (Soomets et al., 2000). This led to the identification of Tp10 which, upon deleting the first 6 residues of Tp (i.e., sequence 7-27 remaining), was internalised as efficiently as Tp but did not have any effect on the GTPases.

PNA (Lundin et al., 2008) and luciferin (Eiriksdottir et al., 2010) were conjugated to both cysteine-modified Tp and Tp10 via disulfide bonds. siRNA was also electrostatically bound to Tp10 but had little silencing effects when transfected into cells (Lundberg et al., 2007). This was surprising insofar as Tp10 was shown earlier to mediate good levels of plasmid expression. This however resonates with comments made by other researchers (Mahon et al., 2010; unpublished observation) who had observed that a carrier's efficiency in plasmid delivery may not automatically apply to the delivery of the shorter and stiffer siRNA molecules. Earlier studies with fixed cells reported low temperature internalisation of Tp

(Pooga et al., 1998) but more recent observations have linked endocytosis to the uptake of both Tp and Tp10 (Lundin et al., 2008).

4.6 Other notable peptide sequences

VP22 is a 300-residue long peptide derived from the structural protein of HSV-1 and has been used successfully to deliver GFP as a fusion protein (Elliott & O'Hare, 1997). When COS-1 cells were microinjected with plasmids encoding for VP22, an interesting pattern was observed in which a central cell would first express VP22 and exhibit cytosolic staining when probed with anti-VP22 antibodies. The VP22 peptide was then excreted and could infect neighbouring cells before eventually localising to their nuclei. CADY is a 20-residue long peptide evaluated for siRNA delivery (Crombez et al., 2009). It changes from unordered to being α-helical in the presence of lipid vesicles which then drives its internalisation independently of the endosomal pathway (Konate et al., 2010). MPG is a 27-residue peptide designed to have a hydrophobic domain (sequence 1-17) derived from HIV gp41 and a NLS domain (sequence 21-27) derived from SV40 separated by a "trp-ser-gln" unit (Morris et al., 1997). The uptake of MPG/oligonucleotide complexes was shown to be rapid and independent of the endosomal pathway. Other carriers explored for delivery include KALA (Wyman et al., 1997) and EB1 (Lundberg et al., 2007).

Throughout the discussion, various peptides with fusogenic and nuclear localising properties were introduced. SV40 is the classical NLS and different sequences exist. The most commonly used sequence for SV40 is provided in Table 1. Other sequences include "glu-asp-pro-tyr" (Trentin et al., 2005) and "glu-pro-tyr-cys" (Moore et al., 2009) being added onto the C-terminus and an even longer form of SV40 has been described (Eguchi et al., 2001). INF 5 and INF 7 are examples of two commonly used fusogenic peptide and both are derived from the parent HA2 peptide (Plank et al., 1994). GALA is a 30-amino acid long pH-sensitive fusogenic peptide (Subbarao et al., 1987). Upon protonation of its glu residues, its secondary structure changes from unordered at neutral pH to being α-helical in acidic environments. Both the amphipathicity and degree of α-helicity have been correlated with the ability of GALA to interact and destabilise membranes (Parente et al., 1990).

5. Conclusion

This chapter started by discussing the challenges and intracellular barriers associated with the delivery of nucleic acids. Strategies used to overcome these hurdles were next examined, mainly in the context of peptide-derived vectors. It is clear that peptide carriers are not characterised by any typical sequences, although the majority of current designs rely on cationic residues to bind nucleic acids. This strategy, nonetheless, may be problematic during *in vivo* applications. An area that deserves more attention is the development of vectors that can bind nucleic acids using non-electrostatic forces, e.g., by including more hydrophobic residues. The stability and *in vivo* behaviour of such vectors then need to be thoroughly evaluated. Another challenge is to further improve strategies that are already in place to shield the cationic charges, e.g., by attaching PEG chains that are intracellularly cleavable so as to increase the circulation time of the complexes without compromising excessively on transfection efficiency. Advances in either will enable peptides to further realise their potential as a class of non-viral vector.

6. References

Akinrimisi, E. O., Bonner, J. & Ts'o, P. O. P. (1965). Binding of basic proteins to DNA. *Journal of Molecular Biology*, Vol. 11, pp. 128-136.

Akita, H., et al. (2010). Nanoparticles for *ex vivo* siRNA delivery to dendritic cells for cancer vaccines: programmed endosomal escape and dissociation. *Journal of Controlled Release*, Vol. 143, pp. 311-317.

Almeida, P. F. & Pokorny, A. (2009). Mechanisms of antimicrobial, cytolytic, and cell-penetrating peptides: from kinetics to thermodynamics. *Biochemistry*, Vol. 48, pp. 8083-8093.

Astriab-Fisher, A., et al. (2000). Antisense inhibition of P-glycoprotein expression using peptide-oligonucleotide conjugates. *Biochemical Pharmacology*, Vol. 60, pp. 83-90.

Belting, M., Sandgren, S. & Wittrup, A. (2005). Nuclear delivery of macromolecules: barriers and carriers. *Advanced Drug Delivery Reviews*, Vol. 57, pp. 505-527.

Bolton, S. J., et al. (2000). Cellular uptake and spread of the cell-permeable peptide penetratin in adult rat brain. *European Journal of Neuroscience*, Vol. 12, pp. 2847-2855.

Boussif, O., et al. (1995). A versatile vector for gene and oligonucleotide transfer into cells in culture and in vivo: polyethylenimine. *Proceedings of the National Academy of Sciences*, Vol. 92, pp. 7297-7301.

Caesar, C. E. B., et al. (2006). Membrane interactions of cell-penetrating peptides probed by tryptophan fluorescence and dichroism techniques: correlations of structure to cellular uptake. *Biochemistry*, Vol. 45, pp. 7682-7692.

Cavazzana-Calvo, M., et al. (2010). Transfusion independence and HMGA2 activation after gene therapy of human β-thalassaemia. *Nature*, Vol. 467, pp. 318-323.

Chang, K.-L., et al. (2010). Efficient gene transfection by histidine-modified chitosan through enhancement of endosomal escape. *Bioconjugate Chemistry*, Vol. 21, pp. 1087-1095.

Chen, C.-P., et al. (2006). Gene transfer with poly-melittin peptides. *Bioconjugate Chemistry*, Vol. 17, pp. 1057-1062.

Chen, C. & Okayama, H. (1987). High-efficiency transformation of mammalian cells by plasmid DNA. *Molecular and Cellular Biology*, Vol. 7, pp. 2745-2752.

Choi, H. S., et al. (2006). An insight into the gene delivery mechanism of the arginine peptide system: role of the peptide/DNA complex size. *Biochimica et Biophysica Acta*, Vol. 1760, pp. 1604-1612.

Cotten, M., et al. (1993). Chicken adenovirus (CELO virus) particles augment receptor-mediated DNA delivery to mammalian cells and yield exceptional levels of stable transformants. *Journal of Virology*, Vol. 67, pp. 3777-3785.

Crombez, L., et al. (2009). A new potent secondary amphipathic cell–penetrating peptide for siRNA delivery into mammalian cells. *Molecular Therapy*, Vol. 17, pp. 95-103.

Curiel, D. T., et al. (1991). Adenovirus enhancement of transferrin-polylysine-mediated gene delivery. *Proceedings of the National Academy of Sciences*, Vol. 88, pp. 8850-8854.

Decuzzi, P., et al. (2010). Size and shape effects in the biodistribution of intravascularly injected particles. *Journal of Controlled Release*, Vol. 141, pp. 320-327.

Derossi, D., et al. (1994). The third helix of the antennapedia homeodornain translocates through biological membranes. *Journal of Biological Chemistry*, Vol. 269, pp. 10444-10450.

Deshayes, A., Herrera-Estrella, L. & Caboche, M. (1985). Liposome-mediated transformation of tobacco mesophyll protoplasts by an Escherichia coli plasmid. *EMBO Journal*, Vol. 4, pp. 2731-2737.

Diebold, S. S., et al. (1999). Mannose polyethylenimine conjugates for targeted DNA delivery into dendritic cells. *Journal of Biological Chemistry*, Vol. 274, pp. 19087-19094.

Doxsey, S. J., et al. (1985). An efficient method for introducing macromolecules into living cells. *Journal of Cell Biology*, Vol. 101, pp. 19-27.

Dubikovskaya, E. A., et al. (2008). Overcoming multidrug resistance of small-molecule therapeutics through conjugation with releasable octaarginine transporters. *Proceedings of the National Academy of Sciences*, Vol. 105, pp. 12128-12133.

Duchardt, F., et al. (2007). A comprehensive model for the cellular uptake of cationic cell-penetrating peptides. *Traffic*, Vol. 8, pp. 848-866.

Duncan, R. (2006). Polymer conjugates as anticancer nanomedicines. *Nature Reviews Cancer*, Vol. 6, pp. 688-701.

Eguchi, A., et al. (2001). Protein transduction domain of HIV-1 tat protein promotes efficient delivery of DNA into mammalian cells. *Journal of Biological Chemistry*, Vol. 276, pp. 26204-26210.

Eiriksdottir, E., et al. (2010). Cellular internalization kinetics of (luciferin-)cell-penetrating peptide conjugates. *Bioconjugate Chemistry*, Vol. 21, pp. 1662-1672.

Elliott, G. & O'Hare, P. (1997). Intercellular trafficking and protein delivery by a herpesvirus structural protein. *Cell*, Vol. 88, pp. 223-233.

Endoh, T., Sisido, M. & Ohtsuki, T. (2008). Cellular siRNA delivery mediated by a cell-permeant RNA-binding protein and photoinduced RNA interference. *Bioconjugate Chemistry*, Vol. 19, pp. 1017-1024.

Fawell, S., et al. (1994). Tat-mediated delivery of heterologous proteins into cells. *Proceedings of the National Academy of Sciences*, Vol. 91, pp. 664-668.

Felgner, P. L., et al. (1987). Lipofection: a highly efficient, lipid-mediated DNA-transfection procedure. *Proceedings of the National Academy of Sciences*, Vol. 84, pp. 7413-7417.

Ferrari, A., et al. (2003). Caveolae-mediated internalization of extracellular HIV-1 tat fusion proteins visualized in real time. *Molecular Therapy*, Vol. 8, pp. 284-294.

Fire, A., et al. (1998). Potent and specific genetic interference by double-stranded RNA in Caenorhabditis elegans. *Nature*, Vol. 391, pp. 806-811.

Fittipaldi, A., et al. (2003). Cell membrane lipid rafts mediate caveolar endocytosis of HIV-1 tat fusion proteins. *Journal of Biological Chemistry*, Vol. 278, pp. 34141-34149.

Frankel, A. D. & Pabo, C. O. (1988). Cellular uptake of the tat protein from human immunodeficiency virus. *Cell*, Vol. 55, pp. 1189-1193.

Frenkel, V. (2008). Ultrasound mediated delivery of drugs and genes to solid tumors. *Advanced Drug Delivery Reviews*, Vol. 60, pp. 1193-1208.

Funhoff, A. M., et al. (2005). PEG shielded polymeric double-layered micelles for gene delivery. *Journal of Controlled Release*, Vol. 102, pp. 711-724.

Futaki, S., et al. (2001a). Stearylated arginine-rich peptides: a new class of transfection systems. *Bioconjugate Chemistry*, Vol. 12, pp. 1005-1011.

Futaki, S., et al. (2001b). Arginine-rich Peptides: an abundant source of membrane-permeable peptides having potential as carriers for intracellular protein delivery. *Journal of Biological Chemistry*, Vol. 276, pp. 5836-5840.

Gabrielson, N. P. & Pack, D. W. (2006). Acetylation of polyethylenimine enhances gene delivery via weakened polymer/DNA interactions. *Biomacromolecules*, Vol. 7, pp. 2427-2435.

Gao, X. & Huang, L. (1996). Potentiation of cationic liposome-mediated gene delivery by polycations. *Biochemistry*, Vol. 35, pp. 1027-1036.

Godbey, W. T., Wu, K. K. & Mikos, A. G. (1999). Tracking the intracellular path of poly(ethylenimine)/DNA complexes for gene delivery. *Proceedings of the National Academy of Sciences*, Vol. 96, pp. 5177-5181.

Guo, X. D., et al. (2008). Cationic micelles self-assembled from cholesterol-conjugated oligopeptides as an efficient gene delivery vector. *Biomaterials*, Vol. 29, pp. 4838-4846.

Graham, F. L. & Eb, A. J. V. D. (1973). A new technique for the assay of infectivity of human adenovirus 5 DNA. *Virology*, Vol. 52, pp. 456-467.

Gratton, S. E. A., et al. (2008a). Microfabricated particles for engineered drug therapies: elucidation into the mechanisms of cellular internalization of PRINT particles. *Pharmaceutical Research*, Vol. 25, pp. 2845-2852.

Gratton, S. E. A., et al. (2008b). The effect of particle design on cellular internalization pathways. *Proceedings of the National Academy of Sciences*, Vol. 105, pp. 11613-11618.

Green, J. J., et al. (2006). Biodegradable polymeric vectors for gene delivery to human endothelial cells. *Bioconjugate Chemistry*, Vol. 17, pp. 1162-1169.

Green, M. & Loewenstein, P. M. (1988). Autonomous functional domains of chemically synthesized human immunodeficiency virus tat trans-activator protein. *Cell*, Vol. 55, pp. 1179-1188,.

Griesenbach, U. & Alton, E. W. F. W. (2009). On behalf of the UK Cystic Fibrosis Gene Therapy Consortium. Gene transfer to the lung: lessons learned from more than 2 decades of CF gene therapy. *Advanced Drug Delivery Reviews*, Vol. 61, pp. 128-139.

Grunwald, J., et al. (2009). Tat peptide and its conjugates: proteolytic stability. *Bioconjugate Chemistry*, Vol. 20, pp. 1531-1537.

Hacein-Bey-Abina, S., et al. (2003). LMO2-associated clonal T cell proliferation in two patients after gene therapy for SCID-X1. *Science*, Vol. 302, pp. 415-419.

Hollon, T. (2000). Researchers and regulators reflect on first gene therapy death. *Nature Medicine*, Vol. 6, p. 6.

Hossann, M., et al. (2010). Size of thermosensitive liposomes influences content release. *Journal of Controlled Release*, Vol. 147, pp. 436-443.

Hyun, H., et al. (2010). Therapeutic effects of a reducible poly (oligo-D-arginine) carrier with the heme oxygenase-1 gene in the treatment of hypoxic-ischemic brain injury. *Biomaterials*, Vol. 31, pp. 9128-9134.

Ignatovich, I. A., et al. (2003). Complexes of plasmid DNA with basic domain 47–57 of the HIV-1 tat protein are transferred to mammalian cells by endocytosis-mediated pathways. *Journal of Biological Chemistry*, Vol. 278, pp. 42625-42636.

Ivanova, M. M., et al. (1999). Receptor-mediated transport of foreign DNA into preimplantation mammalian embryos. *Molecular Reproduction and Development*, Vol. 54, pp. 112-120.

Joliot, A., et al. (1991). Antennapedia homeobox peptide regulates neural morphogenesis. *Proceedings of the National Academy of Sciences*, Vol. 88, pp. 1864-1868.

Kay, M. A., Glorioso, J. C. & Naldini, L. (2001). Viral vectors for gene therapy: the art of turning infectious agents into vehicles of therapeutics. *Nature Medicine*, Vol. 7, pp. 33-40.

Keck, C. M. & Muller, R. H. (2008). Size analysis of submicron particles by laser diffractometry—90% of the published measurements are false. *International Journal of Pharmaceutics*, Vol. 355, pp. 150-163.

Kim, J.-S., et al. (1998). A new non-viral DNA delivery vector: the terplex system. *Journal of Controlled Release*, Vol. 53, pp. 175-182.

Kircheis, R., et al. (1997). Coupling of cell-binding ligands to polyethylenimine for targeted gene delivery. *Gene Therapy*, Vol. 4, pp. 409-418.

Konate, K., et al. (2010). Insight into the cellular uptake mechanism of a secondary amphipathic cell-penetrating peptide for siRNA delivery. *Biochemistry*, Vol. 49, pp. 3393-3402.

Kong, H. J., et al. (2005). Non-viral gene delivery regulated by stiffness of cell adhesion substrates. *Nature Materials*, Vol. 4, pp. 460-464.

Koping-Hoggard, M., et al. (2004). Improved chitosan-mediated gene delivery based on easily dissociated chitosan polyplexes of highly defined chitosan oligomers. *Gene Therapy*, Vol. 11, pp. 1441-1452.

Kwok, K. Y., et al. (2003). In vivo gene transfer using sulfhydryl cross-linked PEG-peptide/glycopeptide DNA co-condensates. *Journal of Pharmaceutical Sciences*, Vol. 92, pp. 1174-1185.

Lam, A. P. & Dean, D. A. (2010). Progress and prospects: nuclear import of nonviral vectors. *Gene Therapy*, Vol. 17, pp. 439-447.

Lee, L. K., et al. (2003). Biophysical characterization of an integrin-targeted non-viral vector. *Medical Science Monitor*, Vol. 9, pp. BR54-61.

Lee, Y., et al. (2007). Visualization of the degradation of a disulfide polymer, linear poly(ethylenimine sulfide), for gene delivery. *Bioconjugate Chemistry*, Vol. 18, pp. 13-18.

Leonetti, M., Gadzinski, A. & Moine, G. (2010). Cell surface heparan sulfate proteoglycans influence MHC class II-restricted antigen presentation. *Journal of Immunology*, Vol. 185, pp. 3847-3856.

Liang, H., Harries, D. & Wong, G. C. L. (2005). Polymorphism of DNA–anionic liposome complexes reveals hierarchy of ion-mediated interactions. *Proceedings of the National Academy of Sciences*, Vol. 102, pp. 11173-11178.

Lin, C., et al. (2007). Novel bioreducible poly(amido amine)s for highly efficient gene delivery. *Bioconjugate Chemistry*, Vol. 18, pp. 138-145.

Lin, S., et al. (2008). An acid-labile block copolymer of PDMAEMA and PEG as potential carrier for intelligent gene delivery systems. *Biomacromolecules*, Vol. 9, pp. 109-115.

Liu, X., Yang, J. W. & Lynn, D. M. (2008). Addition of "charge-shifting" side chains to linear poly(ethyleneimine) enhances cell transfection efficiency. *Biomacromolecules*, Vol. 9, pp. 2063–2071.

Lundberg, P., et al. (2007). Delivery of short interfering RNA using endosomolytic cell-penetrating peptides. *The FASEB Journal*, Vol. 21, pp. 2664-2671.

Lundin, P., et al. (2008). Distinct uptake routes of cell-penetrating peptide conjugates. *Bioconjugate Chemistry*, Vol. 19, pp. 2535-2542.

Luo, D. & Saltzman, W. M. (2000a). Synthetic DNA delivery systems. *Nature Biotechnology*, Vol. 18, pp. 33-37.

Luo, D. & Saltzman, W. M. (2000b). Enhancement of transfection by physical concentration of DNA at the cell surface. *Nature Biotechnology*, Vol. 18, pp. 893-895.

Macia, E., et al. (2006). Dynasore, a cell-permeable inhibitor of dynamin. *Developmental Cell*, Vol. 10, pp. 839-850.

MacLaughlin, F. C., et al. (1998). Chitosan and depolymerized chitosan oligomers as condensing carriers for in vivo plasmid delivery. *Journal of Controlled Release*, Vol. 56, pp. 259-272.

Mahon, K. P., et al. (2010). Combinatorial approach to determine functional group effects on lipidoid-mediated siRNA delivery. *Bioconjugate Chemistry*, Vol. 21, pp. 1448-1454.

Maiolo-III, J. R., Ottinger, E. A. & Ferrer, M. (2004). Specific redistribution of cell-penetrating peptides from endosomes to the cytoplasm and nucleus upon laser illumination. *Journal of the American Chemical Society*, Vol. 126, pp. 15376-15377.

McKenzie, D. L., et al. (2000). Low molecular weight disulfide cross-linking peptides as nonviral gene delivery carriers. *Bioconjugate Chemistry*, Vol. 11, pp. 901-909.

McManus, J. J., Radler, J. O. & Dawson, K. A. (2004). Observation of a rectangular columnar phase in a DNA-calcium-zwitterionic lipid complex. *Journal of the American Chemical Society*, Vol. 126, pp. 15966-15967.

McNeil, P. L., et al. (1984). A method for incorporating macromolecules into adherent cells. *Journal of Cell Biology*, Vol. 98, pp. 1556-1564.

Merediz, S. A. K., et al. (2000). Ballistic transfer of minimalistic immunologically defined expression constructs for IL4 and CTLA4 into the corneal epithelium in mice after orthotopic corneal allograft transplantation. *Graefe's Archive for Clinical and Experimental Ophthalmology*, Vol. 238, pp. 701-707.

Mével, M., et al. (2010). DODAG; a versatile new cationic lipid that mediates efficient delivery of pDNA and siRNA. *Journal of Controlled Release*, Vol. 143, pp. 222-232.

Meyer, M., et al. (2008). Breathing life into polycations: functionalization with pH-responsive endosomolytic peptides and polyethylene glycol enables siRNA delivery. *Journal of the American Chemical Society*, Vol. 130, pp. 3272-3273.

Midoux, P., et al. (1993). Specific gene transfer mediated by lactosylated poly-L-lysine into hepatoma cells. *Nucleic Acids Research*, Vol. 21, pp. 871-878.

Midoux, P. & Monsigny, M. (1999). Efficient gene transfer by histidylated polylysine/pDNA complexes. *Bioconjugate Chemistry*, Vol. 10, pp. 406-411.

Mitchell, D. J., et al. (2000). Polyarginine enters cells more efficiently than other polycationic homopolymers. *Journal of Peptide Research*, Vol. 56, pp. 318-325.

Mok, H., Park, J. W. & Park, T. G. (2008). Enhanced intracellular delivery of quantum dot and adenovirus nanoparticles triggered by acidic pH via surface charge reversal. *Bioconjugate Chemistry*, Vol. 19, pp. 797-801.

Moore, N. M., Sheppard, C. L. & Sakiyama-Elbert, S. E. (2009). Characterization of a multifunctional PEG-based gene delivery system containing nuclear localization signals and endosomal escape peptides. *Acta Biomaterialia*, Vol. 5, pp. 854-864.

Morris, M. C., et al. (1997). A new peptide vector for efficient delivery of oligonucleotides into mammalian cells. *Nucleic Acids Research*, Vol. 25, pp. 2730-2736.

Moulton, H. M., et al. (2004). Cellular uptake of antisense morpholino oligomers conjugated to arginine-rich peptides. *Bioconjugate Chemistry*, Vol. 15, pp. 290-299.

Nakase, I., et al. (2004). Cellular uptake of arginine-rich peptides: roles for macropinocytosis and actin rearrangement. *Molecular Therapy*, Vol. 10, pp. 1011-1022.

Nayak, S. & Herzog, R. W. (2010). Progress and prospects: immune responses to viral vectors. *Gene Therapy*, Vol. 17, pp. 295-304.

Niidome, T., et al. (1997). Binding of cationic α-helical peptides to plasmid DNA and their gene transfer abilities into cells. *Journal of Biological Chemistry*, Vol. 272, pp. 15307-15312.

Okada, C. Y. & Rechsteiner, M. (1982). Introduction of macromolecules into cultured mammalian cells by osmotic lysis of pinocytic vesicles. *Cell*, Vol. 29, pp. 33-41.

Ott, M. G., et al. (2006). Correction of X-linked chronic granulomatous disease by gene therapy, augmented by insertional activation of *MDS1-EVI1*, *PRDM16* or *SETBP1*. *Nature Medicine*, Vol. 12, pp. 401-409.

Palm-Apergi, C., et al. (2009). The membrane repair response masks membrane disturbances caused by cell-penetrating peptide uptake. *The FASEB Journal*, Vol. 23, pp. 214-223.

Parente, R. A., et al. (1990). Association of a pH-sensitive peptide with membrane vesicles: role of amino acid sequence. *Biochemistry*, Vol. 29, pp. 8713-8719.

Park, T. G., Jeong, J. H. & Kim, S. W. (2006). Current status of polymeric gene delivery systems. *Advanced Drug Delivery Reviews*, Vol. 58, pp. 467-486.

Pelkmans, L. & Helenius, A. (2002). Endocytosis via caveolae. *Traffic*, Vol. 3, pp. 311-320.

Perales, J. C., et al. (1994). Gene transfer in vivo: sustained expression and regulation of genes introduced into the liver by receptor-targeted uptake. *Proceedings of the National Academy of Sciences*, Vol. 91, pp. 4086-4090.

Perez, F., et al. (1992). Antennapedia homeobox as a signal for the cellular internalization and nuclear addressing of a small exogenous peptide. *Journal of Cell Science*, Vol. 102, pp. 717-722.

Plank, C., et al. (1994). The influence of endosome-disruptive peptides on gene transfer using synthetic virus-like gene transfer systems. *Journal of Biological Chemistry*, Vol. 269, pp. 12918-12924.

Pooga, M., et al. (1998). Cell penetration by transportan. *The FASEB Journal*, Vol. 12, pp. 67-77.

Pouton, C. W. & Seymour, L. W. (2001). Key issues in non-viral gene delivery. *Advanced Drug Delivery Reviews*, Vol. 46, pp. 187-203.

Puckett, C. A. & Barton, J. K. (2009). Fluorescein redirects a ruthenium-octaarginine conjugate to the nucleus. *Journal of the American Chemical Society*, Vol. 131, pp. 8738-8739.

Putnam, D. (2006). Polymers for gene delivery across length scales. *Nature Medicine*, Vol. 5, pp. 439-451.

Räägel, H., et al. (2009). CPP–protein constructs induce a population of non-acidic vesicles during trafficking through endo-lysosomal pathway. *Journal of Controlled Release*, Vol. 139, pp. 108-117.

Rejman, J., et al. (2004). Size-dependent internalization of particles via the pathways of clathrin and caveolae-mediated endocytosis. *Biochemical Journal*, Vol. 377, pp. 159-169.

Ren, Y., et al. (2010). Charge density and molecular weight of polyphosphoramidate gene carrier are key parameters influencing its DNA compaction ability and transfection efficiency. *Biomacromolecules*, Vol. 11, pp. 3432-3439.

Richard, J. P., et al. (2005). Cellular uptake of unconjugated tat peptide involves clathrin dependent endocytosis and heparan sulfate receptors. *Journal of Biological Chemistry*, Vol. 280, pp. 15300-15306.

Richard, J. P., et al. (2003). Cell-penetrating peptides: a reevaluation of the mechanism of cellular uptake. *Journal of Biological Chemistry*, Vol. 278, pp. 585-590.

Rimann, M., et al. (2008). Characterization of PLL-g-PEG-DNA nanoparticles for the delivery of therapeutic DNA. *Bioconjugate Chemistry*, Vol. 19, pp. 548-557.

Rodal, S. K., et al. (1999). Extraction of cholesterol with methyl-β-cyclodextrin perturbs formation of clathrin-coated endocytic vesicles. *Molecular Biology of the Cell*, Vol. 10, pp. 961-974.

Rothbard, J. B., et al. (2000). Conjugation of arginine oligomers to cyclosporin A facilitates topical delivery and inhibition of inflammation. *Nature Medicine*, Vol. 6, pp. 1253-1257.

Rothbard, J. B., et al. (2004). Role of membrane potential and hydrogen bonding in the mechanism of translocation of guanidinium-rich peptides into cells. *Journal of the American Chemical Society*, Vol. 126, pp. 9506-9507.

Rothbard, J. B., et al. (2002). Arginine-rich molecular transporters for drug delivery: role of backbone spacing in cellular uptake. *Journal of Medicinal Chemistry*, Vol. 45, pp. 3612-3618.

Roux, I. L., et al. (1993). Neurotrophic activity of the Antennapedia homeodomain depends on its specific DNA-binding properties. *Proceedings of the National Academy of Sciences*, Vol. 90, pp. 9120-9124.

Sahay, G., Alakhova, D. Y. & Kabanov, A. V. (2010). Endocytosis of nanomedicines. *Journal of Controlled Release*, Vol. 145, pp. 182-195.

Saleh, A. F., et al. (2010). Improved Tat-mediated plasmid DNA transfer by fusion to LK15 peptide. *Journal of Controlled Release*, Vol. 143, pp. 233-242.

Sandgren, S., Cheng, F. & Belting, M. (2002). Nuclear targeting of macromolecular polyanions by an HIV-Tat derived peptide role for cell-surface proteoglycans. *Journal of Biological Chemistry*, Vol. 277, pp. 38877-38883.

Schaffer, D. V., et al. (2000). Vector unpacking as a potential barrier for receptor-mediated polyplex gene delivery. *Biotechnology and Bioengineering*, Vol. 67, pp. 598-606.

Schlegel, R. A. & Rechsteiner, M. C. (1975). Microinjection of thymidine kinase and bovine serum albumin into mammalian cells by fusion with red blood cells. *Cell*, Vol. 5, pp. 371-379.

Schwarze, S. R., et al. (1999). In vivo protein transduction: delivery of a biologically active protein into the mouse. *Science*, Vol. 285, pp. 1569-1572.

Semple, S. C., et al. (2010). Rational design of cationic lipids for siRNA delivery. *Nature Biotechnology*, Vol. 28, pp. 172-178.

Seow, W. Y. & Yang, Y.-Y. (2009a). Functional polycarbonates and their self-assemblies as promising non-viral vectors. *Journal of Controlled Release*, Vol. 139, pp. 40-47.

Seow, W. Y. & Yang, Y.-Y. (2009b). A class of cationic triblock amphiphilic oligopeptides as efficient gene delivery vectors. *Advanced Materials*, Vol. 21, pp. 86-90.

Seow, W. Y., Yang, Y.-Y. & George, A. J. T. (2009). Oligopeptide-mediated gene transfer into mouse corneal endothelial cells: expression, design optimization, uptake mechanism and nuclear localization. *Nucleic Acids Research*, Vol. 37, pp. 6276-6289.

Sharma, G., et al. (2010). Polymer particle shape independently influences binding and internalization by macrophages. *Journal of Controlled Release*, Vol. 147, pp. 408-412.

Shen, W.-C. & Ryser, H. J.-P. (1978). Conjugation of poly-L-lysine to albumin and horseradish peroxidase: a novel method of enhancing the cellular uptake of proteins. *Proceedings of the National Academy of Sciences*, Vol. 75, pp. 1872-1876.

Sheridan, C. (2011). Gene therapy finds its niche. *Nature Biotechnology*, Vol. 29, pp. 121-128.

Soomets, U., et al. (2000). Deletion analogues of transportan. *Biochimica et Biophysica Acta*, Vol. 1467, pp. 165-176.

Su, Y., et al. (2009). Roles of arginine and lysine residues in the translocation of a cell-penetrating peptide from ^{13}C, ^{31}P, and ^{19}F solid-state NMR. *Biochemistry*, Vol. 48, pp. 4587-4595.

Subbarao, N. K., et al. (1987). pH-dependent bilayer destabilization by an amphipathic peptide. *Biochemistry*, Vol. 26, pp. 2964-2912.

Suh, J., Paik, H.-J. & Hwang, B. K. (1994). Ionization of poly(ethylenimine) and poly(allylamine) at various pH's. *Bioconjugate Chemistry*, Vol. 22, pp. 318-327.

Tagalakis, A. D., et al. (2011). Integrin-targeted nanocomplexes for tumour specific delivery and therapy by systemic administration. *Biomaterials*, Vol. 32, pp. 1370-1376.

Takayama, K., et al. (2009). Enhanced intracellular delivery using arginine-rich peptides by the addition of penetration accelerating sequences (Pas). *Journal of Controlled Release*, Vol. 138, pp. 128-133.

Thoren, P. E. G., et al. (2004). Membrane binding and translocation of cell-penetrating peptides. *Biochemistry*, Vol. 43, pp. 3471-3489.

Torgersen, M. L., et al. (2001). Internalization of cholera toxin by different endocytic mechanisms. *Journal of Cell Science*, Vol. 114, pp. 3737-3747.

Trentin, D., Hubbell, J. & Hall, H. (2005). Non-viral gene delivery for local and controlled DNA release. *Journal of Controlled Release*, Vol. 102, pp. 263-275.

Tyagi, M., et al. (2001). Internalization of HIV-1 tat requires cell surface heparan sulfate proteoglycans. *Journal of Biological Chemistry*, Vol. 276, pp. 3254-3261.

Urakami, H. & Guan, Z. (2008). Living ring-opening polymerization of a carbohydrate-derived lactone for the synthesis of protein-resistant biomaterials. *Biomacromolecules*, Vol. 9, pp. 592-597.

Vaheri, A. & Pagano, J. S. (1965). Infectious poliovirus RNA: a sensitive method of assay. *Virology*, Vol. 27, pp. 434-436.

Varkouhi, A. K., et al. (2010). Gene silencing activity of siRNA polyplexes based on thiolated N,N,N-trimethylated chitosan. *Bioconjugate Chemistry*, Vol. 21, pp. 2339-2346.

Wadia, J. S., Stan, R. V. & Dowdy, S. F. (2004). Transducible TAT-HA fusogenic peptide enhances escape of TAT-fusion proteins after lipid raft macropinocytosis. *Nature Medicine*, Vol. 10, pp. 310-315.

Wagner, E., et al. (1991). Transferrin-polycation-DNA complexes: the effect of polycations on the structure of the complex and DNA delivery to cells. *Proceedings of the National Academy of Sciences*, Vol. 88, pp. 4255-4259.

Wagner, E., et al. (1992a). Influenza virus hemagglutinin HA-2 N-terminal fusogenic peptides augment gene transfer by transferrin-polylysine-DNA complexes: toward a synthetic virus-like gene-transfer vehicle. *Proceedings of the National Academy of Sciences*, Vol. 89, pp. 7934-7938.

Wagner, E., et al. (1992b). Coupling of adenovirus to transferrin-polylysine/DNA complexes greatly enhances receptor-mediated gene delivery and expression of transfected genes. *Proceedings of the National Academy of Sciences*, Vol. 89, pp. 6099-6103.

Wang, D., et al. (1999). Encapsulation of plasmid DNA in biodegradable poly(D,L-lactic-co-glycolic acid) microspheres as a novel approach for immunogene delivery. *Journal of Controlled Release*, Vol. 57, pp. 9-18.

Wang, H., et al. (2010). Enhancement of TAT cell membrane penetration efficiency by dimethyl sulphoxide. *Journal of Controlled Release*, Vol. 143, pp. 64-70.

Wiradharma, N., Tong, Y. W. & Yang, Y.-Y. (2009). Self-assembled oligopeptide nanostructures for co-delivery of drug and gene with synergistic therapeutic effect. *Biomaterials*, Vol. 30, pp. 3100-3109.

Wojcieszyn, J. W., et al. (1983). Studies on the mechanism of polyethylene glycol-mediated cell fusion using fluorescent membrane and cytoplasmic probes. *Journal of Cell Biology*, Vol. 96, pp. 151-159.

Wojcieszyn, J. W., et al. (1981). Diffusion of injected macromolecules within the cytoplasm of living cells. *Proceedings of the National Academy of Sciences*, Vol. 78, pp. 4407-4410.

Won, Y.-Y., Sharma, R. & Konieczny, S. F. (2009). Missing pieces in understanding the intracellular trafficking of polycation/DNA complexes. *Journal of Controlled Release*, Vol. 139, pp. 88-93.

Wood, K. C., et al. (2008). Tumor-targeted gene delivery using molecularly engineered hybrid polymers functionalized with a tumor-homing peptide. *Bioconjugate Chemistry*, Vol. 19, pp. 403-405.

Wood, K. C., et al. (2005). A family of hierarchically self-assembling linear-dendritic hybrid polymers for highly efficient targeted gene delivery. *Angewandte Chemie International Edition*, Vol. 44, pp. 6704-6708.

Wu, C. H., Wilson, J. M. & Wu, G. Y. (1989). Targeting genes: delivery and persistent expression of a foreign gene driven by mammalian regulatory elements in vivo. *Journal of Biological Chemistry*, Vol. 264, pp. 16985-16987.

Wu, G. Y. & Wu, C. H. (1987). Receptor-mediated in vitro gene transformation by a soluble DNA carrier system. *Journal of Biological Chemistry*, Vol. 262, pp. 4429-4432.

Wyman, T. B., et al. (1997). Design, synthesis, and characterization of a cationic peptide that binds to nucleic acids and permeabilizes bilayers. *Biochemistry*, Vol. 36, pp. 3008-3017.

Yang, S., et al. (2009). Cellular uptake of self-assembled cationic peptide–DNA complexes: multifunctional role of the enhancer chloroquine. *Journal of Controlled Release*, Vol. 135, pp. 159-165.

Ye, J., et al. (2010). Determination of penetratin secondary structure in live cells with raman microscopy. *Journal of the American Chemical Society*, Vol. 132, pp. 980-988.

Yukawa, H., et al. (2010). Quantum dots labeling using octa-arginine peptides for imaging of adipose tissue-derived stem cells. *Biomaterials*, Vol. 31, pp. 4094-4103.

Zauner, W., et al. (1997). Glycerol and polylysine synergize in their ability to rupture vesicular membranes: a mechanism for increased transferrin-polylysine-mediated gene transfer. *Experimental Cell Reasearch*, Vol. 232, pp. 137-145.

Zauner, W., Ogris, M. & Wagner, E. (1998). Polylysine-based transfection systems utilizing receptor-mediated delivery. *Advanced Drug Delivery Reviews*, Vol. 30, pp. 97-113.

Ziegler, A., et al. (2005). The cationic cell-penetrating peptide CPP[TAT] Derived from the HIV-1 protein tat is rapidly transported into living fibroblasts: optical, biophysical, and metabolic evidence. *Biochemistry*, Vol. 44, pp. 138-148.

9

Nano-Particulate Calcium Phosphate as a Gene Delivery System

Babak Mostaghaci[1,2], Arash Hanifi[3],
Brigitta Loretz[1] and Claus-Michael Lehr[1,4]

[1]Dept. of Drug Delivery (DDEL), Helmholtz-Institute for Pharmaceutical Research
Saarland (HIPS), Helmholtz Centre for Infectious Research (HZI)
Saarland University, Saarbruecken
[2]Biomaterials Group, Materials Engineering Department
Isfahan University of Technology, Isfahan
[3]Tissue Imaging and Spectroscopy Lab, Bioengineering Department
Temple University, Philadelphia, PA
[4]Department of Biopharmaceutics and Pharmaceutical Technology
Saarland University, Saarbruecken
[1,4]Germany
[2]Iran
[3]USA

1. Introduction

Four decades ago, calcium phosphate systems were introduced for in-vitro gene delivery applications. Recently, many studies have been conducted regarding the different applications of these systems in delivering genes to different cell types for therapeutic purposes. Although there are important limitations of using calcium phosphates in gene delivery, there is a high interest in using this type of gene delivery system. This is because of the significant biocompatibility of calcium phosphates, easy synthesis methods of this system, and intrinsic characteristics of calcium phosphates that increase the transfection efficiency. The combination of these properties are rarely seen in other gene delivery systems.

This chapter aims to localise calcium phosphate nanoparticles among the most common non-viral gene delivery systems. It also reviews the history of using calcium phosphates in gene delivery applications and the efforts made to make this system suitable for further clinical applications.

1.1 Non-viral gene delivery

The application of non-viral systems increased considerably after it was shown that using viral systems can result in several problems including difficulty in production, limited opportunity for repeated administrations due to acute inflammatory response, and delayed humoral or cellular immune responses. Insertional mutagenesis is also a potential issue for some viral systems that integrate foreign DNA into the genome (Al-Dosari & Gao, 2009). Although viral systems such as retrovirus, adenovirus, and adeno-associated virus are potentially efficient, non-viral systems have some advantages in that they are less toxic, less immunogenic, and easier to prepare (Nishikawa & Huang, 2001).

A lot of research has been conducted to find suitable non-viral systems. An ideal gene delivery method needs to meet 3 major criteria:

i.   It should protect the transgene against degradation by nucleases in intercellular matrices.

ii.   It should be able to carry the transgene across the cell membrane and into the nucleus of targeted cells.

iii. It should have no detrimental effects (Gao et al., 2007).

Recently, various materials have been introduced as potential gene delivery systems. Three groups of substances are more advantageous in this application. These three groups are:

i.   Cationic polymers (like polyethyleneimine (Kichler et al., 2001; Kircheis et al., 2001; Wightman et al., 2001), dendrimers (Tang et al., 1996; Zinselmeyer et al., 2002; Dufes et al., 2005), chitosan (Lee et al., 1998; Koping-Hoggard et al., 2001; Loretz & Bernkop-Schnurch, 2006) and poly-L-lysine (Trubetskoy et al., 1992; Benns et al., 2000));

ii.   Lipids (like liposomes (Alton et al., 1993; Templeton et al., 1997; Templeton & Lasic, 1999));

iii. Inorganic materials (like calcium phosphates (Liu et al., 2005) and silica nanoparticles (Kneuer et al., 2000; Csogor et al., 2003; Sameti et al., 2003)).

However, some limitations accompany the use of most of these systems including cell toxicity, immune response and low tranfection efficiency.

1.2 Inorganic vectors

Inorganic systems have been used in in-vitro gene delivery for many years, but their clinical application has been developed mostly in the last decade when amino-functionalized silica was introduced. Researchers at Saarland University showed that amino-functionalized silica exhibits good gene tranfection efficiency in addition to its suitable biocompatibility (Kneuer et al., 2000; Csogor et al., 2003; Sameti et al., 2003). Because of this, several studies have been conducted on using amino-funtionalized silica as a gene delivery system (Bharali et al., 2005; Roy et al., 2005; Klejbor et al., 2007; Choi et al., 2008). Research was also conducted on using silica in combination with other polymers for gene delivery. Results demonstrated that making composites of certain polymers with silica nanoparticles could enhance transfection efficiency due to the dense nature of silica nanoparticles (Luo et al., 2004).

There is an increasing interest in mesoporous silica for drug/gene delivery applications because of their higher capacity and of the potential for tailored release of the active molecule. Some studies have been conducted on functionalized or non-functionalized mesoporous silica but the research on using this type of inorganic systems is still ongoing (Park et al., 2008; Slowing et al., 2008).

Some studies have been done on using functionalized gold nanoparticles as a gene delivery system. The results demonstrated the feasibility of using this approach, but further research is needed in this new area (Liang et al., 2010; Niidome et al., 2011).

In addition to calcium phosphate, (their gene delivery application is reviewed in this chapter), other inorganic systems have also been studied regarding in-vitro gene delivery to targeted cells. Silica nanotubes (Namgung et al., 2011), zirconia (Tan et al., 2007), carbon nanotubes (Pantarotto et al., 2004) and layered double hydroxides (Choy et al., 2008) are some examples of these inorganic systems. However, their low transfection efficacy limits their use. Table 1 summarizes inorganic nanoparticles properties.

The following sections discuss calcium phosphates; one of the most important groups of inorganic non-viral gene delivery systems.

2. Calcium phosphate

The work of Graham and Van Der Eb completed in 1973 shows the first application of calcium phosphate in condensation of genetic materials. The brilliant results of their research were that calcium phosphate could condense DNA and increase the transfection efficiency with a relatively simple procedure (Graham & Van Der EB, 1973a). This first research led to vast application of this technology in in-vitro gene delivery because of the demonstrated easy preparation method and proper results.

In order to have a better understanding of calcium phosphate gene delivery properties, first we shall have a look at the structure and characteristics of the calcium phosphate family.

2.1 Calcium phosphates family

Calcium phosphate-based bioceramics have been used in medicine and dentistry for decades. Applications include dental implants, percutaneous devices, periodontal treatment, alveolar ridge augmentation, orthopedics, maxillofacial surgery, otolaryngology and spinal surgery (Hench, 1991).

Bone is a natural nano-composite composed of organic (40%) and inorganic (60%) components. The inorganic constituent of bone is made up of biological apatites, which provide strength to the skeleton and act as a storehouse for calcium, phosphorus, sodium, and magnesium. These biological apatites are structurally similar, though not identical, to the mineral apatite hydroxyapatite (HAp, $Ca_{10}(PO_4)_6(OH)_2$). Hydroxyapatite is the most ubiquitous and well-known phase of calcium phosphate. It has the Ca/P ratio of 1.67 (Narayan et al., 2004). Different phases of calcium phosphate ceramics are used depending upon whether a resorbable or bioactive material is desired. The stable phases of calcium phosphate ceramics depend considerably upon temperature and the presence of water, either during processing or use in the environment (See Fig. 1) (Hench, 1991).

Going through aforementioned properties, it can be realized that the calcium phosphates family includes several members with different characteristics. Calcium phosphate ratio, Ca/P, has been found as the best way to distinguish among these members. In table 2 these members are shown based on their Ca/P ratio.

2.2 Properties

Calcium phosphates being light in weight, chemically stable and compositionally similar to the mineral phase of the bone are preferred as bone graft materials in hard tissue engineering. They are composed of ions commonly found in physiological environment, which make them highly biocompatible. Many research works demonstrated the biocompatibility of calcium phosphates in-vitro and in-vivo. In addition, these bioceramics are also resistant to microbial attack, pH changes, and solvent conditions (Thamaraiselvi & Rajeswari, 2004; Kalita et al., 2007). Degradation properties are very important, especially in the application of calcium phosphates related to drug delivery. It has been shown that

Kind of nanoparticle	Chemical Composition	Typical Size Range	Solubility in μgL^{-1}	Comments
Cadmium Sulfide	CdS	2–5 nm	0.69 ngL^{-1}	toxic, fluorescent, semiconducting
Calcium Phosphate	$Ca_{10}(PO_4)_6OH_2$ (hydroxyapatite)	10–100 nm	6.1 mg L^{-1}	biodegradable, biocompatible; may be made fluorescent by incorporation of lanthanides; cations and anions may be substituted
Carbon Nanotubes	C_n	diameter of a few nm and length of a few mm	0	Not biodegradable, hollow; may be covalently functionalized to improve solubility and may be loaded with molecules
Cobalt-Platinum	$CoPt_3$	3–10 nm	≈ 0	ferromagnetic or superparamagnetic; toxic in uncoated form
Gold	Au	1–50 nm	≈ 0	easily covalently functionalized, for example, with thiols
Iron Oxide (Magnetite)	Fe_3O_4	5–20 nm	≈ 0	ferromagnetic or superparamagnetic; harmful for cells in uncoated form; solubility increases with falling pH
Layered Double Hydroxide	$Mg_6Al_2(CO_3)(OH)_{16}\cdot4 H_2O$ (hydrotalcite)	50–200 nm	moderate, increases below pH 5–6	high selective anion exchange capacity; biodegradable in slightly acidic environment; cations can be substituted
Nickel	Ni	5–100 nm	≈ 0	immunogenic, toxic
Silica	$SiO_2 \cdot nH_2O$	3–100 nm	ca. 120 mg $SiO_2 L^{-1}$ (for silica particles)	Biodegradable; available also in micro- or mesoporous form (e.g., zeolites); easily functionalizable, for example, by chlorosilanes
Silver	Ag	5–100 nm	≈ 0	Bactericidal; dissolution product (Ag^+) potentially harmful for cells
Zinc Oxide	ZnO	3–60 nm	1.6 to 5 mg L^{-1}	fluorescent, semiconducting
Zinc Sulfide	ZnS	3–50 nm	67 ngL^{-1}	fluorescent, semiconducting

Table 1. Some key properties of inorganic nanoparticles which are used for transfection in cell biology (Reprinted from (Sokolova & Epple, 2008)).

different crystalline phases of calcium phosphate present different degradation properties. Table 3 summarizes the solubility properties and stability pH range of calcium phosphate.

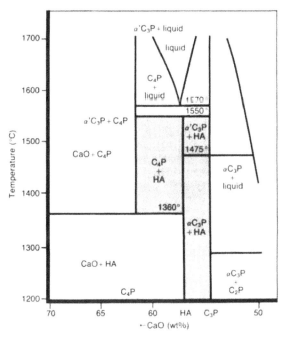

Fig. 1. Calcium phosphate phase equilibrium diagram with 500 mmHg partial pressure of water. Shaded area is the processing range to yield HAp (Hench, 1991).

Ca/P	Name	Formula
2	Tetracalcium phosphate	$Ca_4O(PO4)_2$
1.67	Hydroxyapatite	$Ca_{10}O(PO4)_6(OH)_2$
N/A*	Amorphous calcium phosphate	$Ca_{10-x}H_{2x}(PO4)_6(OH)_2$
1.50	Tricalcium phosphate (α, β, γ)	$Ca_3(PO_4)_2$
1.33	Octacalcium phosphate	$Ca_8H_2(PO_4)_6.5H_2O$
1	Dicalcium phosphate dihydrate	$CaHPO_4.2H_2O$
1	Dicalcium phosphate	$CaHPO_4$
1	Calcium pyrophosphate (α, β, γ)	$Ca_2P_2O_7$
1	Calcium pyrophosphate dihydrate	$Ca_2P_2O_7.2H_2O$
0.7	Heptacalcium phosphate	$Ca_7(P_5O_{16})_2$
0.67	Tetracalcium dihydrogen phosphate	$Ca_4H_2P_6O_{20}$
0.5	Monocalcium phosphate monohydrate	$Ca(H_2PO_4)_2.H_2O$
0.5	Calcium metaphosphate (α, β, γ)	$Ca(PO_3)_2$

*N/A = not applicable

Table 2. Various calcium phosphates with their respective Ca/P atomic ratios (Reprinted from (Vallet-Regi & Gonzalez-Calbet, 2004)).

Phases	Solubility at 25 °C, -log (K_{sp})	pH Stability Range in aqueous solution at 25 °C
Hydroxyapatite (HAp)	116.8	9.5-12
β-Tricalcium Phosphate (β-TCP)	28.9	Cannot be precipitated from aqueous solutions.
α-Tricalcium Phosphate (α-TCP)	25.5	Cannot be precipitated from aqueous solutions.
Tetracalcium Phosphate (TTCP)	38-44	Cannot be precipitated from aqueous solutions.
Dicalcium Phosphate Dehydrate (DCPD)	6.59	2.0 – 6.0
Dicalcium Phosphate Anhydrate (DCPA)	6.90	Stable at temperatures above 100 °C
Amorphous Calcium Phosphate (ACP)	Cannot be measured precisely. However, the following values were reported: 25.7 ± 0.1 (pH 7.40), 29.9 ± 0.1 (pH 6.00), 32.7 ± 0.1 (pH 5.28)	Always metastable. The composition of a precipitate depends on the solution pH value and composition.
Calcium-deficient Hydroxyapatie (CDHA)	≈ 85.1	6.5-9.5

Table 3. Solubility and pH stability of different phases of calcium phosphates (Reprinted from (Kalita et al., 2007)).

2.3 Calcium phosphate nanoparticles

With the introduction of smaller calcium phosphate particles, it has become possible to use them in advanced fields of biomedicine. Calcium phosphate nanoparticles, with a size about 100 nm, are highly biocompatible. These particles are able to penetrate the outer membrane of cells and bacteria. Calcium phosphate nanoparticles could be utilized in different fields of biomedicine such as drug delivery, gene delivery, and imaging (Epple et al., 2010). Also, to produce high quality HAp bioceramics for artificial bone substitution, ultrafine HAp powder is usually employed. Nano-HAp powder results in easy handling, casting, and sintering leading to an excellent sintered body in the bioceramics preparation process (Cao et al., 2005).

3. Calcium phosphate nanoparticles as gene delivery vector

3.1 Historical view

Previously, it is mentioned that the first use of calcium phosphate in gene delivery application was conducted by Graham and Van Der EB in 1973. In this study, calcium phosphate was used for transfecting cells with Adenovirus 5 DNA to assay infectivity. (Graham & Van Der EB, 1973a). They diluted Adenovirus 5 DNA in a buffer containing Na_2HPO_4. Then, calcium chloride was added and the mixture was incubated with KB Cells. Using labeled DNA they concluded that by adding the calcium precursor in the experiment, the uptake of DNA increased and DNA showed a better stability against enzymatic degradation (Fig. 2). It was reported that this technique gave a 100 fold increase in efficiency over the DEAE-dextran method for human adenovirus DNA.

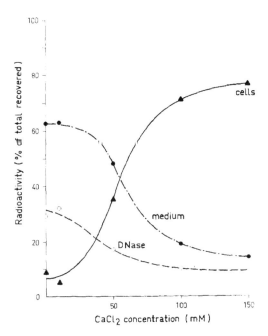

Fig. 2. Effect of $CaCl_2$ on adsorption of ^{14}C-Ad5 DNA to KB cells. KB cells were exposed to MEM-Tris containing DNA plus $CaCl_2$ at various concentrations. The curves represent the fraction of radioactivity recovered in the medium (●), in the DNase digest (○), or in the SDS lysate of the cells (▲) (Graham & Van Der EB, 1973a).

With the same methodology, this group conducted another study to transform rat kidney cells with the DNA of human adenovirus 5. In Fig. 3 the transfected area is clearly visible as contained small, round, densely packed cells characteristic of adenovirus transformation. This work claimed that the "calcium technique" was a suitable system to study transformation by adenovirus DNA and the efficiency of transformation, though not high, appeared to be reasonably reproducible (Graham & Van Der EB, 1973b).

In another study, Graham, Veldhuisen and Wilkie used the aforementioned technique to investigate the infectivity of herpes simplex virus type I (HSV-I) (Graham et al., 1973). In 1975, Abrahams and Van Der EB made a transformation of rat kidney cells and mouse 3T3 cells by DNA from Simian Virus 40 using "calcium technique". They stated that this technique for in-vitro transformation was reproducible (Abrahams & Van Der Eb, 1975). Later, Van Der EB and Graham successfully used "calcium technique" to determine the ability to transform primary baby rat kidney (BRK) cells with specific fragments of human adenoviruses 2 and 5 DNAs (Van Der EB et al., 1977).

In 1976, Stow and Wilkie reported that treatment of cells with dimethyl sulphoxide (DMSO) after injection with "Herpes Simplex Virus DNA"/calcium phosphate complex could lead to a significant increase in the number of plaques obtained. These researchers proposed that DMSO could initiate the plaque formation. It was interesting that in other method (DEAE-dextran) using DMSO did not exhibit that significant enhancement (Fig. 4) (Stow & Wilkie, 1976).

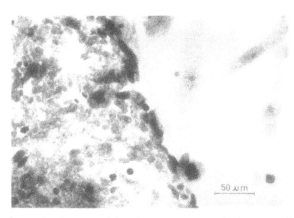

Fig. 3. Part of transformed colony resulting from exposure of primary rat kidney cells to Adenovirus 5 DNA+ CaCl$_2$ 22 days previously. Three normal cells can be seen to the right of the photograph. Giemsa stain (Graham & Van Der EB, 1973b).

During the 1980's, the calcium phosphate method for in-vitro gene delivery had become a common method. In 1981, some of the parameters that affect the transformation procedure by calcium phosphate system had been investigated by Corsaro and Pearson (Corsaro & Pearson, 1981). First, to confirm the work of Stow and Wilkie in 1976, they performed a study on the effect of rinsing the complex of DNA/calcium phosphate with DMSO. They also added an additional variable to this experiment which was the exposure time of DNA/calcium phosphate complex to cells. They claimed that when suboptimal DNA exposure time is applied (e.g. 4-12 hours), the DMSO rinse increases the transformation frequency. However, rinsing with DMSO had no effect when the optimal condition was utilized. They concluded that exposure to DMSO offers no significant advantage.

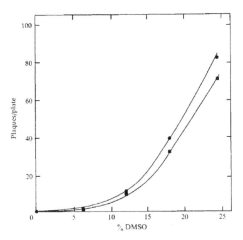

Fig. 4. The effect of DMSO concentration on the enhancement of HSV-I DNA infectivity. Varying concentration of DMSO dissolved in HeBS (●) or eagle's medium (■) (Stow & Wilkie, 1976).

Regarding the formation of DNA/calcium phosphate precipitates, they found that it is critical to add the solution of DNA/$CaCl_2$ to the HEPES-phosphate buffer rather than in the reverse order. Also, they claimed that it is important to add the solution drop-wise, rather than directly (Corsaro & Pearson, 1981).

In 1982, a research group at Yale University conducted research on the mechanism for entry of DNA/calcium phosphate complex in to mammalian cells by electron microscopy and fluorescent dyes (Loyter et al., 1982a; Loyter et al., 1982b).

Electron microscopy and filter hybridization studies revealed that most of the DNA strands enter by phagocytosis. The effect of different drugs and respiratory inhibitors on the entry of DNA was also investigated (Table 4, Fig. 5). Results showed phagocytosis of DNA is inhibited both by respiratory inhibitors and drugs, such as Colcemid, which disassemble microtubules. They concluded that the uptake of DNA/calcium phosphate resembles "receptor mediated" phagocytosis. Also it was seen that ATP-depleted and cold treated cells were not able to adsorb the complex. Thus the authors claimed that the phagocytosis of DNA/calcium phosphate complex is an energy- and temperature-dependent process (Loyter et al., 1982a).

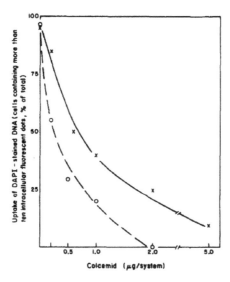

Fig. 5. Effect of increasing concentration of Colcemid on the entry of DAPI-stained DNA/calcium phosphate complexes into Ltk- cells (Loyter et al., 1982a).

These researchers also claimed that the pH of the formation of the DNA/calcium phosphate complexes is crucial for successful gene transfer. Studies on the effect of pH and DNA concentration on the entry of fluorescent dye-labeled DNA into cells showed that only during the calcium phosphate complexes formation in the pH rang of 7.1 to 7.5 could fluorescent spots be visualized in the cytoplasm of recipient cells. For the complexes formed above pH = 7.5 no entry to cells could be detected (Fig. 6A).

On the other hand, the DNA/calcium phosphate ratio is important on the adsorption of the complexes. When higher concentrations of DNA was utilized with the constant concentration of calcium phosphate, adsorption was not affected, whereas the appearance of cytoplasmic florescence was drastically reduced (Fig. 6B) (Loyter et al., 1982b).

System	Effect of DNA Entry
Drugs	
Cytochalasin B (1-4 μg/ml)	No effect
Colcemid (5 μg/ml)	Complete inhibition
DMSO (10%, 10-30 min)	No effect
Respiratory inhibitors	
2 deoxyglucose	Partial inhibition
NaN₃	Partial inhibition
NaF	Partial inhibition
NaF + 2 deoxyglucose	Complete inhibition
NaN₃ + 2 deoxyglucose	Complete inhibition

Table 4. The effect of various drugs and respiratory inhibitors on introduction of DNA into Ltk⁻ Aprt⁻ cells (Reproduced from (Loyter et al., 1982a)).

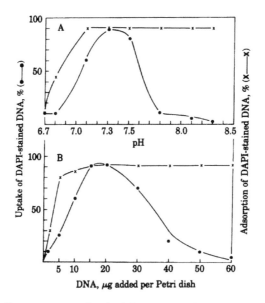

Fig. 6. Adsorption (cells containing adsorbed fluorescent dots) and uptake (cells containing more than 10 intracellular fluorescent dots) of DAPI-stained DNA as a function of the pH of the DNA/calcium phosphate complex (A) and DNA concentration in DNA/calcium phosphate complex (B) (Loyter et al., 1982b).

One of the limitations of calcium phosphate systems in gene delivery applications is that most of the input DNA is degraded before it reaches the nucleus of the cell, where gene expression and DNA replication take place. In 1983, Luthman and Magnusson conducted research on increasing the efficiency of transfection by inhibiting the lysosomal degradation using Chloroquine as a lysosomotropic compound. For this purpose they used a conventional procedure for transfection with calcium phosphate, but they added Chloroquine to the growth medium of the cells. In Fig. 7 the effect of Chloroquine concentration on transfection efficiency using DNA/calcium phosphate complexes can be seen. The authors concluded that when Chloroquine treatment was effective, it increased the fraction of cells that could be successfully transfected. They claimed that this conclusion was supported by the results of experiments in which cells were transfected with linear forms of viral DNA. In that case, in Chloroquine treated cells, the number of DNA molecules which had re-circularized and were able to replicate was much larger than untreated cells (Luthman & Magnusson, 1983).

With the same approach, in 1984 a research group in Norway used different inhibitors of intracellular degradation (such as 3-methyl adenine, NH_4Cl, FCPP and etc.) and claimed that the frequency of transformation was increased due to increasing the cytoplasmic level of exogenous DNA (Table 5) (Ege et al., 1984).

In 1987, Chen and Okayama introduced a new method for gene delivery with calcium phosphate systems. The aim of their work was the formation of DNA/calcium phosphate complexes gradually in medium during incubation with cells. They found that in this method the crucial factors that affect the transfection efficiency are the pH of the buffer used for calcium phosphate precipitation (optimized pH was 6.95) and the CO_2 level during the incubation of DNA with cells. They also found that the amount and the form of DNA are important factors. It was observed that circular DNA has better efficiency than linear DNA but, the reason for this phenomenon was not clear at that time. The authors claimed that the efficiency of their method is comparable to the efficiency of other common transfection systems of that time (Chen & Okayama, 1987).

In 1990 Orrantia and Chang investigated the intracellular distribution of DNA after the DNA/calcium phosphate complexes move into the cells. Results showed that only a small fraction of internalized DNA could be found in the nucleus, the target place for gene delivery. In the enriched nuclear fraction, the mouse cells retained 6.4% of internalized DNA while the human cells retained only 2.2% (Fig. 8).

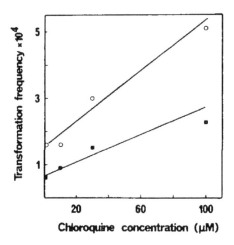

Fig. 7. Effect of Chloroquine concentration on transfection efficiency. Rat-1 cultures were transfected by co-precipitating calcium phosphate and polyoma DNA, 20 ng (■) and 100 ng (o) (Luthman & Magnusson, 1983).

Addition	Concentration	Transformation Frequency after 6 hours
None, no DNA		0
None, DNA alone		4
DNA + glycerol	17 %	10
DNA + DMSO	20 %	22
DNA + NH₄Cl	20 mM	64
DNA + FCPP	1 μM	50
DNA + Procaine	10 mM	3
DNA + chloroquine	100 μM	5
DNA + monensin	5 mM	1
DNA + 3-methyl adenine	5 mM	46

Table 5. Effect of different compounds on the transformation frequency of rat 2 *tk⁻* cells transfected with pAGO DNA 6 hours after incubation of the indicated compounds with the cells (reproduced from (Ege et al., 1984)).

The authors concluded that transfection with DNA/calcium phosphate is a procedure with low efficiency partly because most of the endocytosed DNA is quickly degraded and excreted to the cytosol (Orrantia & Chang, 1990).

In 1994, O'Mahoney and Adams modified the calcium phosphate transfection procedure described by Chen and Okayama in 1987 and claimed that they reached a reliable and reproducible method with high transfection efficiency. They claimed that the critical factor in this method is the standing time of the DNA/$CaCl_2$/BES-buffered saline prior to addition to cultured cells. They concluded that in the optimal condition it is possible to reach 100% efficiency (Omahoney & Adams, 1994).

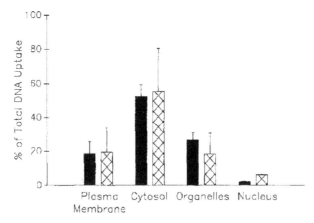

Fig. 8. Distribution of internalized DNA in subcellular fractions from human and mouse cells. Cultured Cells were transfected with ^{32}P-labeled high-molecular-weight DNA/calcium phosphate for 4 h. ■: Human primary fibroblast cells, ⊠: Transformed mouse Ltk- cells (Orrantia & Chang, 1990).

In 1996, a research group in Taiwan conducted some research works on electrochemical properties of DNA/calcium phosphate complexes. The study focused on the variation of zeta potential with changes in pH for calcium phosphate and DNA/calcium phosphate complexes. The point of zero charge (pzc) and isoelectric point (iep) were found to be at pH 7.09 and 7.0, respectively. With addition of plasmid DNA, both pzc and iep points shifted to higher values of 7.18 and 7.15, respectively (Yang & Yang, 1996a).

In their other research on this topic, they revealed that the pH of the formation of DNA/calcium phosphate complexes and the concentration of DNA within the complexes were the crucial factor for the entry of these complexes to cells. The results of their study showed that optimum transfection efficiency occurred in the region close to the iep of DNA-calcium phosphate co-precipitates of pH 7.15 and close to the maximum flocculation of this colloidal system. The enhanced cell transformation efficiency occurred at pH 7.01. The zeta potentials of the DNA co-precipitates prepared in the absence of DMEM and calf serum were determined to lie between 11 and 21 mV. Preparation within these limits resulted in an efficient internalization of the DNA/calcium phosphate complexes, and for endocytosis to occur (Yang & Yang, 1996b).

In 2004, Jordan and Wurm investigated the methods that were applied previously for gene delivery with calcium phosphate particles by different authors. They stated that all of the numerous variations of the protocol found in the literature are based on the same principle — a spontaneous precipitation that occurs in supersaturated solutions. Although a wide range of conditions will lead to precipitates, high transfection efficiencies are only obtained within a narrow range of optimized parameters that assure certain properties of the precipitate. Finally, they concluded that despite a rapidly growing choice of efficient transfection reagents, this method remains highly attractive due to its highly biocompatible nature (Jordan & Wurm, 2004).

3.2 Current studies

Research on using calcium phosphate nanoparticles for gene delivery application is still continuing. Researchers perform a lot of new experiments to optimize the parameters involved in gene delivery with calcium phosphate nanoparticles. We have tried to review some of these studies in this chapter.

A research group in the University of Duisburg-Essen, proposed a method to prepare multi-shell calcium phosphate/DNA particles. They utilized a simple method to prepare multi-shell calcium phosphate as illustrated in Fig. 9.

They prepared different nanoparticles and showed that with multi-shell calcium phosphate/DNA nanoparticles the transfection efficiency is increased due to the protection of DNA against nuclease enzymes (Fig. 10). Moreover, the authors claimed that in contrast with conventional calcium phosphate, these particles could be stored for weeks without loss of their transfection efficiency (Sokolova et al., 2006).

They also showed that the standard calcium phosphate method selectively unbalanced intracellular calcium homeostasis while it remained at low control levels after transfection using nanoparticles. They concluded that with using DNA-functionalized calcium phosphate nanoparticles, cells are able to cope with the associated calcium uptake and therefore proved their method to be a superior transfection method (Neumann et al., 2009).

Haniti et al. conducted some research on the feasibility of using strontium and magnesium substituted calcium phosphate in gene delivery applications. They prepared the particles via a simple sol-gel route. They obtained some particles with nano-size structure, high specific surface area, and a high dissolution rate (Fig. 11). The zeta potential (Table 6) was increased in comparison with simple calcium phosphate. They concluded that due to increased surface charge and solubility, these novel systems could increase the gene transfection efficiency (Hanifi et al., 2010a; Hanifi et al., 2010b).

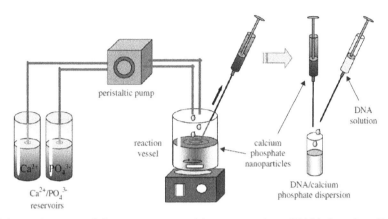

Fig. 9. Schematic set-up of the apparatus used for preparation of DNA-functionalized calcium phosphate nanoparticles. Calcium nitrate and diammonium hydrogen phosphate solutions are mixed in a vessel to form a precipitate. A part of the dispersion is taken with a syringe and mixed with DNA solution in an Eppendorf tube (Sokolova et al., 2006).

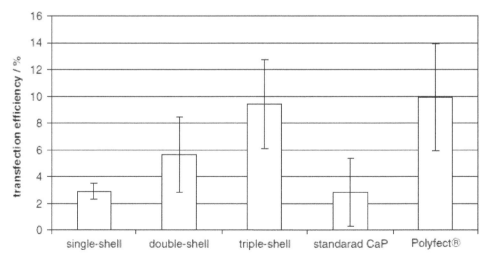

Fig. 10. Comparison of the transfection efficiency of multi-shell calcium phosphate/DNA by different methods. There are significant differences between single-shell and triple-shell (P<0.01) and triple-shell and the standard calcium phosphate methods (P<0.05) (Sokolova et al., 2006).

Recently there has been an approach to incorporate other agents or materials with calcium phosphate to improve its function as a gene delivery system. Stabilizing with bis-phosphonate (Giger et al., 2011), coating with lipids (Zhou et al., 2010), incorporating in alginate hydrogel (Krebs et al., 2010) and association with Adenovirus (Toyoda et al., 2000) are some examples for this approach.

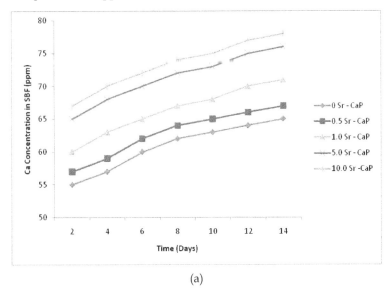

(a)

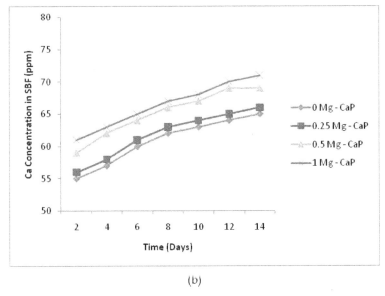

(b)

Fig. 11. Concentration of Ca⁺⁺ ions in SBF solution after predicted period of time. A: Sr-CaP, B: Mg-CaP (Not Published).

Sample composition	Zeta potential (mV)
Sr-Substituted CaP	
0.0Sr-CaP	4.5±0.1
0.5Sr-CaP	5.0±0.2
1.0Sr-CaP	6.1±0.1
5.0Sr-CaP	7.3±0.3
10.0Sr-CaP	7.8±0.2
Mg-Substituted CaP	
0.0Mg-CaP	3.2±0.5
0.25Mg-CaP	6.7±0.4
0.50Mg-CaP	7.5±1
1.0Mg-CaP	8±0.8

Table 6. Surface charge of Sr and Mg substituted calcium phosphate nanoparticles (Reproduce from (Hanifi et al., 2010a; Hanifi et al., 2010b)).

4. Conclusion

Nano-particulate calcium phosphate has shown several interesting advantages in biomedical applications because of its biocompatibility and easy preparation process. The DNA condensation characteristic of nano-particulate calcium phosphate makes it a potential choice for gene therapy system applications. Nano-particulate calcium phosphates are able to condense DNA strands, carry them in the blood, deliver the genetic material to target cells, and move them into cells resulting in reasonable transcription.

Therefore, there is a common agreement among most of the works regarding gene delivery application on utilizing the calcium phosphate to deliver the gene into the nucleus; the final target of gene therapy methods. Because of the advantages of the DNA/calcium phosphate complex, it is one of the highly appealing systems currently studied, although it has been used in in-vitro gene delivery for many years already. The translation of its application into clinical therapy methods requires more work.

Researchers need to solve the instability of calcium phosphate in physiological conditions. If calcium phosphate/DNA complexes degrade in the blood circuit, it cannot be used in most of the clinical gene delivery applications. The other problem is the low transfection efficiency, which currently limits the application of the system. There are controversial reports about the transfection efficiency of calcium phosphate/DNA system, mostly because of instability and the complicated nature of calcium phosphate in solution. Once these problems are overcome by adequate novel technologies, the excellent biocompatibility and biodegradability of calcium phosphate remains as a major advantage.

5. References

Abrahams, P. J. & Van Der Eb, A. J. (1975). In vitro transformation of rat and mouse cells by DNA from simian virus 40. *J Virol*, 16, 1, pp. 206-209

Al-Dosari, M. S. & Gao, X. (2009). Nonviral Gene Delivery: Principle, Limitations, and Recent Progress. *Aaps Journal*, 11, 4, pp. 671-681

Alton, E. W. F. W., Middleton, P. G., Caplen, N. J., Smith, S. N., Steel, D. M., Munkonge, F. M., Jeffery, P. K., Geddes, D. M., Hart, S. L., Williamson, R., Fasold, K. I., Miller, A. D., Dickinson, P., Stevenson, B. J., Mclachlan, G., Dorin, J. R. & Porteous, D. J. (1993). Noninvasive Liposome-Mediated Gene Delivery Can Correct the Ion-Transport Defect in Cystic-Fibrosis Mutant Mice. *Nature Genetics*, 5, 2, pp. 135-142

Benns, J. M., Choi, J. S., Mahato, R. I., Park, J. S. & Kim, S. W. (2000). pH-sensitive cationic polymer gene delivery vehicle: N-Ac-poly(L-histidine)-graft-poly(L-lysine) comb shaped polymer. *Bioconjugate Chemistry*, 11, 5, pp. 637-645

Bharali, D. J., Klejbor, I. Stachowiak, E. K., Dutta, P., Roy, I., Kaur, N., Bergey, E. J., Prasad, P. N. & Stachowiak, M. K. (2005). Organically modified silica nanoparticles: A nonviral vector for in vivo gene delivery and expression in the brain. *Proceedings of the National Academy of Sciences of the United States of America*, 102, 32, pp. 11539-11544

Cao, L. Y., Zhang, C. B. & Huang, H. F. (2005). Synthesis of hydroxyapatite nanoparticles in ultrasonic precipitation. *Ceramics International*, 31, 8, pp. 1041-1044

Chen, C. & Okayama, H. (1987). High-Efficiency Transformation of Mammalian-Cells by Plasmid DNA. *Molecular and Cellular Biology*, 7, 8, pp. 2745-2752

Choi, E. W., Shin, I. S., Lee, C. W. & Youn, H. Y. (2008). The effect of gene therapy using CTLA4Ig/silica-nanoparticles on canine experimental autoimmune thyroiditis. *Journal of Gene Medicine*, 10, 7, pp. 795-804

Choy, J.-H., Park, M. & Oh, J.-M. (2008). Gene and Drug Delivery System with Soluble Inorganic Carriers, In: *NanoBioTechnology : bioinspired devices and materials of the future*, O. Shoseyov and I. Levy, pp. 349-367, Humana Press, Totowa, N.J.

Corsaro, C. M. & Pearson, M. L. (1981). Enhancing the Efficiency of DNA-Mediated Gene-Transfer in Mammalian-Cells. *Somatic Cell Genetics*, 7, 5, pp. 603-616

Csogor, Z., Nacken, M., Sameti, M., Lehr, C. M. & Schmidt, H. (2003). Modified silica particles for gene delivery. *Materials Science & Engineering C-Biomimetic and Supramolecular Systems*, 23, 1-2, pp. 93-97

Dufes, C., Uchegbu, I. F. & Schatzlein, A. G. (2005). Dendrimers in gene delivery. *Advanced Drug Delivery Reviews*, 57, 15, pp. 2177-2202

Ege, T., Reisbig, R. R. & Rogne, S. (1984). Enhancement of DNA-Mediated Gene-Transfer by Inhibitors of Autophagic-Lysosomal Function. *Experimental Cell Research*, 155, 1, pp. 9-16

Epple, M., Ganesan, K., Heumann, R., Klesing, J., Kovtun, A., Neumann, S. & Sokolova, V. (2010). Application of calcium phosphate nanoparticles in biomedicine. *Journal of Materials Chemistry*, 20, 1, pp. 18-23

Gao, X., Kim, K. S. & Liu, D. X. (2007). Nonviral gene delivery: What we know and what is next. *Aaps Journal*, 9, 1, pp. E92-E104

Giger, E. V., Puigmarti-Luis, J., Schlatter, R., Castagner, B., Dittrich, P. S. & Leroux, J. C. (2011). Gene delivery with bisphosphonate-stabilized calcium phosphate nanoparticles. *J Control Release*, 150, 1, pp. 87-93

Graham, F. L. & Van Der EB, A. J. (1973a). New Technique for Assay of Infectivity of Human Adenovirus 5 DNA. *Virology*, 52, 2, pp. 456-467

Graham, F. L. & Van Der EB, A. J. (1973b). Transformation of Rat Cells by DNA of Human Adenovirus-5. *Virology*, 54, 2, pp. 536-539

Graham, F. L., Veldhuis.G & Wilkie, N. M. (1973). Infectious Herpesvirus DNA. *Nature-New Biology*, 245, 148, pp. 265-266

Hanifi, A., Fathi, M. H. & Sadeghi, H. M. M. (2010a). Effect of strontium ions substitution on gene delivery related properties of calcium phosphate nanoparticles. *Journal of Materials Science-Materials in Medicine*, 21, 9, pp. 2601-2609

Hanifi, A., Fathi, M. H., Sadeghi, H. M. M. & Varshosaz, J. (2010b). Mg2+ substituted calcium phosphate nano particles synthesis for non viral gene delivery application. *Journal of Materials Science-Materials in Medicine*, 21, 8, pp. 2393-2401

Hench, L. L. (1991). Bioceramics - from Concept to Clinic. *Journal of the American Ceramic Society*, 74, 7, pp. 1487-1510

Jordan, M. & Wurm, F. (2004). Transfection of adherent and suspended cells by calcium phosphate. *Methods*, 33, 2, pp. 136-143

Kalita, S. J., Bhardwaj, A. & Bhatt, H. A. (2007). Nanocrystalline calcium phosphate ceramics in biomedical engineering. *Materials Science & Engineering C-Biomimetic and Supramolecular Systems*, 27, 3, pp. 441-449

Kichler, A., Leborgne, C., Coeytaux, E. & Danos, O. (2001). Polyethylenimine-mediated gene delivery: a mechanistic study. *Journal of Gene Medicine*, 3, 2, pp. 135-144

Kircheis, R., Wightman, L. & Wagner, E. (2001). Design and gene delivery activity of modified polyethylenimines. *Advanced Drug Delivery Reviews*, 53, 3, pp. 341-358

Klejbor, I., Stachowiak, E. K., Bharali, D. J., Roy, I., Spodnik, I., Morys, J., Bergey, E. J., Prasad, P. N. & Stachowiak, M. K. (2007). ORMOSIL nanoparticles as a non-viral gene delivery vector for modeling polyglutamine induced brain pathology. *Journal of Neuroscience Methods*, 165, 2, pp. 230-243

Kneuer, C., Sameti, M., Haltner, E. G., Schiestel, T., Schirra, H., Schmidt, H. & Lehr, C. M. (2000). Silica nanoparticles modified with aminosilanes as carriers for plasmid DNA. *International Journal of Pharmaceutics*, 196, 2, pp. 257-261

Koping-Hoggard, M., Tubulekas, I., Guan, H., Edwards, K., Nilsson, M., Varum, K. M. & Artursson, P. (2001). Chitosan as a nonviral gene delivery system. Structure-property relationships and characteristics compared with polyethylenimine in vitro and after lung administration in vivo. *Gene Therapy*, 8, 14, pp. 1108-1121

Krebs, M. D., Salter, E., Chen, E., Sutter, K. A. & Alsberg, E. (2010). Calcium phosphate-DNA nanoparticle gene delivery from alginate hydrogels induces in vivo osteogenesis. *J Biomed Mater Res A*, 92, 3, pp. 1131-1138

Lee, K. Y., Kwon, I. C., Kim, Y. H., Jo, W. H. & Jeong, S. Y. (1998). Preparation of chitosan self-aggregates as a gene delivery system. *Journal of Controlled Release*, 51, 2-3, pp. 213-220

Liang, X. J., Guo, S. T., Huang, Y. Y., Jiang, Q. A., Sun, Y., Deng, L. D., Liang, Z. C., Du, Q. A., Xing, J. F., Zhao, Y. L., Wang, P. C. & Dong, A. J. (2010). Enhanced Gene Delivery and siRNA Silencing by Gold Nanoparticles Coated with Charge-Reversal Polyelectrolyte. *Acs Nano*, 4, 9, pp. 5505-5511

Liu, T., Tang, A., Zhang, G. Y., Chen, Y. X., Zhang, J. Y., Peng, S. S. & Cai, Z. M. (2005). Calcium phosphate nanoparticles as a novel nonviral vector for efficient trasfection of DNA in cancer gene therapy. *Cancer Biotherapy and Radiopharmaceuticals*, 20, 2, pp. 141-149

Loretz, B. & Bernkop-Schnurch, A. (2006). In vitro evaluation of chitosan-EDTA conjugate polyplexes as a nanoparticulate gene delivery system. *Aaps Journal*, 8, 4, pp. E756-E764

Loyter, A., Scangos, G., Juricek, D., Keene, D. & Ruddle, F. H. (1982a). Mechanisms of DNA Entry into Mammalian-Cells .2. Phagocytosis of Calcium-Phosphate DNA Coprecipitate Visualized by Electron-Microscopy. *Experimental Cell Research*, 139, 1, pp. 223-234

Loyter, A., Scangos, G. A. & Ruddle, F. H. (1982b). Mechanisms of DNA Uptake by Mammalian-Cells - Fate of Exogenously Added DNA Monitored by the Use of Fluorescent Dyes. *Proceedings of the National Academy of Sciences of the United States of America-Biological Sciences*, 79, 2, pp. 422-426

Luo, D., Han, E., Belcheva, N. & Saltzman, W. M. (2004). A self-assembled, modular DNA delivery system mediated by silica nanoparticles. *Journal of Controlled Release*, 95, 2, pp. 333-341

Luthman, H. & Magnusson, G. (1983). High-Efficiency Polyoma DNA Transfection of Chloroquine Treated-Cells. *Nucleic Acids Research*, 11, 5, pp. 1295-1308

Namgung, R., Zhang, Y., Fang, Q. L., Singha, K., Lee, H. J., Kwon, I. K., Jeong, Y. Y., Park, I. K., Son, S. J. & Kim, W. J. (2011). Multifunctional silica nanotubes for dual-modality gene delivery and MR imaging. *Biomaterials*, 32, 11, pp. 3042-3052

Narayan, R. J., Kumta, P. N., Sfeir, C., Lee, D. H., Olton, D. & Choi, D. W. (2004). Nanostructured ceramics in medical devices: Applications and prospects. *Jom*, 56, 10, pp. 38-43

Neumann, S., Kovtun, A., Dietzel, I. D., Epple, M. & Heumann, R. (2009). The use of size-defined DNA-functionalized calcium phosphate nanoparticles to minimise intracellular calcium disturbance during transfection. *Biomaterials*, 30, 35, pp. 6794-6802

Niidome, T., Pissuwan, D. & Cortie, M. B. (2011). The forthcoming applications of gold nanoparticles in drug and gene delivery systems. *Journal of Controlled Release*, 149, 1, pp. 65-71

Nishikawa, M. & Huang, L. (2001). Nonviral vectors in the new millennium: Delivery barriers in gene transfer. *Human Gene Therapy*, 12, 8, pp. 861-870

Omahoney, J. V. & Adams, T. E. (1994). Optimization of Experimental-Variables Influencing Reporter Gene-Expression in Hepatoma-Cells Following Calcium-Phosphate Transfection. *DNA and Cell Biology*, 13, 12, pp. 1227-1232

Orrantia, E. & Chang, P. L. (1990). Intracellular-Distribution of DNA Internalized through Calcium-Phosphate Precipitation. *Experimental Cell Research*, 190, 2, pp. 170-174

Pantarotto, D., Singh, R., McCarthy, D., Erhardt, M., Briand, J. P., Prato, M., Kostarelos, K. & Bianco, A. (2004). Functionalized carbon nanotubes for plasmid DNA gene delivery. *Angewandte Chemie-International Edition*, 43, 39, pp. 5242-5246

Park, I. Y., Kim, I. Y., Yoo, M. K., Choi, Y. J., Cho, M. H. & Cho, C. S. (2008). Mannosylated polyethylenimine coupled mesoporous silica nanoparticles for receptor-mediated gene delivery. *International Journal of Pharmaceutics*, 359, 1-2, pp. 280-287

Roy, I., Ohulchanskyy, T. Y., Bharali, D. J., Pudavar, H. E., Mistretta, R. A., Kaur, N. & Prasad, P. N. (2005). Optical tracking of organically modified silica nanoparticles as DNA carriers: A nonviral, nanomedicine approach for gene delivery. *Proceedings of the National Academy of Sciences of the United States of America*, 102, 2, pp. 279-284

Sameti, M., Bohr, G., Kumar, M. N. V. R., Kneuer, C., Bakowsky, U., Nacken, M., Schmidt, H. & Lehr, C. M. (2003). Stabilisation by freeze-drying of cationically modified silica nanoparticles for gene delivery. *International Journal of Pharmaceutics*, 266, 1-2, pp. 51-60

Slowing, I. I., Vivero-Escoto, J. L., Wu, C. W. & Lin, V. S. Y. (2008). Mesoporous silica nanoparticles as controlled release drug delivery and gene transfection carriers. *Advanced Drug Delivery Reviews*, 60, 11, pp. 1278-1288

Sokolova, V. & Epple, M. (2008). Inorganic nanoparticles as carriers of nucleic acids into cells. *Angewandte Chemie-International Edition*, 47, 8, pp. 1382-1395

Sokolova, V. V., Radtke, I., Heumann, R. & Epple, M. (2006). Effective transfection of cells with multi-shell calcium phosphate-DNA nanoparticles. *Biomaterials*, 27, 16, pp. 3147-3153

Stow, N. D. & Wilkie, N. M. (1976). Improved Technique for Obtaining Enhanced Infectivity with Herpes-Simplex Virus Type-1 DNA. *Journal of General Virology*, 33, Dec, pp. 447-458

Tan, K., Cheang, P., Ho, I. A. W., Lam, P. Y. P. & Hui, K. M. (2007). Nanosized bioceramic particles could function as efficient gene delivery vehicles with target specificity for the spleen. *Gene Therapy*, 14, 10, pp. 828-835

Tang, M. X., Redemann, C. T. & Szoka, F. C. (1996). In vitro gene delivery by degraded polyamidoamine dendrimers. *Bioconjugate Chemistry*, 7, 6, pp. 703-714

Templeton, N. S. & Lasic, D. D. (1999). New directions in liposome gene delivery. *Molecular Biotechnology*, 11, 2, pp. 175-180

Templeton, N. S., Lasic, D. D., Frederik, P. M., Strey, H. H., Roberts, D. D. & Pavlakis, G. N. (1997). Improved DNA: Liposome complexes for increased systemic delivery and gene expression. *Nature Biotechnology*, 15, 7, pp. 647-652

Thamaraiselvi, T. V. & Rajeswari, S. (2004). Biological Evaluation of Bioceramic Materials - A Review. *Trends Biomater. Artif. Organs*, 18, 1, pp. 9-17

Toyoda, K., Andresen, J. J., Zabner, J., Faraci, F. M. & Heistad, D. D. (2000). Calcium phosphate precipitates augment adenovirus-mediated gene transfer to blood vessels in vitro and in vivo. *Gene Ther*, 7, 15, pp. 1284-1291

Trubetskoy, V. S., Torchilin, V. P., Kennel, S. J. & Huang, L. (1992). Use of N-Terminal Modified Poly(L-Lysine) Antibody Conjugate as a Carrier for Targeted Gene Delivery in Mouse Lung Endothelial-Cells. *Bioconjugate Chemistry*, 3, 4, pp. 323-327

Vallet-Regi, M. & Gonzalez-Calbet, J. M. (2004). Calcium phosphates as substitution of bone tissues. *Progress in Solid State Chemistry*, 32, 1-2, pp. 1-31

Van Der EB, A. J., Mulder, C., Graham, F. L. & Houweling, A. (1977). Transformation with Specific Fragments of Adenovirus Dnas .1. Isolation of Specific Fragments with Transforming Activity of Adenovirus-2 and 5 DNA. *Gene*, 2, 3-4, pp. 115-132

Wightman, L., Kircheis, R., Rossler, V., Carotta, S., Ruzicka, R., Kursa, M. & Wagner, E. (2001). Different behavior of branched and linear polyethylenimine for gene delivery in vitro and in vivo. *Journal of Gene Medicine*, 3, 4, pp. 362-372

Yang, Y. W. & Yang, J. C. (1996a). Characterization of Calcium Phosphate as a Gene Carrier (I): Electrochemical Properties. *Drug Delivery*, 3, pp. 173-179

Yang, Y. W. & Yang, J. C. (1996b). Characterization of Calcium Phosphate as a Gene Carrier (II): Zeta Potential and DNA Transfection. *Drug Delivery*, 3, pp. 181-186

Zhou, C., Yu, B., Yang, X., Huo, T., Lee, L. J., Barth, R. F. & Lee, R. J. (2010). Lipid-coated nano-calcium-phosphate (LNCP) for gene delivery. *Int J Pharm*, 392, 1-2, pp. 201-208

Zinselmeyer, B. H., Mackay, S. P., Schatzlein, A. G. & Uchegbu, I. F. (2002). The lower-generation polypropylenimine dendrimers are effective gene-transfer agents. *Pharmaceutical Research*, 19, 7, pp. 960-967

10

Pyrrole-Imidazole Polyamides for Gene Therapy: Bioanalytical Methods and Pharmacokinetics

Tomonori Kamei[1], Takahiko Aoyama[1], Takahiro Ueno[2],
Noboru Fukuda[2,3], Hiroki Nagase[3,4] and Yoshiaki Matsumoto[1]
[1]*Department of Clinical Pharmacokinetics, School of Pharmacy, Nihon University*
[2]*Department of Medicine, Division of Nephrology and Endocrinology*
Nihon University School of Medicine
[3]*Advanced Research Institute for the Science and Humanities, Nihon University*
[4]*Division of Cancer Genetics, Department of Advanced Medical Science*
Nihon University School of Medicine
Japan

1. Introduction

Pyrrole(Py)-imidazole(Im)(PI) polyamides are small synthetic molecules composed of aromatic rings of N-methylpyrrole and N-methylimidazole amino acids (Trauger et al., 1996). Synthetic polyamides recognize and bind to specific nucleotide sequences in the minor groove of double-helical DNA with high affinity (Pilch et al., 1996). Various sequence-specific DNA-binding PI polyamides have been developed to regulate gene expression by targeting the promoter regions of enhancer and transcription factor-binding elements in vitro (Murty et al., 2004). PI polyamides were first identified from duocarmycin A and distamycin A, which bind in the minor groove of DNA (Tao et al., 1999; Trauger et al., 1996). Sequence-specific DNA recognition by PI polyamide depends on the sequence of side-by-side amino acid pairs. A pair of Py opposite Im targets the CG base pair, whereas Im opposite Py recognizes the GC base pair, and the Py/Py combination binds to both AT and TA base pairs (White et al., 1997). PI polyamides designed to bind to the transcription factors Ets-1, lymphoid-enhancer binding factor 1, and the TATAbox-binding protein DNA binding site have been shown to inhibit virus replication in isolated human peripheral blood lymphocytes (Dickinson et al., 1998).

PI polyamides can easily enter into the nucleus and bind to chromosomal DNA. Many promising observation for gene therapy using PI polyamides have been reported. PI polyamide targeting rat transforming growth factor (TGF)-β_1 has been reported to inhibit the expressions of TGF-β_1 mRNA and protein in the renal cortex of Dahl-S rats. The targeted PI polyamide also reduced glomerulosclerosis and interstitial fibrosis without side effects. These observations indicate that PI polyamides will be effective for TGF-β_1-related diseases, including progressive renal injury (Matsuda et al., 2011; Matsuda et al., 2006). PI polyamides targeting human aurora kinase-A (AURKA) and -B (AURKB) promoters significantly inhibited the promoter activities, and mRNA and protein expression levels of AURKA and

AURKB. They also demonstrated a marked antiproliferative synergy in human tumor cell lines as a result of induction of apoptosis-mediated severe catastrophe of cell-cycle progression (Takahashi et al., 2008). PI polyamides specifically inhibited lectin-like oxidized low-density lipoprotein receptor-1 mRNA expression and apoptosis induced by oxidized low-density lipoprotein and angiotensin II in human umbilical vein endothelial cells (Ueno et al., 2009). From these observations, PI polyamides have been identified as novel candidates for gene therapy.

Pharmacokinetics is the science that studies the behavior of a circulating drug administered to a body, mainly focusing on absorption, distribution, metabolism, and excretion (ADME) of a drug (Jang et al., 2001). The concentration of a drug in a body can be obtained by a bioanalytical method which includes sample extraction and detection of a drug, and the obtained data are analyzed to evaluate the pharmacokinetics of the drug. Needless to say, a robust bioanalytical procedure is crucial for evaluating the appropriate pharmacokinetic profile of a drug.

In this chapter, we show the bioanalytical procedure, pharmacokinetics, and modeling of PI polyamides A and B. PI polyamides A and B are illustrated in Fig. 1. PI polyamide A was composed of Ac-ImPyPy-ImPyPy-β-Dp (β, β-alanine; Dp, N, N-dimethylaminopropylamide). PI polyamide B was composed of Ac-PyPy-β-PyImPy-PyPyPy-β-ImPy-β-Dp. The molecular weights of PI polyamides A and B were calculated from the sum of the standard atomic weights of all the atoms (Wieser, 2006). The molecular weights of PI polyamides A and B are 1035.12 and 1665.78, respectively. PI polyamide B was designed to bind to the activator protein-1 (AP-1)-binding site of the TGF-β_1 promoter, whereas PI polyamide A also, with a hairpin structure, was designed for comparing with other types of PI polyamide with a hairpin structure and a higher molecular weight.

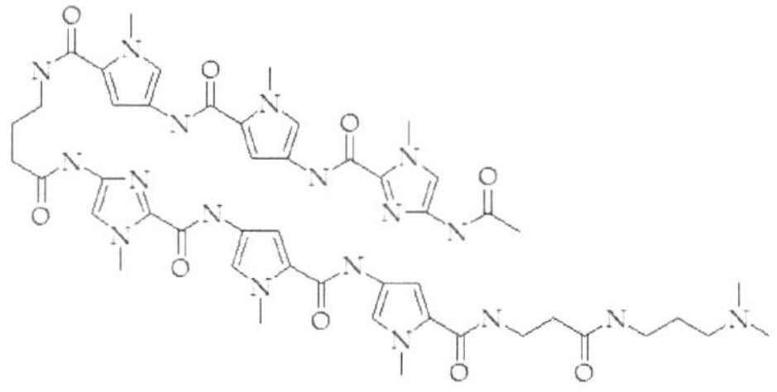

PI polyamide A

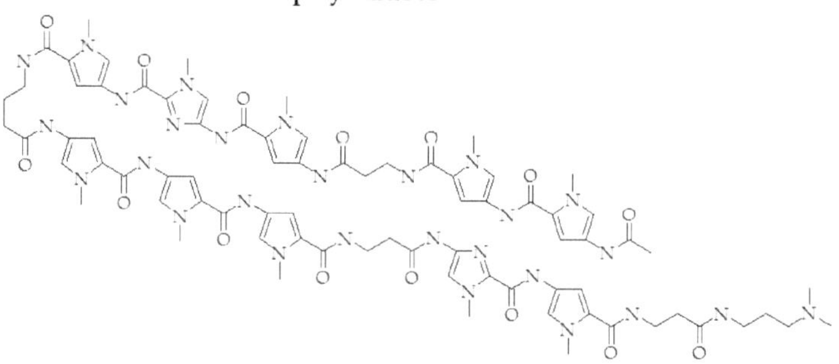

PI polyamide B

Fig. 1. Chemical structures of PI polyamides A and B.

2. Bioanalytics

High-performance liquid chromatography (HPLC) has been used for many years as a useful and conventional tool for the analysis of a drug. Bioanalytical methods by HPLC with UV detection were developed for the determination of PI polyamides A and B in the rat matrix. Sample extraction is one of the important steps and key to success in constructing a robust method. A simple protein precipitation method was developed for the extraction of PI polyamides A and B from rat plasma, whereas solid phase extraction was carried out to extract PI polyamides A and B from rat urine and bile, because a large number of urinary and biliary matrices can interfere with the compounds. It is important to determine the rates of urinary and biliary excretions because these excretions play pivotal roles in the elimination pathway of a drug. The developed methods were successively validated for selectivity, sensitivity, linearity, accuracy, and precision, following the guideline for Bioanalytical Method Validation published by Food and Drug Administration in 2001.

Chromatographic separation was conducted using a reversed-phase TSK-GEL ODS-80T$_M$ (4.6 mm x 150 mm) column maintained at 40 °C. The mobile phase of solvent A was 0.1% acetic acid and that of solvent B was acetonitrile (a linear increase from 0 to 80% B over 10 min (plasma and urine) or 35 min (bile) and an isocratic flow at 60% B for 5 min). The flow rate was set at 1.0 mL/min (plasma and urine) or 0.75 mL/min (bile). The detection wavelength was set at 310 nm. PI polyamides A and B were well separated from the coextracted material under the described chromatographic conditions at approximate retention times of 9.7 (25.0 in bile) and 10.5 min, respectively. The peak shapes were satisfactory and completely resolved from one another. No interference from rat matrices was observed (Fukasawa et al., 2007).

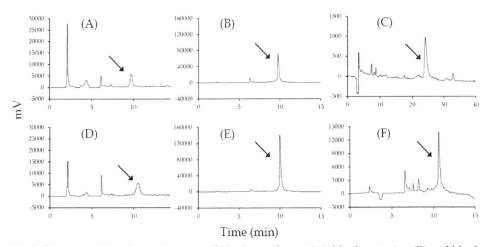

Fig. 2. Representative chromatograms of blank rat plasma (A), blank rat urine (B) and blank rat bile (C) spiked with PI polyamide A, and blank rat plasma (D), blank rat urine (E) and blank rat bile (F) spiked with PI polyamide B. The concentrations of PI polyamides were 5 (A), 20 (B), 1 (C), 5 (D), 20 (E) and 5 (F) µg/ml.

Table 1 shows the intra- and inter-assay precision and accuracy of PI polyamides A and B. The intra- and inter-assay accuracies (RE) were within ± 20% for the lower limit of quantitation (LLOQ) and ± 15% for the other QC samples. The intra- and inter-assay precisions (CV) were also within the acceptable ranges of 20% for the LLOQ and 15% for the other QC samples. The LLOQ was determined as 1 µg/mL for both PI polyamides A and B. All of the methods were successfully applied to evaluate the pharmacokinetics of the PI polyamides (Fukasawa et al., 2009; Fukasawa et al., 2007; Nagashima et al., 2009b).

Matrix		Nominal concentration (µg/mL)	Intra-assay		Inter-assay	
			RE (%)	CV (%)	RE (%)	CV (%)
Plasma	PI polyamide A	1	2.2	5.3	6.7	14.4
		20	1.4	1.4	-8.7	9.7
		100	7.7	3.7	3.6	3.5
	PI polyamide B	1	2.8	10.0	2.2	15.0
		20	-2.5	0.6	-9.2	7.9
		100	3.7	2.6	3.2	3.2
Urine	PI polyamide A	1	13.4	1.2	4.6	7.9
		20	-0.9	0.7	-4.7	3.6
		200	0.4	0.3	-2.6	4.5
	PI polyamide B	1	7.3	1.9	11.9	4.4
		10	1.9	1.2	0.1	2.3
		20	0.4	0.5	0.1	0.8

Table 1. Intra- and inter-assay accuracy and precision for the determination of PI polyamides A and B in rat plasma and urine.

Although HPLC with UV detection is a useful tool for the determination of a drug, the sensitivity is a limitation factor for evaluating pharmacokinetic characteristic for many hours. Recently, liquid chromatography-tandem mass spectrometry (LC-MS/MS) has been used for the determination of a drug, especially when a sensitivity higher than that of HPLC is required. A bioanalytical method for the determination of PI polyamide A in rat plasma was successfully developed and validated by ultra-performance liquid chromatography (UPLC)-MS/MS with electrospray ionization (Nagashima et al., 2009a).

An MS scan was conducted in the positive ion mode to obtain the precursor ion of PI polyamide A. The mass spectra of PI polyamide A showed significant ions at the m/z of 1036, 519, and 346, which corresponds to $[M+H]^+$, $[M+2H]^{2+}$, and $[M+3H]^{3+}$, respectively (Fig. 3). The doubly charged polyamide showed the highest sensitivity during ionization. The product ion spectra of the doubly charged PI polyamide A are shown in Fig. 4. The multiple reaction monitoring (MRM) transition was selected at the m/z of 519 and 288.

Chromatographic separation was performed using an ACQUITY UPLC HSS T3 (1.8 µm, 2.1×50 mm) column with an in-line filter and maintained at 40 °C. The liquid flow rate was set at 0.3 mL/min. The mobile phase of solvent A was acetonitrile/water/acetic acid (5/95/0.1, v/v/v) and that of solvent B was acetonitrile/water/acetic acid (95/5/0.1, v/v/v). The gradient started at the mobile phase A-B (95:5%), changed linearly to A-B (45:55%) until 2 min, washed with A-B (0:100%) until 3.5 min, and equilibrated under the initial condition until 5.5 min. PI polyamide A was well separated from the coextracted material under the described conditions at an approximate retention time of 1.5 min. No interference from rat matrices was observed (Fig. 5).

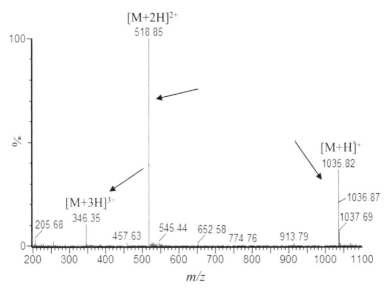

Fig. 3. Representative mass spectra of precursor ions (m/z, 1036 [M+H]+, 519 [M+2H]2+, and 346 [M+3H]3+) of PI polyamide A.

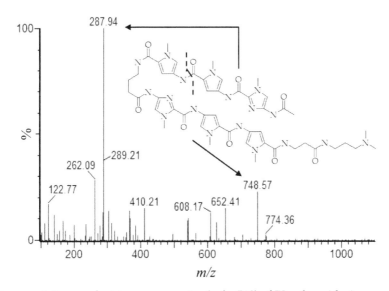

Fig. 4. Representative product ion mass spectra (m/z, 519) of PI polyamide A.

Table 2 shows the intra- and inter-assay precision and accuracy of PI polyamide A. The intra- and inter-assay accuracies (RE) were within ± 20% for the LLOQ and ± 15% for the other QC samples. The intra- and inter-assay precisions (CV) were also within the acceptable ranges of 20% for the LLOQ and 15% for the other QC samples. The LLOQ was

10 ng/mL, which means it has a sufficient sensitivity to evaluate the pharmacokinetics of PI polyamides.

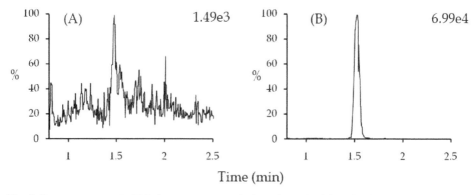

Fig. 5. Representative MRM chromatograms (m/z, 519>288) of (A) blank rat plasma, (B) blank rat plasma spiked with PI polyamide A (10 ng/mL).

Nominal concentration	Intra-assay		Inter-assay	
(ng/mL)	RE (%)	CV (%)	RE (%)	CV (%)
10	-10.6	3.3	3.7	11.2
1000	-11.7	1.5	-2.1	9.2
10000	-0.6	4.6	-5.0	8.9

Table 2. Intra- and inter-assay accuracy and precision for the determination of PI polyamide A in rat plasma.

3. Pharmacokinetics of PI polyamides A and B

3.1 Plasma and lung concentrations of PI polyamides A and B

PI polyamide B significantly inhibited the expressions of TGF-β_1 mRNA and protein in the renal cortex of the Dahl-S rats and reduced the rates of increases in the amounts of urinary protein and albumin in the Dahl-S rats independent of blood pressure at a dose of 1.0 mg (Matsuda et al., 2006). From these observations, the doses of PI polyamides were selected on the basis of 1.0 mg dose of PI polyamide B per rat (about 3.0 mg/kg). PI polyamide B had a lower water solubility than PI polyamide A. The doses of PI polyamides A and B were determined to be in the ranges of 1.3-15.0 mg/kg and 1.0-5.0 mg/kg, respectively.

The mean plasma concentration-time profiles after the intravenous administration of PI polyamide A at 1.3, 2.0, 7.5, and 15.0 mg/kg and after that of PI polyamide B at 1.0, 2.0, 3.0, and 5.0 mg/kg are shown in Fig. 6. The plasma concentrations of PI polyamides A and B declined in a polyexponential manner for the four doses studied. The plasma concentration-time profiles of PI polyamides were analyzed by a non-compartmental method. The area under the plasma concentration-time curve ($AUC_{(0-Tlast)}$) and the area under the first moment curve ($AUMC_{(0-Tlast)}$) were obtained using the linear trapezoidal rule. $AUC_{(Tlast-\infty)}$ and $AUMC_{(Tlast-\infty)}$ were respectively calculated using C_n/λ_z and $t_nC_n/\lambda_z + C_n/\lambda_z{}^2$, where C_n is the last quantifiable concentration. Terminal-phase rate constant (λ_z) was calculated by the regression of the terminal log-linear portion of the plasma concentration curve. Terminal elimination half-life ($t_{1/2}$) was calculated to be $0.693/\lambda_z$. Systemic clearance (CL_t), mean residence time (MRT), and the volume of distribution in the steady state (V_{ss}) were calculated as dose/AUC, AUMC/AUC, and CL_t•MRT, respectively. The plasma concentrations of PI polyamides A and B were extrapolated to time zero (C_0). The maximum plasma concentration (C_{max}) of PI polyamide B was directly obtained from the observed data.

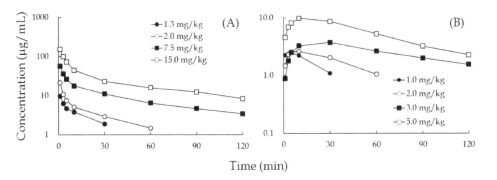

Fig. 6. Mean plasma concentration–time profiles of PI polyamides in rats after intravenous administration. (A) and (B) show PI polyamides A and B.

The pharmacokinetic parameters of PI polyamides A and B obtained in rats using non-compartmental analysis are summarized in Table 3. After the intravenous administration of PI polyamide A at 1.3, 2.0, 7.5, and 15.0 mg/kg, the average $t_{1/2}$, CL_t, and V_{ss} values were in the ranges of 42.3-74.8 min, 4.6-6.4 mL/min/kg, and 244-412 mL/kg, respectively. After the intravenous administration of PI polyamide B at 1.0, 2.0, 3.0, and 5.0 mg/kg, the average $t_{1/2}$, CL_t, and V_{ss} values were in the ranges of 27.5-58.7 min, 7.3-11.9 mL/min/kg, and 407-667 mL/kg, respectively. The CL_t and V_{ss} of PI polyamides A and B showed no significant differences as functions of administration dose. The pharmacokinetics of PI polyamides A and B are linear in the intravenous dose ranges of 1.3-15.0 mg/kg and 1.0-5.0 mg/kg, respectively as revealed by the fact that AUC increased linearly as a function of dose, and CL_t and V_{ss} remained unaltered.

The plasma concentration-time profiles after the intravenous administration of PI polyamide B resembled those after the oral administration. After the intravenous administration of PI polyamide B at 1.0, 2.0, 3.0, and 5.0 mg/kg, C_{max} gradually increased. The concentrations of PI polyamide B in the lungs, liver, heart, kidney and spleen were measured. The mean concentrations of PI polyamide B in the lungs were the highest among those in other tissues, and the mean concentrations 10, 30, and 60 min after injection were 134.7, 97.0, and 73.4 µg/g, respectively. Among various tissues, the concentration of PI polyamide B was observed to be highest in the lungs. The mean lung concentration of PI polyamide B decreased with time.

PI polyamide A

Parameter	Dose			
	1.3 mg/kg	2.0 mg/kg	7.5 mg/kg	15.0 mg/kg
Body weight (kg)	0.267	0.291	0.243	0.26
$t_{1/2}$ (min)	54.8	42.3	74.8	45.3
C_0 (µg/mL)	14.1	22.9	77.1	227.5
AUC (µg min/kg)	259.6	316.8	1528.6	3331.9
Cl (mL/min/kg)	5.6	6.4	5.1	4.6
Vss (mL/kg)	305.8	274.6	411.8	243.7
MRT (min)	68.1	42.6	80.5	54

PI polyamide B

Parameter	Dose			
	1.0 mg/kg	2.0 mg/kg	3.0 mg/kg	5.0 mg/kg
Body weight (kg)	0.313	0.317	0.317	0.317
$t_{1/2}$ (min)	139.1	165.8	207.3	359.3
C_0 (µg/mL)	1.5	4	3.8	4
AUC (µg min/kg)	108.1	205.2	326.8	508.3
Cl (mL/min/kg)	9.9	8.9	9.2	10.3
Vss (mL/kg)	2170.5	1990.1	2602.2	4567
MRT (min)	194.7	222.5	289.7	492.1

Table 3. Mean non-compartmental pharmacokinetic parameters of PI polyamides after intravenous administration at various doses into rats (n = 3).

3.2 Urinary and biliary excretions

Determination of the urinary and biliary excretion rates is crucial for the evaluation of the pharmacokinetics of a drug, because drugs are usually eliminated from the body into urine and/or bile (Ullrich, 1997; van Montfoort et al., 2003). The urinary and biliary excretion rate-time profiles are shown in Figs. 7 and 8, respectively. The urinary excretion rates of PI polyamides A and B showed a linear elimination. The biliary excretion rate of PI polyamide A showed saturation at the early period, while PI polyamide B was not detected in the bile. The cumulative urinary excretion rates of PI polyamides A and B at 48 h were 72.4 ± 11.6 and 4.8 ± 0.5% (mean ± SD, n = 3) of the administered dose, respectively. The cumulative biliary excretion rate of PI polyamide A at 24 h was 4.3 ± 0.4% (n = 4) of the administered dose. These observations indicated that unchanged PI polyamides A and B were slowly eliminated from the body. As observed from the plasma concentration-time profile, it is considered that most of the PI polyamide B remained in the lungs. No peaks of metabolites were detected for all the samples.

The differences in the molecular weights of compounds affect their eliminations (Hirom et al., 1976). The molecular weight thresholds for the excretion of organic cations into rat bile were found to be in the ranges of 200 ± 50 for monovalent organic cations and 500-600 for bivalent organic cations. (Hughes et al., 1973a; b) PI polyamide with a molecular weight of

1422.51 was excreted at 2% into rat urine 24 h after administration and was not detected in rat bile (data not shown). These findings suggested that PI polyamides with high molecular weights tend to be poorly excreted in both rat urine and bile, whereas those with molecular weights less than that of PI polyamide A can be readily eliminated. As described above, the differences in the elimination pathway between PI polyamides A and B may be attributed to the differences in their molecular weights.

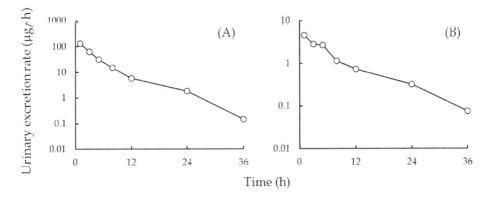

Fig. 7. Urinary excretion rate versus time profile of PI polyamides A (A) and B (B) in rats.

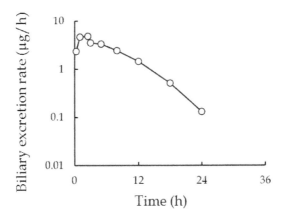

Fig. 8. Biliary excretion rate versus time profile of PI polyamide A in rats.

4 Pharmacokinetic modeling and simulations

4.1 Pharmacokinetic modeling
The plasma concentration-time profiles after the intravenous administration of PI polyamide A was fitted well by a two-compartment model. The estimated pharmacokinetic parameters

using the model are summarized in Table 4. After the intravenous administration of PI polyamide A at 1.3, 2.0, 7.5, and 15.0 mg/kg, the average CL_t and V_{ss} values were in the ranges of 4.9-7.0 mL/min/kg and 245-335 mL/kg, respectively. The CL_t and V_{ss} values estimated using a two-compartment model and a non-compartment model are thought to be identical.

Parameter	Dose			
	1.3 mg/kg	2.0 mg/kg	7.5 mg/kg	15.0 mg/kg
CL_t (mL/min/kg)	5.8	7	5.8	4.9
V_{ss} (mL/kg)	335	250	323	245
V_c (mL/kg)	90.5	89.6	96.6	69.7

Table 4. Estimated pharmacokinetic parameters of PI polyamide A obtained using two-compartment model.

The plasma concentration-time profiles after the intravenous administration of PI polyamide B increased in the early phase and resembled those after the oral administration. The slope of the decline in the lung concentration-time profiles of PI polyamide B was nearly equal to that in the plasma concentration-time profiles of PI polyamide B. To describe the increasing phase of PI polyamide B after the intravenous administration, the lung and plasma concentration-time profiles of PI polyamide B were fitted using a catenary two-compartment model (Fig. 9) (Brown et al., 1981).

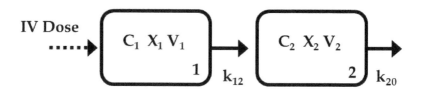

Fig. 9. Pharmacokinetic model of PI polyamide B.

C_1, X_1, and V_1 represent the concentration of PI polyamide B in the lungs, the amount of PI polyamide B in the lungs, and the distribution volume of the lung compartment, respectively. C_2, X_2, and V_2 represent the concentration of PI polyamide B in plasma, the amount of PI polyamide B in plasma, and the distribution volume of the plasma compartment, respectively. The pharmacokinetic parameters were calculated using the NONMEM program.

Figure 10 shows the simulation curves for PI polyamide B based on the catenary two-compartment model. The plasma and lung concentrations were fitted well by the model. The estimated pharmacokinetic parameters after the intravenous administration of PI polyamide B are summarized in Table 5. The estimated coefficients of variation (CV%) were small, the catenary two-compartment model better fitted the concentration-time profile after the intravenous administration of PI polyamide B. The model-estimated clearance (6.8 mL/min/kg) calculated as k_{20} multiplied by V_2 was nearly equal to CL_t (7.3 mL/min/kg). In this study, lung concentrations of first-point were measured at 10 min. It is thought that the concentration in the lungs immediately after the intravenous administration of PI polyamide B is higher than the calculated value. The early-plasma concentration-time profiles after the intravenous administration of a hairpin polyamide-chlorambucil conjugate, duocarmycin, and nitroglycerin are similar to that of PI polyamide B (Alberts et al., 1998; Chou et al., 2008; Wester et al., 1983) Recently, the biodistribution of a hairpin polyamide-chlorambucil conjugate administered into mice has been reported (Chou et al., 2008). The predominant occupancy of the polyamide-chlorambucil conjugate was observed in the lungs, spleen, small intestine, and pancreas 2 and 24 h after the injection. The concentration of polyamide-chlorambucil conjugate in the lungs at 2 h was higher than that of the polyamide-chlorambucil conjugate at 24 h. These findings are consistent with our results. PI polyamide B is distributed in the aorta and localizes in the nuclei of aortic midlayer smooth muscle (Matsuda et al., 2006). The lungs consist of pulmonary alveoli, which are surrounded by capillary vessels. It has been reported that weak basic drugs accumulate in the lungs and that such accumulation is attributable to lysosomal trapping (MacIntyre et al., 1988; Rodgers et al., 2005). A high concentration of PI polyamide B in the lungs was thought to be caused by PI polyamide B being distributed in capillary vessels of the lungs and by PI polyamide B being a weak base compared with PI polyamide with a molecular weight of 1422.51. It is also conceivable that PI polyamide B accumulated in the lungs owing to its high molecular weight, as suggested in a previous study (Wiseman et al., 2000). From these considerations, the proposed catenary two-compartment model may be applicable to describing PI polyamide B in detail.

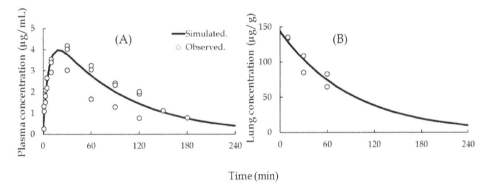

Fig. 10. Model fitted PI polyamide B concentration-time profiles in plasma and lungs. A is plasma concentration–time profiles and B is lung concentration-time profiles. The middle bold line indicates the 50th percentiles for 1000 simulations. Symbols depict the observed data after the intravenous administration of PI polyamide B at 3.0 mg/kg.

4.2 Pharmacokinetic modeling with excretion data in addition to plasma concentration

To predict the plasma concentration-time profile in the elimination phase of PI polyamide A after intravenous administration, two pharmacokinetic models (i.e., one- and two-compartment models with the linear output compartment interpreted as the urine compartment and the non-linear output compartments interpreted as the bile compartment) using the plasma concentration-time profile and cumulative urinary and biliary excretion

Parameter	Estimates
k_{12} (L/min)	0.0109
k_{20} (L/min)	0.1476
V_1 (mL/kg)	20.88
V_2 (mL/kg)	45.86

Table 5. Pharmacokinetic parameters of PI polyamide B from model fitting.

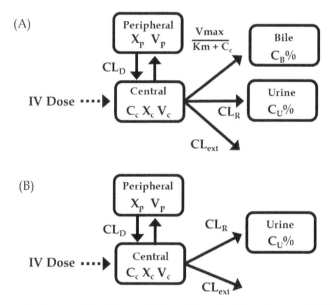

Fig. 11. Scheme of pharmacokinetic model describing the disposition and elimination of PI polyamides A (A) and B (B)

rates of PI polyamide A were tested. A scheme of the two-compartment model, with the linear output compartment interpreted as the urine compartment and the non-linear output compartment interpreted as the bile compartment, is shown in Fig. 11A.

X and V are the amount and volume of distribution in the corresponding compartments designated by the subscripts C, P, U, and B representing central, peripheral, urine, and bile compartments, respectively. CL_D is the distribution clearance, CL_R is the renal clearance, CL_{ext} is the clearance excluding renal and biliary clearances, V_{MAX} is the maximum velocity for excretion into bile, and Km is the Michaelis constant for excretion into bile. Cc represents the plasma concentration of PI polyamide A. $C_U\%$ and $C_B\%$ represent the cumulative urinary and biliary excretion rates (percentage of administered dose), respectively.

The residual error model of the plasma concentration was assumed to be the proportional error model because the plasma concentration was measured by HPLC. The model of the cumulative urinary and biliary excretions was assumed to be the additive error model because the percentage of the administered dose was calculated from the urine and bile concentrations, urine and bile volumes, and administered dose. The choice of model was based on model fitting criteria such as visual inspection of the fitted curves, objective function value of NONMEM (OFV), and CV% of the parameter estimates (Hazra et al., 2007; Matsumoto et al., 2005).

The plasma concentration and cumulative urinary and biliary excretion-time profiles after intravenous administration of PI polyamide A were fitted well by the two-compartment model with the linear output compartment interpreted as the urine compartment and the non-linear output compartment interpreted as the bile compartment (Fig. 12). The 50th percentiles of the model-based prediction for plasma concentrations and cumulative urinary and biliary excretions are presented together with the observed value. To obtain 50th percentiles of the model estimations, 10000 simulations were performed using the estimated model parameters, variability in the estimated parameters, and residual variability of the data. Compared with a one-compartment model using only plasma data, more accurate data can be obtained from the two-compartment model including urine and bile data because PI polyamide A was excreted into urine and bile until at least 36 and 18 h, respectively, after administration. The plasma concentration-time profile in the elimination phase could also be described better using both the linear and non-linear compartments than using plasma data only.

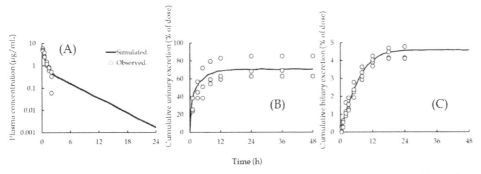

Fig. 12. Plasma concentration–time profile (A), cumulative urinary excretion rate (B), and cumulative biliary excretion rate (C) of PI polyamide A after intravenous administration at 2.0 mg/kg to rats. Each data point represents observed data from three (for plasma and urine) and four rats (for bile). The solid line indicates 50th percentiles from model estimations of 10000 simulations.

To predict the plasma concentration-time profile in the elimination phase of PI polyamide B after intravenous administration, two pharmacokinetic models (i.e., one- and two-compartment models with the linear output compartment interpreted as the urine compartment) using the plasma concentration-time profile and cumulative urinary excretions of PI polyamide B were tested. A scheme of the two-compartment model with the linear output compartment interpreted as the urine compartment is shown in Fig. 11B. The residual error models of the plasma concentration of PI polyamide B were the same as described in the part of PI polyamide A.

The plasma concentration and cumulative urinary excretion-time profiles after intravenous administration of PI polyamide B were fitted well by the two-compartment model with the linear output compartment interpreted as the urine compartment (Fig. 13). The 50th percentiles of the model-based prediction for plasma concentrations and cumulative urinary excretions are presented together with the observed value. To obtain 50th percentiles of the model estimations, 10000 simulations were performed using the estimated model parameters, variability in the estimated parameters, and residual variability of the data.

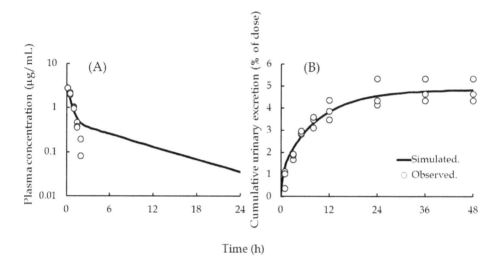

Fig. 13. Plasma concentration–time profile (A) and cumulative urinary excretion (B) of PI polyamide B after intravenous administration at 2.0 mg/kg to rats. Each data point represents observed data from three rats (for plasma and urine). The solid line indicates 50th percentiles from model estimations of 10000 simulations.

To predict the effective dose of PI polyamide B in Dahl-S rats administered at 1 mg every 2 or 3 days for 4 weeks, pharmacokinetic simulations of PI polyamide B were performed using a slightly modified pharmacokinetic model (Nagashima et al., 2009b) by NONMEM program. The average plasma concentrations of PI polyamide B after the administration at 1 mg every 3 and 2 days were 0.18 and 0.28 µg/mL, respectively, which were calculated by the area under the concentration-time curves between 0 and 27 days, divided by 27 days. PI polyamide B did not accumulate following multiple-dose administration.

5. Conclusion

PI polyamides show a remarkable potential for use in non viral gene therapy as many attractive results were obtained. The novel compounds could provide a promising impact on gene therapy for diseases not treatable by current remedies. To obtain the maximum therapeutic effect of the PI polyamide, it is crucial to evaluate the pharmacokinetics of the compounds for designing appropriate dosage regimens. Bioanalytical procedures for PI polyamides A and B were successfully developed and validated by HPLC or LC-MS/MS, and applied to sample assay. The pharmacokinetic profiles of PI polyamides show interesting results, which are thought to be related to their molecular weights (Brown et al.,

1981). It was suggested that the features of various compositions of Py and Im were related to their unique pharmacokinetic profiles. Further examination will be conducted using other PI polyamides that have unique Py and Im combinations for gene therapy.

6. Acknowledgements

This work was supported in part by a Grand-in-Aid from the High-Tech Research Center Project for 2007-2011 and the Academic Frontier Project for 2006-2010 for Private Universities: matching fund subsidy from the Ministry of Education, Culture, Sports, Science and Technology. We thank Takashi Nagashima, Ph.D. and Akiko Fukawasa, Ph.D. for their help.

7. References

Alberts, S. R.; Erlichman, C.; Reid, J. M.; Sloan, J. A.; Ames, M. M.; Richardson, R. L. & Goldberg, R. M. (1998). Phase I study of the duocarmycin semisyntheticderivative KW-2189 given daily for five days every six weeks. *Clin Cancer Res*, Vol. 4, No. 9, pp. 2111-2117, ISSN 1078-0432 (Print) 1078-0432 (Linking).

Brown, P. H.; Krishnamurthy, G. T.; Bobba, V. V. & Kingston, E. (1981). Radiation dose calculation for Tc-99m HIDA in health and disease. *J Nucl Med*, Vol. 22, No. 2, pp. 177-183, ISSN 0161-5505 (Print) 0161-5505 (Linking).

Chou, C. J.; Farkas, M. E.; Tsai, S. M.; Alvarez, D.; Dervan, P. B. & Gottesfeld, J. M. (2008). Small molecules targeting histone H4 as potential therapeutics for chronic myelogenous leukemia. *Mol Cancer Ther*, Vol. 7, No. 4, pp. 769-778, ISSN 1535-7163 (Print) 1535-7163 (Linking).

Dickinson, L. A.; Gulizia, R. J.; Trauger, J. W.; Baird, E. E.; Mosier, D. E.; Gottesfeld, J. M. & Dervan, P. B. (1998). Inhibition of RNA polymerase II transcription in human cells by synthetic DNA-binding ligands. *Proc Natl Acad Sci U S A*, Vol. 95, No. 22, pp. 12890-12895, ISSN 0027-8424 (Print) 0027-8424 (Linking).

Fukasawa, A.; Aoyama, T.; Nagashima, T.; Fukuda, N.; Ueno, T.; Sugiyama, H.; Nagase, H. & Matsumoto, Y. (2009). Pharmacokinetics of pyrrole-imidazole polyamides after intravenous administration in rat. *Biopharm Drug Dispos*, Vol. 30, No. 2, pp. 81-89, ISSN 1099-081X (Electronic) 0142-2782 (Linking).

Fukasawa, A.; Nagashima, T.; Aoyama, T.; Fukuda, N.; Matsuda, H.; Ueno, T.; Sugiyama, H.; Nagase, H. & Matsumoto, Y. (2007). Optimization and validation of a high-performance liquid chromatographic method with UV detection for the determination of pyrrole-imidazole polyamides in rat plasma. *J Chromatogr B Analyt Technol Biomed Life Sci*, Vol. 859, No. 2, pp. 272-275, ISSN 1570-0232 (Print) 1570-0232 (Linking).

Hazra, A.; Pyszczynski, N.; DuBois, D. C.; Almon, R. R. & Jusko, W. J. (2007). Pharmacokinetics of methylprednisolone after intravenous and intramuscular administration in rats. *Biopharm Drug Dispos*, Vol. 28, No. 6, pp. 263-273, ISSN 0142-2782 (Print) 0142-2782 (Linking).

Hirom, P. C.; Millburn, P. & Smith, R. L. (1976). Bile and urine as complementary pathways for the excretion of foreign organic compounds. *Xenobiotica*, Vol. 6, No. 1, pp. 55-64, ISSN 0049-8254 (Print) 0049-8254 (Linking).

Hughes, R. D.; Millburn, P. & Williams, R. T. (1973a). Biliary excretion of some diquaternary ammonium cations in the rat, guinea pig and rabbit. *Biochem J*, Vol. 136, No. 4, pp. 979-984, ISSN 0264-6021 (Print) 0264-6021 (Linking).

Hughes, R. D.; Millburn, P. & Williams, R. T. (1973b). Molecular weight as a factor in the excretion of monoquaternary ammonium cations in the bile of the rat, rabbit and guinea pig. *Biochem J*, Vol. 136, No. 4, pp. 967-978, ISSN 0264-6021 (Print) 0264-6021 (Linking).

Jang, G. R.; Harris, R. Z. & Lau, D. T. (2001). Pharmacokinetics and its role in small molecule drug discovery research. *Med Res Rev*, Vol. 21, No. 5, pp. 382-396, ISSN 0198-6325 (Print) 0198-6325 (Linking).

MacIntyre, A. C. & Cutler, D. J. (1988). The potential role of lysosomes in tissue distribution of weak bases. *Biopharm Drug Dispos*, Vol. 9, No. 6, pp. 513-526, ISSN 0142-2782 (Print) 0142-2782 (Linking).

Matsuda, H.; Fukuda, N.; Ueno, T.; Katakawa, M.; Wang, X.; Watanabe, T.; Matsui, S.; Aoyama, T.; Saito, K.; Bando, T.; Matsumoto, Y.; Nagase, H.; Matsumoto, K. & Sugiyama, H. (2011). Transcriptional inhibition of progressive renal disease by gene silencing pyrrole-imidazole polyamide targeting of the transforming growth factor-beta1 promoter. *Kidney Int*, Vol. 79, No. 1, pp. 46-56, ISSN 1523-1755 (Electronic) 0085-2538 (Linking).

Matsuda, H.; Fukuda, N.; Ueno, T.; Tahira, Y.; Ayame, H.; Zhang, W.; Bando, T.; Sugiyama, H.; Saito, S.; Matsumoto, K.; Mugishima, H. & Serie, K. (2006). Development of gene silencing pyrrole-imidazole polyamide targeting the TGF-beta1 promoter for treatment of progressive renal diseases. *J Am Soc Nephrol*, Vol. 17, No. 2, pp. 422-432, ISSN 1046-6673 (Print) 1046-6673 (Linking).

Matsumoto, Y.; Fujita, T.; Ishida, Y.; Shimizu, M.; Kakuo, H.; Yamashita, K.; Majima, M. & Kumagai, Y. (2005). Population pharmacokinetic-pharmacodynamic modeling of TF-505 using extension of indirect response model by incorporating a circadian rhythm in healthy volunteers. *Biol Pharm Bull*, Vol. 28, No. 8, pp. 1455-1461, ISSN 0918-6158 (Print) 0918-6158 (Linking).

Murty, M. S. & Sugiyama, H. (2004). Biology of N-methylpyrrole-N-methylimidazole hairpin polyamide. *Biol Pharm Bull*, Vol. 27, No. 4, pp. 468-474, ISSN 0918-6158 (Print) 0918-6158 (Linking).

Nagashima, T.; Aoyama, T.; Fukasawa, A.; Watabe, S.; Fukuda, N.; Ueno, T.; Sugiyama, H.; Nagase, H. & Matsumoto, Y. (2009a). Determination of pyrrole-imidazole polyamide in rat plasma by liquid chromatography-tandem mass spectrometry. *J Chromatogr B Analyt Technol Biomed Life Sci*, Vol. 877, No. 11-12, pp. 1070-1076, ISSN 1873-376X (Electronic) 1570-0232 (Linking).

Nagashima, T.; Aoyama, T.; Yokoe, T.; Fukasawa, A.; Fukuda, N.; Ueno, T.; Sugiyama, H.; Nagase, H. & Matsumoto, Y. (2009b). Pharmacokinetic modeling and prediction of plasma pyrrole-imidazole polyamide concentration in rats using simultaneous urinary and biliary excretion data. *Biol Pharm Bull*, Vol. 32, No. 5, pp. 921-927, ISSN 0918-6158 (Print) 0918-6158 (Linking).

Pilch, D. S.; Poklar, N.; Gelfand, C. A.; Law, S. M.; Breslauer, K. J.; Baird, E. E. & Dervan, P. B. (1996). Binding of a hairpin polyamide in the minor groove of DNA: sequence-specific enthalpic discrimination. *Proc Natl Acad Sci U S A*, Vol. 93, No. 16, pp. 8306-8311, ISSN 0027-8424 (Print) 0027-8424 (Linking).

Rodgers, T.; Leahy, D. & Rowland, M. (2005). Tissue distribution of basic drugs: accounting for enantiomeric, compound and regional differences amongst beta-blocking drugs in rat. *J Pharm Sci*, Vol. 94, No. 6, pp. 1237-1248, ISSN 0022-3549 (Print) 0022-3549 (Linking).

Takahashi, T.; Asami, Y.; Kitamura, E.; Suzuki, T.; Wang, X.; Igarashi, J.; Morohashi, A.; Shinojima, Y.; Kanou, H.; Saito, K.; Takasu, T.; Nagase, H.; Harada, Y.; Kuroda, K.; Watanabe, T.; Kumamoto, S.; Aoyama, T.; Matsumoto, Y.; Bando, T.; Sugiyama, H.; Yoshida-Noro, C.; Fukuda, N. & Hayashi, N. (2008). Development of pyrrole-imidazole polyamide for specific regulation of human aurora kinase-A and -B gene expression. *Chem Biol*, Vol. 15, No. 8, pp. 829-841, ISSN 1074-5521 (Print) 1074-5521 (Linking).

Tao, Z. F.; Fujiwara, T.; Saito, I. & Sugiyama, H. (1999). Sequence-specific alkylation of DNA by duocarmycin A and its novel derivatives bearing PY/IM polyamides. *Nucleosides Nucleotides*, Vol. 18, No. 6-7, pp. 1615-1616, ISSN 0732-8311 (Print) 0732-8311 (Linking).

Trauger, J. W.; Baird, E. E. & Dervan, P. B. (1996). Recognition of DNA by designed ligands at subnanomolar concentrations. *Nature*, Vol. 382, No. 6591, pp. 559-561, ISSN 0028-0836 (Print) 0028-0836 (Linking).

Ueno, T.; Fukuda, N.; Tsunemi, A.; Yao, E. H.; Matsuda, H.; Tahira, K.; Matsumoto, T.; Matsumoto, K.; Matsumoto, Y.; Nagase, H.; Sugiyama, H. & Sawamura, T. (2009). A novel gene silencer, pyrrole-imidazole polyamide targeting human lectin-like oxidized low-density lipoprotein receptor-1 gene improves endothelial cell function. *J Hypertens*, Vol. 27, No. 3, pp. 508-516, ISSN 1473-5598 (Electronic) 0263-6352 (Linking).

Ullrich, K. J. (1997). Renal transporters for organic anions and organic cations. Structural requirements for substrates. *J Membr Biol*, Vol. 158, No. 2, pp. 95-107, ISSN 0022-2631 (Print) 0022-2631 (Linking).

van Montfoort, J. E.; Hagenbuch, B.; Groothuis, G. M.; Koepsell, H.; Meier, P. J. & Meijer, D. K. (2003). Drug uptake systems in liver and kidney. *Curr Drug Metab*, Vol. 4, No. 3, pp. 185-211, ISSN 1389-2002 (Print) 1389-2002 (Linking).

Wester, R. C.; Noonan, P. K.; Smeach, S. & Kosobud, L. (1983). Pharmacokinetics and bioavailability of intravenous and topical nitroglycerin in the rhesus monkey: estimate of percutaneous first-pass metabolism. *J Pharm Sci*, Vol. 72, No. 7, pp. 745-748, ISSN 0022-3549 (Print) 0022-3549 (Linking).

White, S.; Baird, E. E. & Dervan, P. B. (1997). On the pairing rules for recognition in the minor groove of DNA by pyrrole-imidazole polyamides. *Chem Biol*, Vol. 4, No. 8, pp. 569-578, ISSN 1074-5521 (Print) 1074-5521 (Linking).

Wieser, M. (2006). Atomic weights of the elements 2005. *Pure Appl. Chem.*, Vol. 78, No. 11, pp. 2051-2066,

Wiseman, G. A.; White, C. A.; Stabin, M.; Dunn, W. L.; Erwin, W.; Dahlbom, M.;
    Raubitschek, A.; Karvelis, K.; Schultheiss, T.; Witzig, T. E.; Belanger, R.; Spies, S.;
    Silverman, D. H.; Berlfein, J. R.; Ding, E. & Grillo-Lopez, A. J. (2000). Phase I/II
    90Y-Zevalin (yttrium-90 ibritumomab tiuxetan, IDEC-Y2B8) radioimmunotherapy
    dosimetry results in relapsed or refractory non-Hodgkin's lymphoma. *Eur J Nucl
    Med*, Vol. 27, No. 7, pp. 766-777, ISSN 0340-6997 (Print) 0340-6997 (Linking).

11

Binding of Protein-Functionalized Entities onto Synthetic Vesicles

Federica De Persiis[1], Ramon Pons[2], Carlotta Pucci[1],
Franco Tardani[1] and Camillo La Mesa[1,3]
[1]Dept. of Chemistry, La Sapienza University, Rome, Italy
[2]Institut de Química Avançada de Catalunya, IQAC-CSIC
[3]SOFT-INFM-CNR Research Centre, La Sapienza University, Rome
[1,3]Italy
[2]Spain

1. Introduction

Mono-disperse silica nano-particles with pending functional acid groups lying on their surface were reacted with coupling agents and, then, with lysozyme, to get protein-functionalized entities. The synthetic procedure reported therein gives tiny amounts of protein functionalized sites; surface coverage by the protein is, thus, moderate. The amount of covalently bound lysozyme was estimated from *UV*-vis methods and resulted to be about <5> molecules per nano-particle. Electro-phoretic mobility experiments indicate the occurrence of significant variations in surface charge density of functionalized nano-particles compared to the original ones and ensure a significant binding efficiency onto reconstructed, or synthetic, vesicles.

Protein-functionalized nano-particles form clusters and are readily re-dispersed by application of shear methods. Thereafter, they remain in disperse form for long times. According to *DLS*, protein-functionalized nano-particles interact with either cationic or cat-anionic synthetic vesicles. Care was made to ensure that nano-particles and vesicles have comparable sizes. The above procedure ensures to determine the fate of the reactive pathways by *DLS*. At room temperature and moderate ionic strength, the binding of protein-functionalized entities onto the aforementioned vesicles is completed in about one hour. The nano-particle vesicle complexes precipitate as fine powders, or form large floating objects, depending on vesicle size, relative concentrations of protein-functionalized particles and their net charge (which is related to the *pH* of the dispersing medium).

The binding efficiency for the above processes is controlled by the overlapping of repulsive and attractive interactions between particles and vesicles. The kinetic pathways relative to the interactions between vesicles and nano-particles were investigated, and significant differences were met in the two cases. Some technological implications of the above systems are preliminarily discussed. For instance, it is stated that interactions between nano-particles and vesicles mimic those occurring between cells and solid particles, or viral vectors, located in the medium surrounding vesicles.

Graphical Abstract

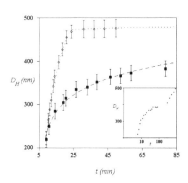
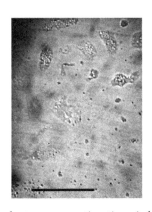

Left, Dependence of the size of nano-particle/vesicle clusters on reaction time, inferred by DLS methods.
Right, Clusters of vesicles and protein-functionalized nano-particles obtained by mixing DDAB vesicles and nano-particles in number ratio 300/1. Images were visualized through a Zeiss optical microscope using normal light. The bar size in the left bottom of the figure is 100 mm large.

Nanotechnologies deal with the synthesis, the characterization, the production and the application of objects and devices operating at the nano-scale level [1]. As a consequence of substantial interest in this field, many scientific journals and books are progressively addressing attention to nano-technologically oriented items. The same holds for the number of patents relative to these subjects. This is because the demand on the possible applications of the above materials is drastically increasing in the last few years. Practical applications are manifold and find use in electronics, in the preparation of magnetic devices, in chemistry (mostly in the field of heterogeneous catalysis), but also in biotechnology and biomedicine.
Materials at the nano-scale are widely different each from the other in chemical composition, size and surface functionalities. Particles properties depend on the preparation procedures and can be tailored accordingly. Nano-particles can be made of metals, oxides, polymers and/or a combination thereof. Properly functionalized particles, such as quantum dots, spheres, disks, filaments, tubes and composite objects (all in the nano-meter size range) find substantial application in the aforementioned fields.
In this contribution, we report on silica nano-particles, onto which a protein, lysozyme, was covalently bound [2,3]. The synthetic part of the work is reported below. The same holds for the characterization of the resulting hybrid composites. A substantial amount of work was needed to ensure the required performances to nano-particles, which were tailored in terms of state of the dispersion, size, stability and net charge. Obviously, the above effects are strongly interrelated each other. The reasons for using protein-functionalized entities arise by the need to have objects at the nano-scale level, characterized by a significant number of bound proteins. Apart from intrinsic interest towards the structural properties of hybrid nano-composites, the advantages of protein-functionalized particles are manifold compared to other bio-medical formulations, since:

i.   the surface area of the resulting nano-composites can be properly controlled,

ii. the number of covalently bound proteins can be modulated accordingly, and,

iii. the conformation of proteins adsorbed therein can be somehow predicted [4].

Silica was used as an anchoring site because of its good bio-compatibility, which is substantially higher compared to polymer-based nano-particles. It is particularly useful since blood and other bio-fluids contain markers adsorbing on the surface of hydrophobic carriers, and indicating to *RES* (the *Reticulum Endothelial System*) the urgency to remove them from the target tissue [5]. Conversely, silica nano-particles (*NPs*) are of friendly use with biological tissues. As most inorganic oxides, SiO_2 is strongly hydrophilic in character. Such property increases its compatibility and ensures a safe circulation in bio-fluids. In addition, it is possible to anchor efficiently proteins or other biologically active substances onto mono-dispersed silica.

Lysozyme was chosen to test the covalent binding efficiency onto nano-particles because of its ubiquitary nature. In the following, we report on anchoring efficiency and do not explicitly account for the effect that *pH*, salts or other substances have on the fate of protein-functionalized *NPs* in biological matrices. The present communication only focuses on the synthesis and characterization of such materials.

In the second part of this contribution the interactions between protein-functionalized silica *NPs* and synthetic vesicles were experienced. The synthetic vesicles dealt with in this contribution are also relatively mono-dispersed, thermodynamically, or kinetically, stable and are characterized, in some cases, by a bi-layer structure [6]. Hence, they can be considered the synthetic analogues of cell membranes. Were the interactions between vesicles and *NPs* effective, the possibility of surface adhesion, or encapsulation, can be realized. Perspectives of these complex systems as composite drug-delivery carriers are, thus, at hand.

We choose different vesicle-forming materials based on a synthetic double-chain surfactant and mixtures of different surface active species. The performances of the former class, based on quaternary ammonium salts, were extensively characterized by Barenholz and coworkers [7,8]. Such species, however, are of questionable utility for biomedical applications, since most quaternary ammonium salts have strong anti-bacterial character. In addition, the vesicles they form are intrinsically meta-stable and progressively coagulate into large entities.

Recently, alternatives to the above lipido-mimetic systems were proposed; they rely on systems obtained by mixing oppositely charged surfactants, or lipids, in due amounts. Such mixtures are currently defined by the acronym cat-anionic. These systems came in use since when Kaler and Khan independently characterized some of them [9,10]. In cat-anionic systems the vesicle size and net charge are tuned by modulating the ratio between the two components, provided one of them is in excess. (N.B. If not, the 1/1 mixtures precipitate out.) It is possible, thus, to get negatively or positively charged vesicles. This can be relevant in case vesicles should selectively interact through electrostatic interactions with proteins [11] or *DNA* [12] and form complexes, or lipo-plexes, with the above substances.

In the following we report on the synthetic procedures we have followed, on the optimization required getting stable dispersions of hybrid protein-silica colloids, and on their interactions with vesicles. For reasons to be discussed later, the characterization of the above protein-silica composite material is based on the combination of optical (*UV-vis* or *CD*), dynamic light scattering, *DLS*, and electro-phoretic mobility methods. Some relevant results are briefly reported in the forthcoming sections. Biomedical applications, which are surely relevant, require dedicated formulation work and need substantial studies on the cyto-toxicity of vesicles, lysozyme-bound *NPs* and of the related adducts. The former systems were previously characterized on this regard by some of us [13], but almost nothing is known on the latter ones.

2. Experimental section

Materials. 3-aminopropyl-(3-oxobutanoic acid)-functionalized silica *NPs*, termed *APOB*, contain significant amounts of carboxylic acids on their surface. They are given from the purveyor (Sigma Aldrich) as 2.5% (w/v) dispersions in dimethylformamide, *DMF*. Their nominal density is 0.927 g ml^{-1} at 25°C [14]. *NPs* were dialyzed against aqueous Borax (50 millimol, pH 8.5) under stirring, sonicated and recovered. The resulting dispersions are relatively stable, since *APOB* nano-particles bear negative charges on their surface.

Hen yolk lysozyme, *LYS*, (Sigma Aldrich) was dialyzed, crystallized, lyophilized and dried over P_2O_5. Its purity was confirmed by ionic conductance, density and viscosity of the corresponding aqueous solutions, at 25.00 °C [15,16].

Sodium dodecylsulfate, *SDS*, cetyltrimethylammonium bromide, *CTAB*, and didodecyl-dimethylammonium bromide, *DDAB*, (Sigma Aldrich) were individually dissolved in ethanol and precipitated by addition of cold acetone. The products were vacuum dried at 70°C. Their purity was confirmed by conductometric determination of the critical micellar concentration, *CMC*, at 25.00 °C. *Pluronic F-127* (Sigma Aldrich), a surface active block co-polymer, forming micelles at high temperatures [17], was used as dispersant, when required.

A water soluble carbodiimide, termed *EDAC*, hydroxysuccynimide, *NHS*, triethylamine, *N(Et)₃*, and glycine, (Sigma Aldrich), were used as such.

3. Materials preparation

LYS-ABOP nano-particles. 20 mg of *APOB* in 50 millimolar kg^{-1} (*mmol*) aqueous Borax were added with 13.0 mg *EDAC*, 10.0 mg *NHS* and 7.27 mg *N(Et)₃*, at 25°C [7], and homogenized upon stirring. 44.13 mg solid *LYS* was added and the reaction proceeded for 5 hours, at 40°C. The reaction between *ABOP* and *LYS* is concomitant to an increase in opalescence of the dispersions, due to both a decreased surface charge density (because of the reaction of *COOH* groups with *EDAC*), and to protein covalent binding. The final dispersion was centrifuged at 12000 rpm for 10 minutes, at 4°C. Thereafter, 10 mmol glycine was added, to quench un-reacted groups that were eventually bound onto *NPs*. The latter procedure significantly reduces the dispersion turbidity. A summary of the whole synthetic procedure, in four stages, is sketched in *Scheme 1*, where are indicated the different preparation steps.

Prolonged sonication, dialysis, with pH and/or ionic strength adjustment significantly tailors the average size of *NPs* and reduces their size. Substantial characterization is required to ensure the attainment of equilibrium conditions, since the size of particles increases with aging, *Figure 1*. The dispersions were extensively dialyzed against the buffer, until no more lysozime, *EDAC* and/or *NHS* was determined in the supernatant. To avoid the occurrence of clusters, the dispersions must be sheared [18] or forced to flow in tilted long syringe steel needles [19], as indicated in *Figure 2A*.

Synthesis of Lys-ABOP nano-particles:
a reactive scheme

Step 1

   P-NH-R-COOH $\xrightarrow[\substack{Borax\ 50\ mmol \\ pH\ 8.5}]{dialysis}$ **P-NH-R-COOH**

     (in DMF)   *(in Borax buffer)*

Step 2

   P-NH-R-COOH $\xrightarrow[\text{Borax 50 mmol, 25°C}]{}$ **Active**

     (in Borax buffer)

Step 3

   Active + Lyso $\xrightarrow[\text{Borax 50 mmol}]{10\ mmol\ Glycine}$ **Lys-ABOP nano-particles**

Step 4

Dialisys + pH conditioning + ionic strength control
+ centrifugation

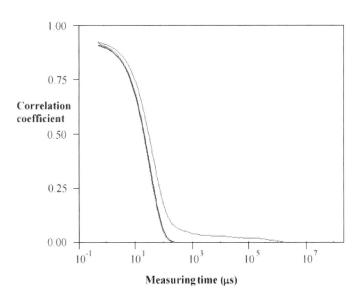

Fig. 1. Plots of the correlation coefficient (in arbitrary units) versus the measuring time, in μs, for a 0.20 wt/vol % dispersion of Lysozyme-ABOP nano-particles (in 50 mmol Borax buffer, pH 8.5, at 25°C) one day after preparation, in blue, one week, in orange, and one month, in cyan.

When particles are subjected to shear forces during flow, large aggregates break down. This procedure decreases the size of *LYS/ABOP* NPs, *Figure 2B*.

Cat-anionic vesicles were prepared by mixing 6.00 *mmol* aqueous *SDS* with 6.00 *mmol CTAB*, in due proportions. Optimal sizes and surface charge density occur when the mole ratio between *SDS* and *CTAB* is in the range 1.5-2.5. The dispersions are milky, because multi-lamellar, and size-poly-disperse, vesicles occur. It was formerly observed, however, that heating them to temperatures close to 50°C reduces the average size of multi-lamellar vesicles, with formation of truly bi-layered entities [20]. Thereafter, vesicles remain in such state for over two months, even when they are kept at room temperature.

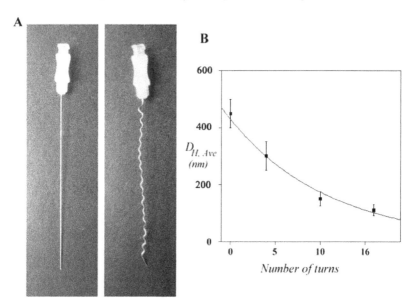

Fig. 2. A; View of iron steel needles, tilted to increase the number of turns. B; Reduction in size of 0.12 w/v % LYS-ABOP nano-particles obtained by coupling (and dispersed in 50 mmol Borax, pH 8.5, at 25°C) when forced to flow in tilted needles. Data are reported as average particles size (nm) versus number of turns in the needle. Each sample was forced to flow in the needles for 50 times.

DDAB vesicles are multi-layered entities and their properties were tailored by extrusion and/or thermal cycling. Both vesicular dispersions were thermally equilibrated at 25.0°C soon after the preparation procedures and controlled over a long-time scale. Temperatures lower than 20°C were avoided, since they imply partial surfactant precipitation in the *SDS-CTAB* system.

4. Methods

Dynamic Light Scattering. A Zeta Nanosizer unit, Malvern, performed measurements at 632.8 nm, in back scattering mode (*BSM*), at 173°. This configuration minimizes multiple scattering and allows measuring poly-disperse systems. The unit performances were checked by standard procedures [21]. Thermal equilibrium was controlled by a Peltier unit, at

25.0°C. The dispersions were passed through 0.80 μm Millipore filters and equilibrated at 25.0° or 37.0°C for some minutes. Correlation fits of the light scattering intensity were elaborated by *CONTIN* algorithms [22]. The auto-correlation decay function, $g_1(\tau)$, determined the self-diffusion coefficient, and the hydrodynamic radii were evaluated by the Stokes-Einstein equation ($D_{app} = K_BT/6\pi\eta R_H$). The uncertainty on vesicles sizes is to 10-20 nm, depending on their size.

ζ-*potential measurements.* ζ-potential methods determined the surface charge density, σ, of particles moving under the effect of an applied electric field, $\bar{E}$ [23]. A laser-Doppler utility performed measurements, at 25.0°C, in cells equipped with gold electrodes. The scattered light passing in the medium, subjected to the action of E, shifts in frequency compared to unperturbed conditions. Data manipulation of the signal gives the ζ-potential ($\zeta = 4\pi\sigma\tau/\varepsilon^\circ$, where τ the double layer thickness and ε° the static dielectric constant of the medium). The uncertainty on ζ-potentials is 0.5-1.0 mV. Data are reported in *Figure 3.*

Ionic Conductivity. The electrical conductance, κ *(S cm^{-1}),* was determined by a Wayne-Kerr impedance bridge, at 1 *KHz,* using a Daggett-Krauss cell thermostated to 25.00±0.01°C.

CD. Measurements were run on a Jasco J-715 unit, working with 1 nm resolution. 0.100 cm quartz cells were used. Spectra are the average of three independent runs in the 190-300 nm range. Signals due to native *LYS,* at 208 and 222 nm, respectively, were determined.

UV-Vis Light Absorbance. Light absorption spectra, *A,* were recorded in the range 190-300 nm by a Jasco V-570 unit, at 25.0±0.1 °C; the cell path length was 0.100 cm.

Microscopy. Optical microscopy, in normal or polarized light, was performed through a Zeiss optical microscope.

Density. The particles density was determined by a DMA-60 Anton Paar vibrating densimeter, and thermally controlled by a water circulation bath working at 25.00 ± 0.01 °C.

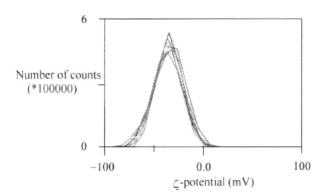

Fig. 3. Plot of ζ-potential values for different dispersions of nominal concentration in LYS-ABOP nano-particles equal to 0.12 w/v %. Measurements were run in 50 mmol Borax, at 25.0°C. Data are reported as number of counts (*10^5) vs. measured ζ-potential value.

5. Results and discussion

Nano-particles characterization. Nano-particles made of *LYS* and *APOB* (termed as *LYS-ABOP*) were characterized by *DLS, CD, UV-vis* and ζ-potential methods. A substantial amount of work was required to stabilize the resulting dispersions, because of their tendency to agglomerate and/or phase separate. The optimal conditions for an effective stabilization (i.e. stirring, temperature, *pH* and/or ionic strength) were determined. The surface charge density, σ, plays a pivotal role in the stability of these dispersions and depends on the medium ionic strength. In buffers with 50 mmol Borax and 10 mmol *NaCl* the dispersions remain stable for about two weeks; usually, they were used one day after preparation. Care was taken to get macroscopic homogeneity and to avoid the presence of clusters or sediments.

In the characterization by *DLS*, a proper selection of the elaborating functions, taking into account the particles sizes and poly-dispersity, was necessary. The cumulant method was applied and the scattering equation, $g_1(t)$, was expressed as a power-law series, according to the well-known relation

$$\ln g_1(t) = \sum_{n=1}^{\infty} \Gamma_n \frac{(-t)^n}{n!} = -\Gamma_1 t + \frac{1}{2!}\Gamma_2 t^2 - \frac{1}{3!}\Gamma_3 t^3 + \ldots\ldots\ldots \tag{1}$$

Eq. (1) gives information on the average value of the distribution function, (that is $\Gamma_1 = <\Gamma>$ $= q^2<D_{app}>$), and on poly-dispersity index, *PdI* (Γ_2/Γ_1^2). Minor terms are also present.

Even when the particles number is moderate, a prolonged aging of the dispersions must be avoided, since a significant shift of the correlation functions is observed, *Figure 1*. That is, both Γ_1 (related to the particles self-diffusion, D_{app}) and Γ_2 (related to *PdI*) depend on aging. This implies the presence of reactive terms. Data were analyzed accounting for the diffusive contributions pertinent to nano-particles and for the respective reactive terms, respectively. The results are expressed in terms of the relation

$$I_2(t) = \left[|I_1(0)|^2 + |I_1(t)|^2 \right] \tag{2}$$

where $I_2(t)$, $I_1(0)$ and $I_1(t)$ are the scattering intensity at time t, the original value at time zero and the reactive part, respectively.

DLS data were interpreted according to Berne and Pecora [24]. Attractive terms, due to particles coagulation, and electrostatic ones, due to the presence of repulsive or attractive forces between colloid entities, are introduced in the time-dependent scattering functions. The relation contains a reactive term, related to the formation of large particles, and is balanced by a flux, in which mobility and diffusive terms are accounted for [24]. Accordingly,

$$\left(\frac{\partial c_a}{\partial t} \right) + \nabla \bullet J_a = k_b c_b - k_a c_a \tag{3}$$

where (dc_a/dt) indicates the production, or disappearance, of particles with time. The second term in the right hand side of the equation is expressed as

$$J_a = \mu_a \overline{E} c_a - D_{app,a} \nabla c_a \tag{4}$$

where μ_a is the electro-phoretic mobility of a class of particles, at concentration c_a, under the effect of and applied electric field, $\overline{E}$, and D_{app} is the self diffusion times the concentration gradient, ∇c_a. K_a and K_b are the kinetic constants of reactants, a, and products, b, respectively.

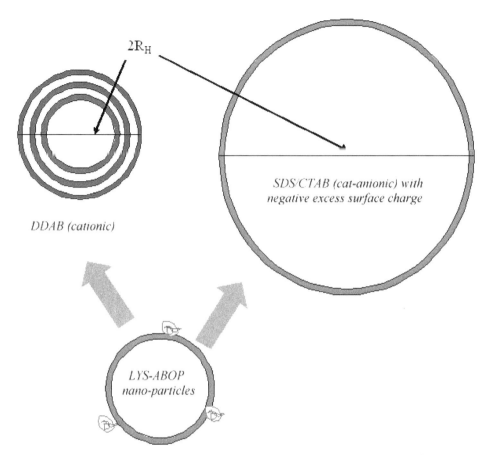

Fig. 4. In the top is reported a schematic representation of vesicle structure. On the upper left is reported a picture relative to multi-lamellar DDAB vesicles (in red/cyan colors, to distinguish the different layers), on the upper right the one related to bi-layered SDS/CTAB vesicles (in blue color). Sizes scale with the average hydrodynamic vesicle radius, inferred from DLS. In the bottom is indicated a cartoon of ABOP nano-particles with surface-bound LYS molecules. As before, regions in red indicate the dominance of positive charges (around the protein), when the blue color of the corona indicates an excess of negative charges.

The above approach helps determining the kinetic features of interactions between different *LYS-ABOP* particles. It will also be used to account for the interactions taking place between vesicles and *LYS-ABOP*. It is expected that attractions are experienced in the interaction between *LYS-ABOP* and cat-anionic vesicles (bearing a negative charge), and repulsions in the other case, *Figure 4*.

DLS alone does not allow to asses any firm statement on lysozyme binding, since the sizes of functionalized *NPs* is only slightly higher than before the reaction. That's why combination of optical absorbance with *DLS*, *CD* and electro-phoretic mobility is helpful.

The former method quantifies the amount of *ABOP*-bound protein (in native or denatured state) and whether binding is effective. The second gives information on the conformational state of *LYS*. Electro-phoretic mobility, finally, indicates an effective surface modification of silica upon protein binding. Binding will reduce in modulus the ζ-potential values, as observed.

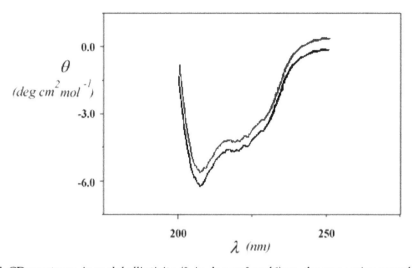

Fig. 5. CD spectrum, in molal ellipticity (θ, in deg cm^2 mol^{-1}) vs. the measuring wavelength (λ, in nm) of LYS-ABOP nano-particles, in grey color, compared to the corresponding value for bulk LYS, in black. The signal intensities were rescaled to allow for a comparison. In both cases data refer to pH 8.5, with 50.0 mmol Borax buffer, and 25.0° C. The former was upward shifted, to avoid overlapping.

Optical absorbance, performed in the 220-230 nm range, determined the presence and number of *LYS* molecules bound onto *ABOP* particles. The average value is <5±1> molecules. The uncertainty is high since the number of *NPs* in the medium is low, and scattering effects reduce the datum quality. *CD* data, *Figure 5*, indicate that the conformation of covalently bound protein is very close to its native form. Thus, the presence of bound protein was inferred by optical absorbance (and elemental analysis, as well), whereas a conformation close to the native one was inferred by *CD*.

Finally, the ζ-potential of *LYS-ABOP* particles decreases from -36 mV of the bare ones to -20, in case of protein-bound entities. Data indicate a significant *LYS* binding and surface modification, but a significant reduction of surface charge density compared to the native particles. This is because some *COOH* units are linked with *LYS* and the charge density of the particle as a whole is substantially reduced. The reduction in ζ-potential also explains why *LYS-ABOP* adducts are less kinetically stable compared to bare *ABOP*.

The optimal conditions leading to stabilization are fulfilled for *pH* values between 7.0 and 8.5. Below *pH* 7.0 the particles sizes increase significantly and such conditions were avoided. Substantial amounts of salt must be used to stabilize the dispersions in such *pH* conditions.

A scheme representing all particles considered here is in *Figure 4*. There is indicated the structure of vesicles and *LYS-ABOP* complexes, with charge distribution in evidence. It is expected that the charge distribution is responsible for interactions with both negatively or positively charged vesicles. It is expected that the kinetic features inherent to vesicle-*LYS-ABOP* particles interactions should behave accordingly.

The analysis of kinetic data, performed by *DLS* methods, is essentially based on the supposed dominance of electrostatic interactions between particles. Were this hypothesis absolutely unrealistic, different kinetic approaches should be considered. For instance the elecctro-phoretic term in the flux equation should be critically reconsidered. Very presumably, however, binding is due to the combined effect of dominant electrostatic contributions plus hydrophobic and ancillary (osmotic?) ones into an as yet undefined mechanism.

Kinetic features. Processes related to vesicles-*NPs* interactions are dealt with in this part. Dispersions of *DDAB* and (*SDS-CTAB*), at the same nominal concentration in lipid, were mixed with tiny amounts of *LYS-ABOP* particles. The number ratio between the latter and vesicles is moderate. This allows measuring the kinetic features inherent to the interactions between *LYS-ABOP* NPs and vesicles. An eye-view to the results, *Figure 6* and *Figure 7*, indicates that the interactive processes can be rationalized on volume fraction statistics. The kinetic pathways scale with the *VES-NP* number ratio. Vesicles sizes are different each from the other, but are reasonably close to *NPs*. That means that changes in size of the scattering entities are mostly due to vesicles-*NPs* adducts. The respective kinetic pathways and the size of particles obtained at the end of the respective reactive processes are different in the two cases. In the [*DDAB*+(*LYS-ABOP*)] system sizes at equilibrium are lower compared to the [(*SDS-CTAB*)+(*LYS-ABOP*)] one. These effects are a sound indication of clustering between

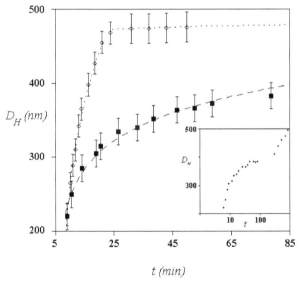

t (min)

Fig. 6. Kinetics of vesicle-NP interaction inferred from DLS plots of average particles size, D_H, as a function of measuring time, t (min), for two different vesicles to LYS-ABOP nano-particles number ratios. Data refer to systems buffered with 50 mmol Borax, at 25°C. Black symbols refer to a number ratio between NP's and cat-anionic SDS-CTAB vesicles (having mole ratio between the two of 1.7/1.0) equal to 1/60 and 1/150 in the other case. In the inset is reported the long term behavior observed in the former system.

objects similar in size, driven by electrostatic interactions between the two entities. Differences in the size of super-colloids formed in these mixtures are the consequences of the interaction mechanisms and result in significant changes in size and shape (presumably) of the resulting entities. Similar features were observed in the [DDAB+(LYS-ABOP)] system, *Figure 7*. There a marked tendency to sedimentation is observed after the interactions took place. Presumably, part of the observed decrease in size may be due to sedimentation processes, occurring at the early stages of the process.

The interactions between *DDAB* and *LYS-ABOP NP*'s show a different kinetic behavior compared to the former system, with a significant increase in size at low times, followed by a substantial decrease at long ones. This behavior is controlled by the net charge of the reacting objects and indicates that electrostatic terms are significant. According to *Figure 7*, there is a pronounced redistribution of particles sizes after about 40 minutes. Such features are, very presumably, related to a structural rearrangement and eventual rupture of vesicle-*NP* adducts with time.

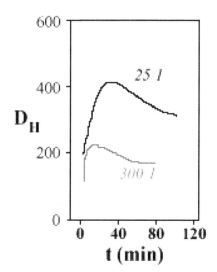

Fig. 7. Plot of the average vesicle/Lys-ABOP adducts size (in nm) with time, in minutes, upon interaction between DDAB vesicles and LYS-ABOP nano-particles. The nominal number ratio between the colloidal objects is indicated in the figure. Experimental conditions refer to the same pH and temperature values reported above.

It is also possible that adducts sedimentation takes place after some time. In words, the formation of composites colloids implies a progressive saturation mechanism in case of *SDS-CTAB* vesicles. Conversely, a significantly different behavior occurs in the *DDAB* containing system. This is put in evidence by the macroscopic appearance of the super-colloid entities formed in this way. In some instances sediments are found at the bottom of vials, in others large floating particles are observed in the medium. That means that the super-colloids formed upon interaction between vesicles and nano-particles differ each from the other in packing density and surface charge, to mind but a few effects.

According to *Figure 8*, for instance, it is evident that entities made of *DDAB* and *LYS-ABOP* particles do form small aggregates, held together by significant forces, presumably electrostatic in nature. According to optical microscopy, it results that these composite objects are made of different sub-domains, differing each from the other in optical appearance and color. Apparently, there is no significant relation between the average stoichiometry of adducts made by vesicles and nano-particles and that pertinent to mother solution. In words, there is no direct proportionality between number of particles in the medium and composition of the precipitates.

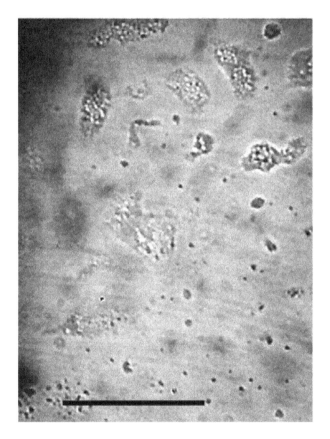

Fig. 8. Vesicle- PFNP clusters, obtained by mixing DDAB and PFNP in number ratios 300/1 and recovering the precipitates. They are visualized through a Zeiss Optical Microscope using normal light. The bar size in the bottom is 100 μm large.

6. Conclusions

The results reported here indicate the possibility to get *"hybrid"* colloid composites from the interactions between *LYS-NPs* complexes and vesicles. The reported results refer to the phenomenological aspects of the interaction process, as it was inferred from *DLS*. Very presumably, the observed features are related to structural rearrangements and to eventual rupture of vesicle-*NP* adducts with time. In one case, apparently, the sedimentation of adducts takes place after some time. In others, large floating objects are present in the dispersing medium.

Depending on the forces active between vesicles and *LYS-NPs*, it is possible that the kinetics of adducts formation follows different pathways. In the case of *SDS-CTAB* cat-anionic vesicles (bearing a substantial negative charge), the interaction mechanism obeys a pseudo first-order mechanism, controlled by the number ratio between the components. In the interaction between *DDAB* vesicles and *LYS-NPs*, conversely, the situation is more cumbersome to be rationalized. In this latter case, it is presumed that the interaction mechanism implies the formation of a transient state (characterized by a maximum in *DLS* plots); after some time the mixed colloid particles rearrange and change in size and shape. It is also possible that the large increase in size observed in this system is due to the incipient nucleation of particles, which precipitate after some time.

Some questions are still under debate on the biological implications of the above systems. However, when *LYS-ABOP* particles interact with cells, it is expected that the reactive behavior (mostly the one relative to surface adsorption) will be close to that reported in case of cat-anionic surfactant mixtures. In fact, cells are negatively charged and are generally composed by mixtures of oppositely charged lipids. On this regard, thus, cat-anionic systems are much more effective as bio-mimetic models compared to other currently used lipid dispersions. It must be also considered that the mechanisms controlling the pynocytosis of particles adsorbed onto cells require the deformation of the latter. In fact, vesicles made by different lipids are more prone to be deformed and envaginate [25], as a consequence of local changes in composition associated to adsorption of charged and bulky entities onto them. This implies the migration of the lipid components in the bi-layer and induces a local deformation of vesicles, making possible particles uptake into cells. More dedicated investigation is required to clarify such aspects.

Another relevant question deals with use of the above systems in modeling bio-mimetic processes. In nature there are cases of interactions between "*hard*" and "*soft*" particles, as, for instance, in the interactions between viruses and other viral vectors and cells [26,27]. From such a point of view, the ones presented here are excellent mimetic models of the above interactions, because viruses are generally covered with enzymes attaching onto the surface of cells and tissues. Preparing nano-particles sharing some properties in common to viruses (having, for instance, a similar surface coverage) would help understanding the physical grounds underlying the interactions between viruses and cells.

7. Acknowledgments

This work was made possible through a financial support from La Sapienza University. F.D.P. wishes to acknowledge the Ministry of Education for financing her stay in Barcelona, where she completed the characterization of the above mixtures.

Financial support from MICIN CTQ2010-14897, Generalitat de Catalunya, through the 2009SGR1331 grant and COST Action Project on Chemistry at Interfaces, D36, are gratefully acknowledged.

Thanks to A. Scipioni, Dept. of Chemistry at La Sapienza, for help in performing *CD* spectra, and for fruitful discussions on some aspects of the manuscript. Thanks also to G. Risuleo,

Dept. of Molecular Biology at La Sapienza, for suggestions on the biological implications of these systems.

8. References

[1] F. Feng, F. Le, L. An, S. Wang, Y. Li, D. Zhu, *Adv. Mater.*, 2008, *20*, 2959.

[2] H.K. Valo; P.H. Laaksonen; L.J. Peltonen; M.B. Linder; J.T. Hirvonen; T.J. Laaksonen, *ACS Nano*, 2010, *4*, 1750.

[3] C. Mateo; J.M. Palomo; G. Fernàndez-Lorente; J.M. Guisàn; R. Fernàndez-Lafuente, *Enzyme Microbial Technol.*, 2007, *40*, 1451.

[4] J.L. Brash; T.A. Horbett, *ACS Symp. Ser. (Proteins at Interfaces)*, 1995, Vol. *602*, p. 1.

[5] E. Soussan; S. Cassel; M. Blanzat; I. Rico-Lattes, *Angew. Chem. Int. Ed.*, 2009, *48*, 274.

[6] C. Letizia, P. Andreozzi, A. Scipioni, C. La Mesa, A. Bonincontro, E. Spigone, *J. Phys. Chem. B*, 2007, *111*, 898.

[7] J. Szebeni; L. Baranyi; S. Savay; J. Milosevits; R. Bunger; P. Laverman; J.M. Metselaar; G. Storm; A. Chanan-Khan; L. Liebes; F.M. Muggia; R. Cohen; Y. Barenholz; C.R. Alving, *J. Liposome Res.*, 2002, *12*, 165.

[8] D. Simberg; S. Weisman; Y. Talmon; Y. Barenholz, *Crit. Rev. Ther. Drug Carrier Syst.*, 2004, *21*, 257.

[9] H.T. Jung; B. Coldren; J.A. Zasadzinski,; D.J. Iampietro; E.W. Kaler, *Proc. Nat. Acad. Sci. U.S.A.*, 2001, *98*, 1353.

[10] E.F. Marques; O. Regev; A. Khan; B. Lindman, *Adv. Colloid Interface Sci.*, 2003, *100-102*, 83.

[11] A. Bonincontro; E. Spigone; M. Ruiz Peña; C. Letizia; C. La Mesa, *J. Colloid Interface Sci.*, 2006, *304*, 342.

[12] A. Bonincontro; C. La Mesa; C. Proietti; G. Risuleo, *Biomacromolecules*, 2007, 8, 1824.

[13] C. Aiello; P. Andreozzi; C. La Mesa; G. Risuleo, *Colloids Surf. B: Biointerfaces*, 2010, *78*, 149.

[14] T.H. Galow; K. Boal; V.M. Rotello, *Adv. Mater.*, 2000, *12*, 576.

[15] A. Zielenciewicz, *J. Therm. Anal. Calor.* 2001, *65*, 467.

[16] K. Monkos, *Biochim. Biophys. Acta: Prot. Struct. Mol. Enzymol.*, 1997, *1339*, 304.

[17] G. Gente; A. Iovino; C. La Mesa, *J. Colloid Interface Sci.*, 2004, *274*, 458.

[18] A. Budhian; S.J. Siegel; K.I. Winey, *Intern. J. Pharmaceutics*, 2007, *336*, 367.

[19] F. De Persiis; P. Andreozzi; C. La Mesa; R. Pons, *submitted*.

[20] P. Andreozzi; S.S. Funari; C. La Mesa; P. Mariani; M.G. Ortore; R. Sinibaldi; F. Spinozzi, *J. Phys. Chem. B*, 2010, *114*, 8056.

[21] P. Andreozzi; A. Bonincontro; C. La Mesa, *J. Phys. Chem. B*, 2008, *112*, 3339.

[22] S. W. Provencher, *Comput. Phys. Comm.* 1982, *27*, 213.

[23] A.W. Adamson, *Physical Chemistry of Surfaces*, 5th ed.; Wiley & Sons: New York, 1990; Chapt. *V*, p. 203.

[24] J.B. Berne; R. Pecora, *Dynamic Light Scattering*; Wiley & Sons: New York, 1976; Chapt. *VI*, p. 96.

[25] D. Fennel Evans; H. Wennerstroem, *The Colloidal Domain: where Physics, Chemistry, Biology and Technology meet*, VCH Publishers, Inc.; New York, 1994, Chapt. *VI*, p. 239.

[26] M.F. Hagan, *J. Chem. Phys.*, 2009, *130*, 114902/1.

[27] X. Huang; L.M. Bronstein; J. Retrum; C. Dufort; I. Tsvetkova; S. Aniagyei; B. Stein; G. Stucky; M. McKenna; N. Remmes; D. Baxter; C.C. Kao; B. Dragnea, *Nano Lett.*, 2007, *7*, 2407.

12

Targeting TRAIL Receptors with Genetically-Engineered CD34+ Hematopoietic Stem Cells

Carmelo Carlo-Stella, Arianna Giacomini, Silvia L. Locatelli
Cristiana Lavazza and Alessandro M. Gianni
Medical Oncology, Fondazione IRCCS Istituto Nazionale Tumori and
University of Milano
Italy

1. Introduction

Dysregulated apoptosis plays a key role in the pathogenesis and progression of neoplastic disorders, allowing tumor cells to survive beyond their normal life-span, and to eventually acquire chemo-radioresistance (Laconi et al., 2000; Pommier et al., 2004). Thus, targeting either the intrinsic or the extrinsic pathways of apoptosis represent attractive therapeutic strategies for restoring apoptosis sensitivity of malignant cells, or activating agonists of apoptosis (Waxman & Schwartz, 2003). Due to the ability of death receptor ligands to induce cell death, there has been considerable interest in the physiological roles and therapeutic potential of these cytokines as anti-cancer agents. Death receptor ligands of the tumor necrosis factor α (TNFα) superfamily are type II transmembrane proteins that signal to target cells upon cell-cell contact, or after protease-mediated release to the extracellular space (Ashkenazi, 2002). Members of this family, including Fas ligand (FasL), TNFα, and tumor necrosis factor-related apoptosis-inducing ligand (TRAIL), stand out because of their ability to induce cell death (Wajant, 2003; Wiley et al., 1995).

2. Soluble TRAIL

Unlike other apoptosis-inducing TNF family members, soluble TRAIL appears to be inactive against normal healthy tissue (Ashkenazi et al., 1999; Lawrence et al., 2001). A variety of preclinical data clearly show that soluble TRAIL is a cancer cell-specific molecule exerting a remarkable antitumor activity both in vitro (Ashkenazi et al., 1999; Gazitt, 1999; Jin et al., 2004; Mitsiades et al., 2001; Pollack et al., 2001; Rieger et al., 1998) as well as in vivo in athymic nude mice or in non-obese diabetic/severe combined immunodeficient (NOD-SCID) mice (Ashkenazi et al., 1999; Daniel et al., 2007; Kelley et al., 2001).

The physiological functions of TRAIL are not yet fully understood, but mouse gene knockout studies indicate that this agent has an important role in antitumor surveillance by immune cells, mediates thymocyte apoptosis, and is important in the induction of autoimmune diseases (Cretney et al., 2002; Lamhamedi-Cherradi et al., 2003; Smyth et al., 2003).

TRAIL signals by interacting with its receptors. So far, five receptors have been identified, including the two agonistic receptors TRAIL-R1 (Pan et al., 1997b) and TRAIL-R2 (Walczak et al., 1997), and the three antagonistic receptors (Sheridan et al., 1997) TRAIL-R3 (Pan et al.,

1997a), TRAIL-R4 (Degli-Esposti et al., 1997), and osteoprotegerin (OPG) (Emery et al., 1998). Both TRAIL-R1 and TRAIL-R2 are type I transmembrane proteins containing a cytoplasmic death domain (DD) motif that engage apoptotic machinery upon ligand binding (Almasan & Ashkenazi, 2003), whereas the other three receptors either act as decoys or transduce antiapoptotic signals (Wang & El-Deiry, 2003). TRAIL-R3 and TRAIL-R4 have close homology to the extracellular domains of agonistic receptors. TRAIL-R4 has a truncated, nonfunctional cytoplasmic DD, while TRAIL-R3 exists on the plasma membrane as a glycophospholipid-anchored protein lacking the cytosolic tail. The physiological relevance of OPG as a soluble receptor for TRAIL is unclear, but a recent study suggests that cancer-derived OPG may be an important survival factor in hormone-resistant prostate cancer cells (Holen et al., 2002).

3. TRAIL-induced apoptosis signaling

Soluble TRAIL forms homotrimers that bind three receptor molecules, each at the interface between two of its subunits. A Zn atom bound to cysteine residues in the trimeric ligand is essential for trimer stability and optimal biologic activity. Binding of TRAIL to the extracellular domain of agonistic receptors results in trimerization of the receptors and clustering of the intracellular DDs, which leads to the recruitment of the adaptor molecule Fas-associated protein with death domain (FADD). Subsequently, FADD recruits initiator caspase-8 and -10, leading to the formation of the death-inducing signaling complex (DISC), where initiator caspases are autoactivated by proteolysis. Once they become enzymatically active, caspase-8 and/or -10 are released from the DISC and signal through two different proteolytic pathways that converge on caspase-3 and lead to cellular disassembly (Kaufmann & Steensma, 2005). In type I cells, activation of initiator caspases upon death receptors ligation is sufficient to directly activate downstream effector caspases, such as caspase-3 and/or -7 (Scaffidi et al., 1998). This extrinsic pathway is independent of the mitochondria and is not blocked by overexpression of Bcl-2. In type II cells, the commitment from death receptor ligation to apoptosis is less direct (Scaffidi et al., 1998). The amount of initially cleaved caspase-8 and/or -10 is not enough to directly trigger effector caspases activation. Consequently, apoptotic signaling requires an amplification loop by mithocondrial pathway engagement through caspase 8-mediated cleavage of Bid (BH3 interacting death domain agonist), which, in turn, induces the cytosolic Bcl-2 family member Bax (Bcl-2-associated X protein) and/or the loosely bound mitochondrial homolog Bak (Bcl-2 antagonist/killer) to insert into the mitochondrial membrane, where they contribute to the mitochondrial release of cytochrome c (Lucken-Ardjomande & Martinou, 2005). In the cytosol, cytochrome c binds the adaptor protein Apaf-1 (apoptotic protease activating factor 1) to form an apoptosome with recruitment and activation of the apoptosis-initiating caspase-9, which proteolytically activates additional caspase-3. These events are further amplified by apoptogenic factors released from the mitochondrial space, including Smac/DIABLO (second mitochondrial activator of caspases/direct IAP-binding protein with low pI) (Verhagen & Vaux, 2002).

4. Enhancing the antitumor efficacy of soluble TRAIL

Despite very promising preclinical in vitro and in vivo antitumor evidences, phase I/II clinical trials have demonstrated limited antitumor activity of soluble TRAIL likely due to its short half-life and the consequent short exposure of tumor cells to the molecule (Ashkenazi et al., 2008). Because of soluble TRAIL's short half-life (Ashkenazi et al., 1999; Kelley et al., 2001; Walczak et al., 1999), it seems unlikely that the recommended soluble TRAIL dose of 8 mg/kg body weight will allow adequate exposure of tumor cells at high drug concentrations (Ashkenazi et al., 2008). Strategies to enhance the therapeutic activity of soluble TRAIL include combining it with conventional chemotherapy (Ballestrero et al., 2004) or with new agents such as histone deacetylase inhibitors that upregulate TRAIL-R1 and/or TRAIL-R2 (Inoue et al., 2004).

Gene therapy approaches have also been proposed to enhance TRAIL-mediated tumor cell targeting. Recently, a TRAIL expressing adenoviral vector (Ad-TRAIL) has been shown to cause direct tumor cell killing, as well as a potent bystander effect through presentation of TRAIL by transduced normal cells (Lee et al., 2002). Thus, using Ad-TRAIL might be an alternative to systemic delivery of soluble TRAIL possibly resulting in better tumor cell targeting and increased tumoricidal activity (Armeanu et al., 2003; Griffith et al., 2000; Griffith & Broghammer, 2001; Kagawa et al., 2001; Lee et al., 2002). However, systemic Ad-TRAIL-based gene therapy requires efficient infection of target tumor cells as well as avoidance of immune clearance, and is limited by several safety and toxicity issues related to intravenous adenovector administration (Harrington et al., 2002). Intratumoral injection of TRAIL-encoding adenovectors has been successfully explored in a number of experimental models; however, this approach results in local antitumor activity and has little, if any, value in the treatment of disseminated tumors.

Alternatively, cell-based vehiculation of the full-length, membrane-bound (m)TRAIL (Griffith et al., 2009) has been proposed to achieve an optimal systemic delivery. Indeed, genetically modified stem/progenitor cells represent an innovative approach for delivery of anticancer molecules (Harrington et al., 2002; Introna et al., 2004). Due to their homing properties, systemically injected stem/progenitor cells could infiltrate both primary and metastatic tumor sites, thus allowing tumor-specific targeting (Burger & Kipps, 2006; Jin et al., 2006; Kaplan et al., 2007; Kucia et al., 2005; Loebinger et al., 2009; Najbauer et al., 2007; Rafii et al., 2002), and potentially overcoming limitations inherent to the pharmacokinetic profile of soluble drugs (Aboody et al., 2008; Griffith et al., 2009; Sasportas et al., 2009). Neural or mesenchymal stem cell-mediated mTRAIL delivery has been investigated in solid tumors (Grisendi et al., 2010; Kim et al., 2008; Loebinger et al., 2009; Menon et al., 2009; Mohr et al., 2008; Uzzaman et al., 2009).

In order to optimize the use of TRAIL-encoding adenovectors for the treatment of systemic tumors, we have recently investigated a cell-based approach using mobilized CD34+ hematopoietic cells transduced with a replication-deficient Ad-TRAIL (CD34-TRAIL+) encoding a full-length mTRAIL under the control of the CMV promoter (Carlo-Stella et al., 2006; Griffith et al., 2000). Several lines of evidence support the use of gene-modified CD34+ cells as optimal vehicles of antitumor molecules. In fact, CD34+ cells are already widely used in the clinical setting. Additionally, they can migrate from the bloodstream into tumor tissues due to the expression of adhesion receptors that specifically interact with counter-receptors on endothelial cells in the tumor microenvironment (Burger & Kipps, 2006; Kaplan et al., 2005; Verfaillie, 1998). Moreover, up-regulation of inflammatory chemo-attractants in the tumor microenvironment provides with a permissive milieu that potentially allows for homing of systemically delivered CD34-TRAIL+ cells and efficient tumor targeting (Jin et al., 2006). Using a multiplicity of infection (MOI) of 500, the transduction protocol optimized for the transduction of CD34+ cells consistently results in a transduction efficiency higher than 80% (range 70% - 96%), a high level expression of mTRAIL, and a cell viability ≥85%. Flow cytometry analysis of CD34-TRAIL+ cells shows significant levels of transgene expression for at least 96 hours after transduction, and Western blot analysis reveals the presence of 32- and 55-kDa proteins, which are the expected products for full-length monomer and dimer TRAIL, respectively (Carlo-Stella et al., 2006).

5. Antitumor activity of mTRAIL-expressing cells

The antitumor activity of CD34-TRAIL+ cells has been investigated in a variety of localized and disseminated tumor models in NOD/SCID mice. Using a localized, subcutaneous multiple myeloma model (KMS-11 cell line), intravenously-injected mTRAIL-expressing cells significantly reduced tumor growth over controls as well as soluble TRAIL.[1] In fact, compared with untreated controls, both CD34-TRAIL+ cells and soluble TRAIL significantly inhibited tumor growth by day 28 after tumor injection, when tumor volumes were reduced by 38% (P < .05) and 31% (P < .05), respectively. However, on day 35, CD34-TRAIL+ cells induced a 40% reduction in tumor growth over controls (4.2 ± 1.2 vs 7.0 ± 2.0 g, P < .001), whereas a 29% reduction of tumor growth was detected in mice receiving soluble TRAIL (5.0 ± 1.7 g vs 7.0 ± 2.0 g, P < .001) (Lavazza et al., 2010). Even more importantly, an efficient antitumor activity of intravenously injected mTRAIL-expressing CD34+ cells was also detected in NOD/SCID mice bearing disseminated, systemic multiple myeloma and non-Hodgkin lymphoma xenografts (Carlo-Stella et al., 2006; Carlo-Stella et al., 2007; Carlo-Stella et al., 2008). Using KMS-11 as model system, treatment of advanced-stage disease with CD34-TRAIL+ cells resulted in a significant increase of median survival over controls (83 vs 55 days, P ≤ 0.0001), with 28% of NOD/SCID mice alive and disease-free at the end of the 150-day observation period (Carlo-Stella et al., 2006).[2]

6. In vivo homing of CD34-TRAIL+ cells

Homing properties of transduced cells in healthy tissues as well as tumor nodules were extensively investigated in tumor-bearing NOD/SCID mice who received a single

---

[1] Six- to eight-week-old female NOD/SCID mice with body weight of 20 to 25 g were purchased from Charles River (Milano, Italy, EU). Mice were housed under standard laboratory conditions according to our institutional guidelines. Animal experiments were performed according to the Italian laws (D.L. 116/92 and following additions), and were approved by the institutional Ethical Committee for Animal Experimentation. KMS-11 cells (5 × 10⁶ cells/mouse) were inoculated subcutaneosuly in the left flank of each mouse. When tumor reached approximately 7 - 10 mm in diameter (usually 10–12 days after tumor inoculation), mice were randomly assigned to planned treatments consisting of daily injections of either CD34-TRAIL+ cells or mock-transduced CD34+ cells (1 × 10⁶ cells/mouse/injection/day, intravenous, days 12–15), or a 4-day course of recombinant soluble TRAIL (30 mg/kg/day, intraperitoneal, days 12–15). Mice were checked twice weekly for tumor appearance, tumor dimensions, body weight, and toxicity. Tumor volumes were measured with calipers and their weights calculated using the formula: $(a \times b^2)/2$, where a and b represented the longest and shortest diameters, respectively. Mice were followed up for 3 weeks after the end of the treatments. The endpoint of the subcutaneous model was tumor weight. Each experiment was performed on at least two separate occasions, using five mice per treatment group.

[2] KMS-11 (0.5 × 10⁶ cells/mouse) cell line was inoculated intravenously. CD34-mock or CD34-TRAIL+ cells (1 × 10⁶ cells/mouse/injection) were inoculated intravenously weekly for 4 weeks starting either on day 7 (early-stage tumor model), or 14 (advanced-stage tumor model) after tumor cell injection.

intravenous injection of CD34-TRAIL+ cells (3×10^6 cells/mouse) (Lavazza et al., 2010). Tumor and healthy tissue sections were immunostained with an anti-human CD45 antibody and digitally recorded to count transduced cells on entire tissue sections.[3] Early following injection, transduced cells were detected at high frequencies in the lung, liver and spleen (**Figure 1**). CD34-TRAIL+ cells progressively decreased and were no longer detectable in these tissues 24 hours after injection. Bone marrow CD34-TRAIL+ cells peaked 5 hours after injection and were detectable up to 24 hours. Low frequencies of transduced cells were detected within tumors as early as 30 minutes following injection. They progressively increased and peaked 48 hours post-injection when on average 188 ± 25 CD45+ cells per 10^5 tumor cells (i.e., $0.2 \pm 0.03\%$) were recorded (**Figure 1**). Overall, kinetics data suggest that transduced cells transiently circulate through healthy tissues, whereas they are preferentially recruited within tumor nodules, allowing to hypothesize that homing signals by tumor endothelial cells actively promote intratumor homing of transduced cells.

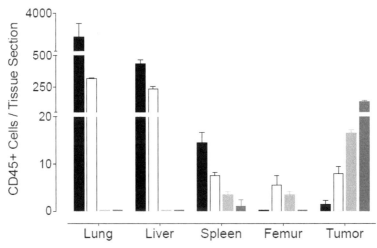

Fig. 1. Tissue kinetics of CD34-TRAIL+ cells. Lung, liver, spleen, femur, and tumor nodules were harvested from tumor-bearing NOD/SCID mice 0.5 (■), 5 (□), 24 (▨), and 48 (■) hours after a single intravenous injection of CD34-TRAIL+ cells (3×10^6 cells/mouse). Shown is the quantification of CD34-TRAIL+ cells on digitally acquired tissue sections stained with anti-CD45. Frequency of CD34-TRAIL+ cells is expressed as the mean ($\pm$ SD) number of CD45+ cells per tissue section.

---

[3] Images of tissue sections were acquired at 20× magnification with an automatic high-resolution scanner (dotSlide System, Olympus, Tokyo, Japan) and subdivided into a collection of non-overlapping red, green, and blue (RGB) images in TIFF format (final resolution 3.125 pixels/μm). Image analysis was carried out using the open-source ImageJ software (http://rsb.info.nih.gov/ij/). Routines for image analysis were coded in ImageJ macro language and executed on RGB images without further treatment. Per each experimental condition, at least three sections from different tumor nodules or healthy tissues were analyzed. Intratumor frequency of CD34-TRAIL+ cells was expressed as the number of CD45+ cells per total cells per tisue section. Total cells were counted by the ImageJ internal function for particle analysis, whereas CD45+ cells were manually counted in all images from whole scanning of histochemically stained tissue sections.

7. Vascular signals involved in tumor homing

This issue was investigated by evaluating the expression of homing receptors on tumor vasculature. Confocal microscopy[4] revealed that 30% of tumor vessels expressed high levels of VCAM-1 on the luminal surface (**Figure 2$_{b-c}$**) (Jin et al., 2006), whereas SFD-1 was ubiquitously expressed on tumor vessels and tumor cells (**Figure 2$_{e-f}$**). Thus, α4β1 integrins and the CXCR4 chemokine (De Raeve et al., 2004; Peled et al., 1999) seem to play a critical role in regulating intratumor homing of mTRAIL-expressing cells. To further investigate the functional relevance of SDF-1/CXCR4 and VCAM-1/VLA-4 pathways in mediating tumor homing of transduced cells, inhibitory experiments with an anti–VCAM-1 antibody and the CXCR4 antagonist AMD3100 were performed.[5] As compared to controls, tumor homing of CD34-TRAIL+ cells was significantly reduced in mice administered with anti–VCAM-1 antibody [0.2 ± 0.03% vs 0.09 ± 0.01% (P = .001)] or the CXCR4 antagonist AMD3100 (Fricker et al., 2006) [0.2 ± 0.03% vs 0.05 ± 0.006% (P = .0003)]. Tumor vasculature was also analyzed for the expression of TRAIL-R2 receptor. Indeed, confocal microscopy revealed that approximately 8 - 12% of tumor endothelial cells expressed TRAIL-R2 receptor on their luminal surface (**Figure 2$_{h-i}$**), suggesting that mechanisms other than SDF-1/CXCR4 and VCAM-1/VLA-4, such as the mTRAIL/TRAIL-R2 interactions, might be involved in regulating intratumor homing as well as functional activity of CD34-TRAIL+ cells (Lavazza et al., 2010).

8. CD34-TRAIL+ cells induce tumor cell apoptosis and hemorrhagic necrosis

Tumor-homing of CD34-TRAIL+ cells is associated with significant levels of tumor cell apoptosis (Carlo-Stella et al., 2006). To obtain an objective quantification of apoptosis, a computer-aided image analysis using ImageJ software was performed.[6] As compared to controls, TUNEL+ cells were increased by 8- (2.4 ± 1.4% vs 0.3 ± 0.3%, P < .0001) and 4-fold (1.2 ± 0.7% vs 0.3 ± 0.3%, P < .0001) following treatment with CD34-TRAIL+ cells and soluble TRAIL, respectively (**Figure 3A**). Interestingly, apoptotic effects of CD34-TRAIL+ cells resulted significantly more potent than those exerted by soluble TRAIL (P < .0001). Additionally, TUNEL staining of tumor sections from untreated, mock- and soluble TRAIL-

---

[4] Cryosections were fixed with cold acetone, rinsed with PBS, and then blocked with 2% BSA. Sections were first incubated with the appropriate primary antibody, including mouse anti-human stromal cell-derived factor-1 (SDF-1) (R&D Systems), rat anti-mouse VCAM-1 (Southern Biotech), or hamster anti-mouse TRAIL-R2 (BD Pharmingen). After washing, sections were incubated with the appropriate Alexa Fluor 568-conjugated secondary antibody (Invitrogen). Biotinylated tumor vessels were revealed with Alexa Fluor 488-conjugated streptavidin (Invitrogen). Sections were examined under an epifluorescent microscope equipped with a laser confocal system (MRC-1024, Bio-Rad Laboratories). Image processing was carried out using LaserSharp computer software (Bio-Rad Laboratories).

[5] To inhibit intratumor homing of CD34-TRAIL+ cells, mice received either one single intraperitoneal dose of anti–VCAM-1 (vascular cell adhesion molecule-1) antibody (clone M/K-2; Southern Biotech, Birmingham, AL, USA) at 0.5 mg/mouse, 3 hours before cell administration, or two doses of AMD3100 (5 mg/kg, subcutaneous, 1 hour prior to and 3 hours after cell administration).

[6] The number of total and TUNEL+ cells per section was counted as follows. Briefly, the dynamic range of images was expanded to full by contrast enhancement, and cells were identified by appropriate filtering in the red, green, and blue (RGB) channels. Resulting black and white images were combined to represent only pixels selected in every color channel. For each image, both total and TUNEL+ cells were counted by the ImageJ internal function for particle analysis.

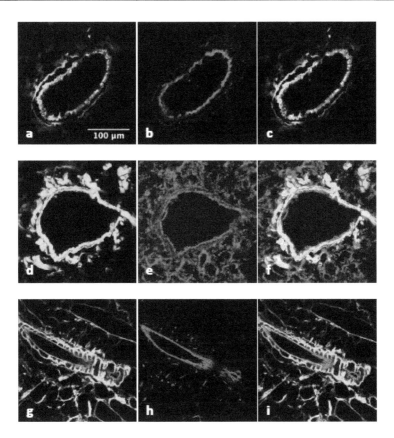

Fig. 2. Vascular molecules involved in intratumor homing of CD34-TRAIL+ cells. Confocal microscopy analysis of intratumor recruiting signals was carried out on 4-μm cryosections from in vivo biotinylated tumors. Cryosections were stained with Alexa Fluor 488-conjugated streptavidin (*green*) to detect tumor vasculature (*a, d, g*). Cryosections were also stained with anti–VCAM-1 (*b*), anti–SDF-1 (*e*), or anti–TRAIL-R2 (*h*) followed by the appropriate Alexa Fluor 568-conjugated secondary antibody for indirect detection of the corresponding antigen (*red*). Merged images demonstrate VCAM-1 (*c*), SDF-1 (*f*), or TRAIL-R2 (*i*) expression by endothelial cells. Objective lens, 40×.

treated mice revealed a homogeneous mass of viable cells with necrotic areas accounting only for 1.4 ± 1.0%, 1.8 ± 1%, and 2.9 ± 1% of total tissue, respectively (**Figure 3B**). In contrast, tumors from CD34-TRAIL-treated mice displayed a significant increase of necrotic areas as compared to controls, with percentages of necrotic areas per tissue section ranging from 6% to 18%, and a mean 8-fold increase over controls (11 ± 3.8% vs 1.4 ± 1.0%, $P < .0001$), and 4-fold increase over soluble TRAIL-treated mice (11 ± 3.8% vs 2.9 ± 1%, $P = .0001$) (**Figure 3B**). Pharmacological inhibition of intratumor recruitment of CD34-TRAIL+ cells using AMD3100, or anti-VCAM-1 antibody significantly reduced necrotic areas by 37% ($P = .02$) and 56% ($P = .002$), respectively (**Figure 3C**), suggesting that intratumor recruitment of CD34-TRAIL+ cells specifically triggered tumor necrosis.

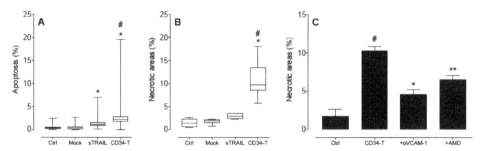

Fig. 3. Pro-apoptotic and necrotic effects of CD34-TRAIL+ cells. NOD/SCID mice bearing subcutaneous tumor nodules 10 mm in diameter were randomly assigned to receive CD34-TRAIL+ cells, mock-transduced CD34+ cells (3×10^6 cells/mouse, intravenous), recombinant soluble TRAIL (500 µg/mouse, IP), or control vehicle. (A) Percentages of apoptotic cells in tumors from untreated or treated animals were computationally calculated on digitally acquired images (objective lens, 20×) using ImageJ. At least three sections from different animals were analyzed. The boxes extend from the 25th to the 75th percentiles, the lines indicate the median values, and the whiskers indicate the range of values. * P < .0001, compared to controls. # P < .0001, compared to soluble TRAIL. (B) Quantification of necrotic areas by ImageJ analysis on tissue sections stained with TUNEL. At least six sections from different animals were analyzed per treatment group. * P < .0001, compared to controls. # P = .0001, compared to soluble TRAIL. (C) Anti–VCAM-1 and AMD3100 reduced tumor necrosis in mice treated with CD34-TRAIL+ cells. # P < .0001, compared to control. * P = .002, compared with CD34-TRAIL+ cells. ** P = .02, compared with CD34-TRAIL+ cells.

A distinctive and prominent feature of tumors treated with CD34-TRAIL+ cells was represented by hemorrhagic phenomena within necrotic areas close to damaged vessels which were detected by immunohistochemical staining with glycophorin A (**Figure 4A**). Hemorrhagic phenomena exactly matched TUNEL+ necrotic areas and closely associated with apoptotic endothelial cells (**Figure 4B$_L$**). In striking contrast, apoptotic vessels and hemorrhagic phenomena could not be detected neither in tumors from mice treated with soluble TRAIL (**Figure 4B$_K$** and **4A**), nor in healthy tissues (**Figure 5**), suggesting a tumor-restricted antivascular activity by CD34-TRAIL+ cells.

9. Antivascular effects of CD34-TRAIL+ cells

To better understand the relationship between the antitumor effects of CD34-TRAIL+ cells and apoptosis of endothelial cells, an extensive vascular analysis[7] was performed on

---

[7] Tumor vasculature was analyzed on cryosections using the open-source ImageJ software (http://rsb.info.nih.gov/ij/) from in vivo biotinylated mice stained with HRP-conjugated streptavidin. To calculate endothelial area, i.e., the percentage of tissue section occupied by endothelium, endothelial cells were identified by contrast enhancement and appropriate filtering. Background signal was removed considering only structures larger than an arbitrary minimal value. To analyze vessel wall thickness, we manually selected rectangular regions of RGB input images containing at least a hollow vessel. An automatic routine computed vessel thickness according to the formula: Thickness = 2 × (vessel area)/[(vessel perimeter) + (lumen perimeter)]. At first, endothelial tissue was identified applying a threshold on the blue channel and obtaining a binary image representative of its

histological sections from tumors treated with transduced cells and subsequently in vivo biotinylated to detect tumor vasculature (Lavazza et al., 2010; Rybak et al., 2005). In untreated mice, tumor vasculature was abundant, tortuous, and evenly distributed throughout the tumor (**Figure 6A**). In striking contrast, in NOD/SCID mice treated with CD34-TRAIL+ cells, viable tumor cells surrounding necrotic areas appeared deficient in capillaries and small-caliber blood vessels, which were less tortuous and had fewer branches and sprouts (**Figure 6A**). Globally, mean percentages of endothelial areas from control and mock-treated tumors were 8.8 ± 5.6% and 8.2 ± 3.3%, respectively (**Figure 6B**). Administration of soluble TRAIL did not affect endothelial area compared to controls (8.1 ± 2.9% vs 8.8 ± 5.6%, P = ns). In contrast, a single intravenous injection of 3 × 10⁶ CD34-TRAIL+ cells caused a 37% decrease of endothelial area compared to control (5.6 ± 3.2% vs 8.8 ± 5.6%, P < .0001) (**Figure 6B**). Additionally, blood vessels from tumors treated with CD34-TRAIL+ cells were thicker than those observed in untreated or soluble TRAIL-treated animals (**Figure 6A**). Based on these findings, we isolated images of transversally oriented vessels in streptavidin-HPR stained sections and calculated vessel wall thickness by processing images with ImageJ and specifically written macros. As shown in **Figure 6C**, wall thickness was 1.7-fold increased compared to control (5.5 ± 1.4 vs 3.2 ± 0.8 μm, P < .0001), whereas no increases emerged after soluble TRAIL administration (3.3 ± 0.7 vs 3.2 ± 0.8 μm).

10. Conclusions

Experimental data obtained in a variety of preclinical models of both localized and disseminated disease strongly suggest that TRAIL-expressing CD34+ cells can efficiently vehiculate mTRAIL within the tumors where they exert potent antivascular and antitumor activities resulting in a significant reduction of tumor growth. Analysis of tumor nodules obtained 48 hours after a single administration of transduced cells showed that TRAIL-expressing cells were 2-fold more effective than soluble TRAIL in inducing apoptosis of tumor cells. Broad necrotic events, involving up to 18% of tumor tissue, were detected only after administration of CD34-TRAIL+ cells and were associated with a hemorrhagic component which was not detectable after soluble TRAIL administration. Hemorrhagic

---

distribution. Then, the lumen of each vessel in the image was identified as a non-endothelial area, ringed by endothelial tissue and greater than an arbitrary threshold. This procedure rejected smaller artifacts and allowed for recognition of hollow vessels even when erythrocytes or other cells occupied the lumen. Subsequently, we identified the endothelium surrounding a given lumen by an iterative procedure. At first, we subdivided the binary representation of stained tissue into areas by means of a watershed algorithm. Then we selected only those regions adjacent to the lumen, obtaining a minimal image of the vessel wall. This minimal image was used to compute a working thickness according to the previously stated formula. Then, to avoid arbitrary removal of bona fide portions of the walls, we calculated a theoretical vessel contour expanding the lumen outline by a number of pixels equivalent to the working thickness. We next turned back to the watershedded image of endothelium distribution, selecting only those areas connected with the new, theoretical contour. Inclusion of the new regions in the minimal image produced the final vessel image. Both images were saved to allow for manual appreciation of proper vessel identification. At last, the final vessel thickness was calculated after assessment of the final vessel area and external perimeter. Per each parameter, the accuracy and appropriate cut-off levels were determined by comparing processed images to the RGB originals. In all instances, automatic routines were validated by comparing results with those obtained by visual counting of up to 10% of the total images by two independent pathologists.

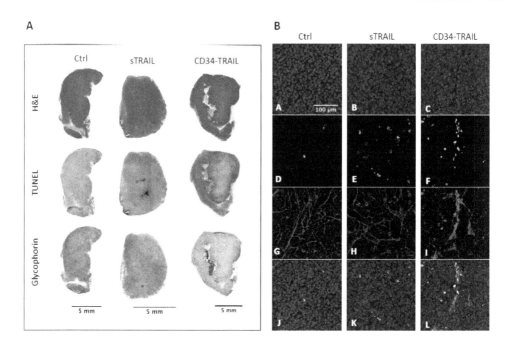

Fig. 4. Tumor hemorrhagic necrosis and endothelial cell apoptosis induced by CD34-TRAIL+ cells. NOD/SCID mice bearing subcutaneous tumor nodules 10 mm in diameter were randomly assigned to receive CD34-TRAIL+ cells, recombinant TRAIL (500 µg/mouse, IP), or control vehicle. Tumors were harvested forty-eight hours after treatment. (**A**) Hematoxylin and eosin (H&E), TUNEL and glycophorin A staining were performed. Objective lens, 2×. (**B**) Just before sacrifice NOD/SCID mice were intravenously injected with sulfo-NHS-LC-biotin to biotinylate tumor vasculature. Representative confocal images of tumors from untreated and treated animals processed by triple immunofluorescence staining. (*A–C*) Cell nuclei were detected in blue by TO-PRO-3; (*D–F*) apoptotic cells were detected in green by TUNEL staining; (*G–I*) tumor endothelial cells were detected in red by Alexa 568-conjugated streptavidin. (*J–L*) After merging of single-color images, apoptotic nuclei (*green*) were detectable throughout tumor parenchyma after treatment with either soluble TRAIL or CD34-TRAIL+ cells, whereas endothelial cells with apoptotic nuclei (*yellow*) could be detected only in CD34-TRAIL+ cell–treated animals. Objective lens, 40×.

necrosis was localized near TUNEL+ blood vessels, suggesting that apoptosis of tumor endothelial cells represents an early event triggered by CD34-TRAIL+ cells. Overall, these findings support the hypothesis that CD34-TRAIL+ cells exert their cytotoxic activity not only by targeting parenchymal tumor cells but also by targeting tumor vasculature (Carlo-Stella et al., 2006; Lavazza et al., 2010). Indeed, the vascular-disrupting activity of mTRAIL might represent a major concern in view of clinical applications. Notwithstanding the intratumor vascular-disrupting activity of mTRAIL, extensive analysis of healthy tissues failed to detect any evidence of hemorrhagic necrosis, suggesting that vascular damage was tumor-restricted.

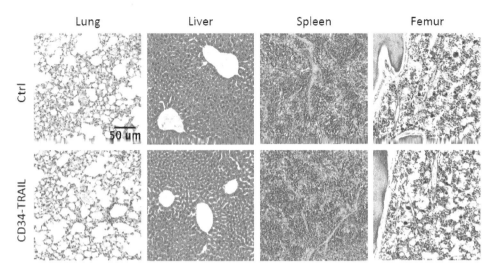

Fig. 5. Tissue and vascular toxicity in healthy tissue after CD34-TRAIL+ cells administration. NOD/SCID mice bearing subcutaneous tumor nodules received a single intravenous injection of CD34-TRAIL+ cells (3 × 10⁶ cells/mouse), or control vehicle. Forty-eight hours after treatment, lung, liver, spleen, and femur were harvested and analyzed. Hematoxylin and eosin staining demonstrated the absence of tissue or vascular damage. Representative histological images are shown. Objective lens, 10x.

Increasing evidences suggest that recruitment of CD34+ cells in the tumor microenvironment is due to homing signals similar to those found in the bone marrow hematopoietic niches (Jin et al., 2006; Kaplan et al., 2007; Rafii et al., 2002; Wels et al., 2008). Both SDF-1/CXCR4 and VCAM-1/VLA-4 pathways play a key role in regulating bone marrow homing of transplanted hematopoietic stem cells (Aiuti et al., 1997; Peled et al., 1999) as well as intratumor recruitment of CXCR4-expressing cells and neovascularization during acute ischemia and tumor growth (Burger & Kipps, 2006; Jin et al., 2006; Petit et al., 2007). Kinetics data obtained in our models clearly show that intravenously injected transduced cells circulate in normal tissues up to 24 hours, but they progressively and preferentially home at tumor sites where they can be detected up to 48 hours after injection. Lack of intratumor detection of CD34-TRAIL+ cells beyond 48 hours after injection (data not shown) may be due to destruction of mTRAIL-expressing cells in the context of antitumor activities (i.e., disruption of tumor vasculature, hemorrhagic necrosis, tumor necrosis, etc.). Pharmacological manipulation of adhesion receptor expression using either AMD3100 or anti–VCAM-1 antibodies significantly reduced both the frequency and the antitumor efficacy of CD34-TRAIL+ cells strongly suggesting that SDF-1 and VCAM-1 expressed by tumor vasculature efficiently recruit transduced CD34+ cells within tumors by challenging their trafficking and homing properties. The role of additional binding systems, such as mTRAIL/TRAIL-R2, in mediating tumor tropism of CD34-TRAIL+ cells may be hypothesized on the basis of our data. Binding of CD34-TRAIL+ cells to TRAIL-R2 expressed by tumor vasculature could significantly contribute to initiation of a cascade of events that induce early endothelial damage, leading to extensive tumor cell death (Arafat et al., 2000).

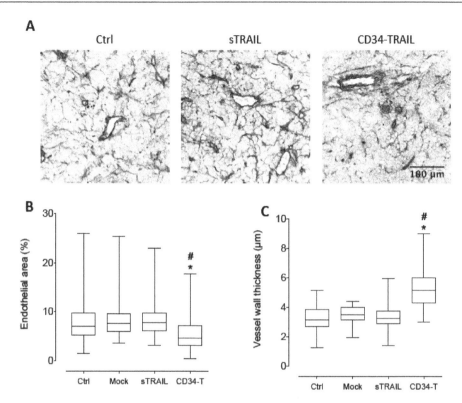

Fig. 6. Antivascular effects of CD34-TRAIL+ cells. NOD/SCID mice bearing subcutaneous tumor nodules 10 mm in diameter were randomly assigned to receive CD34-TRAIL+ cells, mock-transduced CD34+ cells (3 × 10⁶ cells/mouse, intravenous), recombinant soluble TRAIL (500 µg/mouse, IP), and control vehicle. (**A**) Forty-eight hours after treatment, NOD/SCID mice were intravenously injected with 0.2 mL of sulfo-NHS-LC-biotin (5 mg/mL) to biotinylate tumor vasculature. Tumors were then excised, and biotinylated endothelium was revealed by HRP-streptavidin and 3,3'-diaminobenzidine for light microscopy analysis. Representative histological images of in vivo biotinylated mice receiving the different treatments are shown. (**B**) Sections were analyzed using ImageJ for quantification of vascular parameters. Endothelial area was calculated on whole tissue sections as (streptavidin-HRP stained area)/(total tissue area) × 100. * P < .0001, compared to controls. # P < .0001, compared to soluble TRAIL . (**C**) Vessel wall thickness was calculated on transversally oriented vessels. * P < .0001, compared to controls. # P < .0001, compared to soluble TRAIL .

In conclusion, under our experimental conditions the use of transduced CD34+ cells as a vehicle of mTRAIL resulted in an antitumor effect greater than that exerted by soluble TRAIL, likely because of an antivascular action. Our findings appear to be of outstanding interest in the context of the increasing need for therapeutic strategies targeting not only tumor cells but also the tumor microenvironment (De Raeve et al., 2004; Joyce, 2005; Rafii et al., 2002). Finally, the clinical feasibility of such a systemic CD34+ cell-based gene therapy approach could be exploited to develop effective autologous or allogeneic anticancer treatments.

11. Acknowledgements

This work was supported in part by grants from Special Program Molecular Clinical Oncology of Associazione Italiana per la Ricerca sul Cancro (Milano, Italy), Ministero dell'Istruzione, dell'Università e della Ricerca (MIUR, Rome, Italy), Ministero della Salute (Rome, Italy), Alleanza Contro il Cancro (Rome, Italy), and the Michelangelo Foundation for Advances in Cancer Research and Treatment (Milano, Italy).

12. References

Aboody, K.S., Najbauer, J., and Danks, M.K. (2008). Stem and progenitor cell-mediated tumor selective gene therapy. *Gene Ther,* Vol.15, No.10, (May 2008), pp. 739-752

Aiuti, A., Webb, I.J., Bleul, C., Springer, T., and Gutierrez-Ramos, J.C. (1997). The chemokine SDF-1 is a chemoattractant for human CD34+ hematopoietic progenitor cells and provides a new mechanism to explain the mobilization of CD34+ progenitors to peripheral blood. *J Exp Med,* Vol.185, No.1, (Jan 6 1997), pp. 111-120

Almasan, A., and Ashkenazi, A. (2003). Apo2L/TRAIL: apoptosis signaling, biology, and potential for cancer therapy. *Cytokine Growth Factor Rev,* Vol.14, No.3-4, (Jun-Aug 2003), pp. 337-348

Arafat, W.O., Casado, E., Wang, M., Alvarez, R.D., Siegal, G.P., Glorioso, J.C., Curiel, D.T., and Gomez-Navarro, J. (2000). Genetically modified CD34+ cells exert a cytotoxic bystander effect on human endothelial and cancer cells. *Clin Cancer Res,* Vol.6, No.11, (Nov 2000), pp. 4442-4448

Armeanu, S., Lauer, U.M., Smirnow, I., Schenk, M., Weiss, T.S., Gregor, M., and Bitzer, M. (2003). Adenoviral gene transfer of tumor necrosis factor-related apoptosis-inducing ligand overcomes an impaired response of hepatoma cells but causes severe apoptosis in primary human hepatocytes. *Cancer Res,* Vol.63, No.10, (May 15 2003), pp. 2369-2372

Ashkenazi, A., Pai, R.C., Fong, S., Leung, S., Lawrence, D.A., Marsters, S.A., Blackie, C., Chang, L., McMurtrey, A.E., Hebert, A., DeForge, L., Koumenis, I.L., Lewis, D., Harris, L., Bussiere, J., Koeppen, H., Shahrokh, Z., and Schwall, R.H. (1999). Safety and antitumor activity of recombinant soluble Apo2 ligand. *J. Clin. Invest.,* Vol.104, No.2, (July 15 1999), pp. 155-162

Ashkenazi, A. (2002). Targeting death and decoy receptors of the tumour-necrosis factor superfamily. *Nat Rev Cancer,* Vol.2, No.6, (Jun 2002), pp. 420-430

Ashkenazi, A., Holland, P., and Eckhardt, S.G. (2008). Ligand-based targeting of apoptosis in cancer: the potential of recombinant human apoptosis ligand 2/Tumor necrosis factor-related apoptosis-inducing ligand (rhApo2L/TRAIL). *J Clin Oncol,* Vol.26, No.21, (Jul 20 2008), pp. 3621-3630

Ballestrero, A., Nencioni, A., Boy, D., Rocco, I., Garuti, A., Mela, G.S., Van Parijs, L., Brossart, P., Wesselborg, S., and Patrone, F. (2004). Tumor necrosis factor-related apoptosis-inducing ligand cooperates with anticancer drugs to overcome chemoresistance in antiapoptotic Bcl-2 family members expressing jurkat cells. *Clin Cancer Res,* Vol.10, No.4, (Feb 15 2004), pp. 1463-1470

Burger, J.A., and Kipps, T.J. (2006). CXCR4: a key receptor in the crosstalk between tumor cells and their microenvironment. *Blood,* Vol.107, No.5, (Mar 1 2006), pp. 1761-1767

Carlo-Stella, C., Lavazza, C., Di Nicola, M., Cleris, L., Longoni, P., Milanesi, M., Magni, M., Morelli, D., Gloghini, A., Carbone, A., and Gianni, A.M. (2006). Antitumor activity of human CD34+ cells expressing membrane-bound tumor necrosis factor-related apoptosis-inducing ligand. *Human gene therapy,* Vol.17, No.12, (Dec 2006), pp. 1225-1240

Carlo-Stella, C., Lavazza, C., Locatelli, A., Vigano, L., Gianni, A.M., and Gianni, L. (2007). Targeting TRAIL Agonistic Receptors for Cancer Therapy. *Clin Cancer Res,* Vol.13, No.8, (Apr 15 2007), pp. 2313-2317

Carlo-Stella, C., Lavazza, C., Carbone, A., and Gianni, A.M. (2008). Anticancer cell therapy with TRAIL-armed CD34+ progenitor cells. *Adv Exp Med Biol,* Vol.610, (2008), pp. 100-111

Cretney, E., Takeda, K., Yagita, H., Glaccum, M., Peschon, J.J., and Smyth, M.J. (2002). Increased susceptibility to tumor initiation and metastasis in TNF-related apoptosis-inducing ligand-deficient mice. *J Immunol,* Vol.168, No.3, (Feb 1 2002), pp. 1356-1361

Daniel, D., Yang, B., Lawrence, D.A., Totpal, K., Balter, I., Lee, W.P., Gogineni, A., Cole, M.J., Yee, S.F., Ross, S., and Ashkenazi, A. (2007). Cooperation of the proapoptotic receptor agonist rhApo2L/TRAIL with the CD20 antibody rituximab against non-Hodgkin lymphoma xenografts. *Blood,* Vol.110, No.12, (Dec 1 2007), pp. 4037-4046

De Raeve, H., Van Marck, E., Van Camp, B., and Vanderkerken, K. (2004). Angiogenesis and the role of bone marrow endothelial cells in haematological malignancies. *Histol Histopathol,* Vol.19, No.3, (Jul 2004), pp. 935-950

Degli-Esposti, M.A., Dougall, W.C., Smolak, P.J., Waugh, J.Y., Smith, C.A., and Goodwin, R.G. (1997). The novel receptor TRAIL-R4 induces NF-kappaB and protects against TRAIL-mediated apoptosis, yet retains an incomplete death domain. *Immunity,* Vol.7, No.6, (Dec 1997), pp. 813-820

Emery, J.G., McDonnell, P., Burke, M.B., Deen, K.C., Lyn, S., Silverman, C., Dul, E., Appelbaum, E.R., Eichman, C., DiPrinzio, R., Dodds, R.A., James, I.E., Rosenberg, M., Lee, J.C., and Young, P.R. (1998). Osteoprotegerin is a receptor for the cytotoxic ligand TRAIL. *J Biol Chem,* Vol.273, No.23, (Jun 5 1998), pp. 14363-14367

Fricker, S.P., Anastassov, V., Cox, J., Darkes, M.C., Grujic, O., Idzan, S.R., Labrecque, J., Lau, G., Mosi, R.M., Nelson, K.L., Qin, L., Santucci, Z., and Wong, R.S. (2006). Characterization of the molecular pharmacology of AMD3100: a specific antagonist of the G-protein coupled chemokine receptor, CXCR4. *Biochem Pharmacol,* Vol.72, No.5, (Aug 28 2006), pp. 588-596

Gazitt, Y. (1999). TRAIL is a potent inducer of apoptosis in myeloma cells derived from multiple myeloma patients and is not cytotoxic to hematopoietic stem cells. *Leukemia,* Vol.13, No.11, (Nov 1999), pp. 1817-1824

Griffith, T.S., Anderson, R.D., Davidson, B.L., Williams, R.D., and Ratliff, T.L. (2000). Adenoviral-mediated transfer of the TNF-related apoptosis-inducing ligand/Apo-2 ligand gene induces tumor cell apoptosis. *J Immunol,* Vol.165, No.5, (Sep 1 2000), pp. 2886-2894

Griffith, T.S., and Broghammer, E.L. (2001). Suppression of tumor growth following intralesional therapy with TRAIL recombinant adenovirus. *Mol Ther*, Vol.4, No.3, (Sep 2001), pp. 257-266

Griffith, T.S., Stokes, B., Kucaba, T.A., Earel, J.K., Jr., VanOosten, R.L., Brincks, E.L., and Norian, L.A. (2009). TRAIL gene therapy: from preclinical development to clinical application. *Curr Gene Ther*, Vol.9, No.1, (Feb 2009), pp. 9-19

Grisendi, G., Bussolari, R., Cafarelli, L., Petak, I., Rasini, V., Veronesi, E., De Santis, G., Spano, C., Tagliazzucchi, M., Barti-Juhasz, H., Scarabelli, L., Bambi, F., Frassoldati, A., Rossi, G., Casali, C., Morandi, U., Horwitz, E.M., Paolucci, P., Conte, P., and Dominici, M. (2010). Adipose-derived mesenchymal stem cells as stable source of tumor necrosis factor-related apoptosis-inducing ligand delivery for cancer therapy. *Cancer Research*, Vol.70, No.9, (May 1 2010), pp. 3718-3729

Harrington, K., Alvarez-Vallina, L., Crittenden, M., Gough, M., Chong, H., Diaz, R.M., Vassaux, G., Lemoine, N., and Vile, R. (2002). Cells as vehicles for cancer gene therapy: the missing link between targeted vectors and systemic delivery? *Hum Gene Ther*, Vol.13, No.11, (Jul 20 2002), pp. 1263-1280

Holen, I., Croucher, P.I., Hamdy, F.C., and Eaton, C.L. (2002). Osteoprotegerin (OPG) is a survival factor for human prostate cancer cells. *Cancer Res*, Vol.62, No.6, (Mar 15 2002), pp. 1619-1623

Inoue, S., Macfarlane, M., Harper, N., Wheat, L.M., Dyer, M.J., and Cohen, G.M. (2004). Histone deacetylase inhibitors potentiate TNF-related apoptosis-inducing ligand (TRAIL)-induced apoptosis in lymphoid malignancies. *Cell Death Differ*, Vol.11 Suppl 2, (December 2004), pp. S193-206

Introna, M., Barbui, A.M., Golay, J., and Rambaldi, A. (2004). Innovative cell-based therapies in onco-hematology: what are the clinical facts ? *Haematologica*, Vol.89, No.10, (Oct 2004), pp. 1253-1260

Jin, H., Aiyer, A., Su, J., Borgstrom, P., Stupack, D., Friedlander, M., and Varner, J. (2006). A homing mechanism for bone marrow-derived progenitor cell recruitment to the neovasculature. *J Clin Invest*, Vol.116, No.3, (Mar 1 2006), pp. 652-662

Joyce, J.A. (2005). Therapeutic targeting of the tumor microenvironment. *Cancer Cell*, Vol.7, No.6, (Jun 2005), pp. 513-520

Kagawa, S., He, C., Gu, J., Koch, P., Rha, S.-J., Roth, J.A., Curley, S.A., Stephens, L.C., and Fang, B. (2001). Antitumor activity and bystander effects of the tumor necrosis factor-related apoptosis-inducing ligand (TRAIL) gene. *Cancer Res*, Vol.61, No.8, (April 1, 2001 2001), pp. 3330-3338

Kaplan, R.N., Riba, R.D., Zacharoulis, S., Bramley, A.H., Vincent, L., Costa, C., MacDonald, D.D., Jin, D.K., Shido, K., Kerns, S.A., Zhu, Z., Hicklin, D., Wu, Y., Port, J.L., Altorki, N., Port, E.R., Ruggero, D., Shmelkov, S.V., Jensen, K.K., Rafii, S., and Lyden, D. (2005). VEGFR1-positive haematopoietic bone marrow progenitors initiate the pre-metastatic niche. *Nature*, Vol.438, No.7069, (Dec 8 2005), pp. 820-827

Kaplan, R.N., Psaila, B., and Lyden, D. (2007). Niche-to-niche migration of bone-marrow-derived cells. *Trends Mol Med*, Vol.13, No.2, (Feb 2007), pp. 72-81

Kaufmann, S.H., and Steensma, D.P. (2005). On the TRAIL of a new therapy for leukemia. *Leukemia*, Vol.19, No.12, (Dec 2005), pp. 2195-2202

Kelley, S.K., Harris, L.A., Xie, D., Deforge, L., Totpal, K., Bussiere, J., and Fox, J.A. (2001). Preclinical studies to predict the disposition of Apo2L/tumor necrosis factor-related apoptosis-inducing ligand in humans: characterization of in vivo efficacy, pharmacokinetics, and safety. *J Pharmacol Exp Ther,* Vol.299, No.1, (Oct 2001), pp. 31-38

Kim, S.M., Lim, J.Y., Park, S.I., Jeong, C.H., Oh, J.H., Jeong, M., Oh, W., Park, S.H., Sung, Y.C., and Jeun, S.S. (2008). Gene therapy using TRAIL-secreting human umbilical cord blood-derived mesenchymal stem cells against intracranial glioma. *Cancer Res,* Vol.68, No.23, (Dec 1 2008), pp. 9614-9623

Kucia, M., Reca, R., Miekus, K., Wanzeck, J., Wojakowski, W., Janowska-Wieczorek, A., Ratajczak, J., and Ratajczak, M.Z. (2005). Trafficking of normal stem cells and metastasis of cancer stem cells involve similar mechanisms: pivotal role of the SDF-1-CXCR4 axis. *Stem Cells,* Vol.23, No.7, (Aug 2005), pp. 879-894

Laconi, E., Pani, P., and Farber, E. (2000). The resistance phenotype in the development and treatment of cancer. *Lancet Oncol,* Vol.1, (Dec 2000), pp. 235-241

Lamhamedi-Cherradi, S.E., Zheng, S.J., Maguschak, K.A., Peschon, J., and Chen, Y.H. (2003). Defective thymocyte apoptosis and accelerated autoimmune diseases in TRAIL-/-mice. *Nat Immunol,* Vol.4, No.3, (Mar 2003), pp. 255-260

Lavazza, C., Carlo-Stella, C., Giacomini, A., Cleris, L., Righi, M., Sia, D., Di Nicola, M., Magni, M., Longoni, P., Milanesi, M., Francolini, M., Gloghini, A., Carbone, A., Formelli, F., and Gianni, A.M. (2010). Human CD34+ cells engineered to express membrane-bound tumor necrosis factor-related apoptosis-inducing ligand target both tumor cells and tumor vasculature. *Blood,* Vol.115, No.11, (Mar 18 2010), pp. 2231-2240

Lawrence, D., Shahrokh, Z., Marsters, S., Achilles, K., Shih, D., Mounho, B., Hillan, K., Totpal, K., DeForge, L., Schow, P., Hooley, J., Sherwood, S., Pai, R., Leung, S., Khan, L., Gliniak, B., Bussiere, J., Smith, C.A., Strom, S.S., Kelley, S., Fox, J.A., Thomas, D., and Ashkenazi, A. (2001). Differential hepatocyte toxicity of recombinant Apo2L/TRAIL versions. *Nat Med,* Vol.7, No.4, (Apr 2001), pp. 383-385

Lee, J., Hampl, M., Albert, P., and Fine, H.A. (2002). Antitumor activity and prolonged expression from a TRAIL-expressing adenoviral vector. *Neoplasia (New York, N.Y.),* Vol.4, No.4, (2002), pp. 312-323

Loebinger, M.R., Eddaoudi, A., Davies, D., and Janes, S.M. (2009). Mesenchymal stem cell delivery of TRAIL can eliminate metastatic cancer. *Cancer Res,* Vol.69, No.10, (May 15 2009), pp. 4134-4142

Lucken-Ardjomande, S., and Martinou, J.C. (2005). Newcomers in the process of mitochondrial permeabilization. *J Cell Sci,* Vol.118, No.Pt 3, (Feb 1 2005), pp. 473-483

Menon, L.G., Kelly, K., Wei Yang, H., Kim, S.K., Black, P.M., and Carroll, R.S. (2009). Human Bone Marrow Derived Mesenchymal Stromal Cells Expressing S-TRAIL as a Cellular Delivery Vehicle for Human Glioma Therapy. *Stem Cells,* (May 28 2009), pp.

Mitsiades, C.S., Treon, S.P., Mitsiades, N., Shima, Y., Richardson, P., Schlossman, R., Hideshima, T., and Anderson, K.C. (2001). TRAIL/Apo2L ligand selectively induces apoptosis and overcomes drug resistance in multiple myeloma: therapeutic applications. *Blood,* Vol.98, No.3, (2001/8/1 2001), pp. 795-804

Mohr, A., Lyons, M., Deedigan, L., Harte, T., Shaw, G., Howard, L., Barry, F., O'Brien, T., and Zwacka, R. (2008). Mesenchymal Stem Cells expressing TRAIL lead to tumour growth inhibition in an experimental lung cancer model. *J Cell Mol Med,* (Mar 28 2008), pp.

Najbauer, J., Danks, M., Schmidt, N., Kim, S., and Aboody, K. (2007). Neural stem cell-mediated therapy of primary and metastatic solid tumors. *Progress in Gene Therapy, Autologous and Cancer Stem Cell Gene Therapy. World Scientific: Singapore,* (2007), pp.

Pan, G., Ni, J., Wei, Y.F., Yu, G., Gentz, R., and Dixit, V.M. (1997a). An antagonist decoy receptor and a death domain-containing receptor for TRAIL. *Science,* Vol.277, No.5327, (Aug 8 1997a), pp. 815-818

Pan, G., O'Rourke, K., Chinnaiyan, A.M., Gentz, R., Ebner, R., Ni, J., and Dixit, V.M. (1997b). The receptor for the cytotoxic ligand TRAIL. *Science,* Vol.276, No.5309, (Apr 4 1997b), pp. 111-113

Peled, A., Petit, I., Kollet, O., Magid, M., Ponomaryov, T., Byk, T., Nagler, A., Ben-Hur, H., Many, A., Shultz, L., Lider, O., Alon, R., Zipori, D., and Lapidot, T. (1999). Dependence of human stem cell engraftment and repopulation of NOD/SCID mice on CXCR4. *Science,* Vol.283, No.5403, (Feb 5 1999), pp. 845-848

Petit, I., Jin, D., and Rafii, S. (2007). The SDF-1-CXCR4 signaling pathway: a molecular hub modulating neo-angiogenesis. *Trends Immunol,* Vol.28, No.7, (Jul 2007), pp. 299-307

Pollack, I.F., Erff, M., and Ashkenazi, A. (2001). Direct stimulation of apoptotic signaling by soluble Apo2L/tumor necrosis factor-related apoptosis-inducing ligand leads to selective killing of glioma cells. *Clinical Cancer Research,* Vol.7, No.5, (2001), pp. 1362-1369

Pommier, Y., Sordet, O., Antony, S., Hayward, R.L., and Kohn, K.W. (2004). Apoptosis defects and chemotherapy resistance: molecular interaction maps and networks. *Oncogene,* Vol.23, No.16, (Apr 12 2004), pp. 2934-2949

Rafii, S., Lyden, D., Benezra, R., Hattori, K., and Heissig, B. (2002). Vascular and haematopoietic stem cells: novel targets for anti-angiogenesis therapy? *Nat Rev Cancer,* Vol.2, No.11, (Nov 2002), pp. 826-835

Rieger, J., Naumann, U., Glaser, T., Ashkenazi, A., and Weller, M. (1998). APO2 ligand: a novel lethal weapon against malignant glioma? *FEBS Lett,* Vol.427, No.1, (May 1 1998), pp. 124-128

Rybak, J.N., Ettorre, A., Kaissling, B., Giavazzi, R., Neri, D., and Elia, G. (2005). In vivo protein biotinylation for identification of organ-specific antigens accessible from the vasculature. *Nat Methods,* Vol.2, No.4, (Apr 2005), pp. 291-298

Sasportas, L.S., Kasmieh, R., Wakimoto, H., Hingtgen, S., van de Water, J.A., Mohapatra, G., Figueiredo, J.L., Martuza, R.L., Weissleder, R., and Shah, K. (2009). Assessment of therapeutic efficacy and fate of engineered human mesenchymal stem cells for cancer therapy. *Proc Natl Acad Sci U S A,* Vol.106, No.12, (Mar 24 2009), pp. 4822-4827

Scaffidi, C., Fulda, S., Srinivasan, A., Friesen, C., Li, F., Tomaselli, K.J., Debatin, K.M., Krammer, P.H., and Peter, M.E. (1998). Two CD95 (APO-1/Fas) signaling pathways. *Embo J,* Vol.17, No.6, (Mar 16 1998), pp. 1675-1687

Sheridan, J.P., Marsters, S.A., Pitti, R.M., Gurney, A., Skubatch, M., Baldwin, D., Ramakrishnan, L., Gray, C.L., Baker, K., Wood, W.I., Goddard, A.D., Godowski, P., and Ashkenazi, A. (1997). Control of TRAIL-induced apoptosis by a family of signaling and decoy receptors. *Science,* Vol.277, No.5327, (Aug 8 1997), pp. 818-821

Smyth, M.J., Takeda, K., Hayakawa, Y., Peschon, J.J., van den Brink, M.R., and Yagita, H. (2003). Nature's TRAIL--on a path to cancer immunotherapy. *Immunity*, Vol.18, No.1, (Jan 2003), pp. 1-6

Uzzaman, M., Keller, G., and Germano, I.M. (2009). In vivo gene delivery by embryonic-stem-cell-derived astrocytes for malignant gliomas. *Neuro Oncol*, Vol.11, No.2, (Apr 2009), pp. 102-108

Verfaillie, C.M. (1998). Adhesion Receptors as Regulators of the Hematopoietic Process. *Blood*, Vol.92, No.8, (October 15, 1998 1998), pp. 2609-2612

Verhagen, A.M., and Vaux, D.L. (2002). Cell death regulation by the mammalian IAP antagonist Diablo/Smac. *Apoptosis*, Vol.7, No.2, (Apr 2002), pp. 163-166

Wajant, H. (2003). Death receptors. *Essays Biochem*, Vol.39, (2003), pp. 53-71

Walczak, H., Degli-Esposti, M.A., Johnson, R.S., Smolak, P.J., Waugh, J.Y., Boiani, N., Timour, M.S., Gerhart, M.J., Schooley, K.A., Smith, C.A., Goodwin, R.G., and Rauch, C.T. (1997). TRAIL-R2: a novel apoptosis-mediating receptor for TRAIL. *Embo J*, Vol.16, No.17, (Sep 1 1997), pp. 5386-5397

Walczak, H., Miller, R.E., Ariail, K., Gliniak, B., Griffith, T.S., Kubin, M., Chin, W., Jones, J., Woodward, A., Le, T., Smith, C., Smolak, P., Goodwin, R.G., Rauch, C.T., Schuh, J.C., and Lynch, D.H. (1999). Tumoricidal activity of tumor necrosis factor-related apoptosis-inducing ligand in vivo. *Nat Med*, Vol.5, No.2, (Feb 1999), pp. 157-163

Wang, S., and El-Deiry, W.S. (2003). TRAIL and apoptosis induction by TNF-family death receptors. *Oncogene*, Vol.22, No.53, (Nov 24 2003), pp. 8628-8633

Waxman, D.J., and Schwartz, P.S. (2003). Harnessing apoptosis for improved anticancer gene therapy. *Cancer Res*, Vol.63, No.24, (Dec 15 2003), pp. 8563-8572

Wels, J., Kaplan, R.N., Rafii, S., and Lyden, D. (2008). Migratory neighbors and distant invaders: tumor-associated niche cells. *Genes Dev*, Vol.22, No.5, (Mar 1 2008), pp. 559-574

Wiley, S.R., Schooley, K., Smolak, P.J., Din, W.S., Huang, C.P., Nicholl, J.K., Sutherland, G.R., Smith, T.D., Rauch, C., and Smith, C.A. (1995). Identification and characterization of a new member of the TNF family that induces apoptosis. *Immunity*, Vol.3, No.6, (Dec 1995), pp. 673-682

Permissions

The contributors of this book come from diverse backgrounds, making this book a truly international effort. This book will bring forth new frontiers with its revolutionizing research information and detailed analysis of the nascent developments around the world.

We would like to thank Xu-bo Yuan, for lending his expertise to make the book truly unique. He has played a crucial role in the development of this book. Without his invaluable contribution this book wouldn't have been possible. He has made vital efforts to compile up to date information on the varied aspects of this subject to make this book a valuable addition to the collection of many professionals and students.

This book was conceptualized with the vision of imparting up-to-date information and advanced data in this field. To ensure the same, a matchless editorial board was set up. Every individual on the board went through rigorous rounds of assessment to prove their worth. After which they invested a large part of their time researching and compiling the most relevant data for our readers. Conferences and sessions were held from time to time between the editorial board and the contributing authors to present the data in the most comprehensible form. The editorial team has worked tirelessly to provide valuable and valid information to help people across the globe.

Every chapter published in this book has been scrutinized by our experts. Their significance has been extensively debated. The topics covered herein carry significant findings which will fuel the growth of the discipline. They may even be implemented as practical applications or may be referred to as a beginning point for another development. Chapters in this book were first published by InTech; hereby published with permission under the Creative Commons Attribution License or equivalent.

The editorial board has been involved in producing this book since its inception. They have spent rigorous hours researching and exploring the diverse topics which have resulted in the successful publishing of this book. They have passed on their knowledge of decades through this book. To expedite this challenging task, the publisher supported the team at every step. A small team of assistant editors was also appointed to further simplify the editing procedure and attain best results for the readers.

Our editorial team has been hand-picked from every corner of the world. Their multi-ethnicity adds dynamic inputs to the discussions which result in innovative outcomes. These outcomes are then further discussed with the researchers and contributors who give their valuable feedback and opinion regarding the same. The feedback is then collaborated with the researches and they are edited in a comprehensive manner to aid the understanding of the subject.

Apart from the editorial board, the designing team has also invested a significant amount of their time in understanding the subject and creating the most relevant covers. They scrutinized every image to scout for the most suitable representation of the subject and create an appropriate cover for the book.

The publishing team has been involved in this book since its early stages. They were actively engaged in every process, be it collecting the data, connecting with the contributors or procuring relevant information. The team has been an ardent support to the editorial, designing and production team. Their endless efforts to recruit the best for this project, has resulted in the accomplishment of this book. They are a veteran in the field of academics and their pool of knowledge is as vast as their experience in printing. Their expertise and guidance has proved useful at every step. Their uncompromising quality standards have made this book an exceptional effort. Their encouragement from time to time has been an inspiration for everyone.

The publisher and the editorial board hope that this book will prove to be a valuable piece of knowledge for researchers, students, practitioners and scholars across the globe.

List of Contributors

Hu-Lin Jiang and Myung-Haing Cho
College of Veterinary Medicine, Seoul National University, Korea

You-Kyoung Kim and Chong-Su Cho
Department of Agricultural Biotechnology and Research Institute for Agriculture and Life Sciences, Seoul National University, Korea

Myung-Haing Cho
Department of Nanofusion Technology, Graduate School of Convergence Science and Technology, Seoul National University, Korea
Advanced Institute of Convergence Technology, Seoul National University, Korea
Graduate Group of Tumor Biology, Seoul National University, Korea
Center for Food Safety and Toxicology, Seoul National University, Korea

Qin Shi, Mohamed Benderdour and Julio C. Fernandes
Orthopedic Research Laboratory, Hôpital du Sacré-Coeur de Montréal, Université de Montréal, Canada

Marcio J. Tiera
Departamento de Quimica e Ciencias Ambientais, UNESP-Universidade Estadual, Paulista-Brazil, Brazil

Xiaoling Zhang and Kerong Dai
The key laboratory of Stem Cell Biology, Institute of Health Sciences, Shanghai Jiao Tong University School of Medicine (SJTUSM) & Shanghai, Institutes for Biological Sciences (SIBS), Chinese Academy of Sciences (CAS), China

Xuan Zhou, Yu Ren, Xubo Yuan, Peiyu Pu and Chunsheng Kang
Department of Neurosurgery, Laboratory of Neuro-Oncology, Tianjin Medical University, Tianjin research center of basic medical science, Tianjin medical university, First Department of Head and Neck Cancer, Tianjin Medical University Cancer Institute & Hospital, School of Materials Science & Engineering, Tianjin University, China

Roderick A. Slavcev, Shawn Wettig and Tranum Kaur
School of Pharmacy, University of Waterloo, Ontario, Canada

Andrea Beyerle and Tobias Stoeger
Comprehensive Pneumology Center, Institute of Lung Biology and Disease, Helmholtz Zentrum, München, Germany

Andrea Beyerle, Thomas Kissel and Tobias Stoeger
Department of Pharmaceutics and Biopharmacy, Philipps-University Marburg, Germany

Yadollah Omidi, Vala Kafil and Jaleh Barar
Research Center for Pharmaceutical Nanotechnology, Faculty of Pharmacy, Tabriz University of Medical Sciences, Tabriz, Iran

Hugo Peluffo
Department of Histology and Embryology, Faculty of Medicine, University of the Republic (UDELAR) and Neurodegeneration Laboratory, Institut Pasteur de Montevideo, Uruguay

Wei Yang Seow and Andrew JT George
Imperial College London, England, United Kingdom

Babak Mostaghaci, Brigitta Loretz and Claus-Michael Lehr
Dept. of Drug Delivery (DDEL), Helmholtz-Institute for Pharmaceutical Research, Saarland (HIPS), Helmholtz Centre for Infectious Research (HZI), Saarland University, Saarbruecken, Germany

Babak Mostaghaci
Biomaterials Group, Materials Engineering Department, Isfahan University of Technology, Isfahan, Iran

Arash Hanifi
Tissue Imaging and Spectroscopy Lab, Bioengineering Department, Temple University, Philadelphia, PA, USA

Claus-Michael Lehr
Department of Biopharmaceutics and Pharmaceutical Technology, Saarland University, Saarbruecken, Germany

Tomonori Kamei, Takahiko Aoyama and Yoshiaki Matsumoto
Department of Clinical Pharmacokinetics, School of Pharmacy, Nihon University, Japan

Takahiro Ueno and Noboru Fukuda
Department of Medicine, Division of Nephrology and Endocrinology, Nihon University School of Medicine, Japan

Noboru Fukuda and Hiroki Nagase
Advanced Research Institute for the Science and Humanities, Nihon University, Japan

Hiroki Nagase
Division of Cancer Genetics, Department of Advanced Medical Science, Nihon University School of Medicine, Japan

Federica De Persiis, Carlotta Pucci, Franco Tardani and Camillo La Mesa
Dept. of Chemistry, La Sapienza University, Rome, Italy

Ramon Pons
Institut de Química Avançada de Catalunya, IQAC-CSIC, Spain

Camillo La Mesa
SOFT-INFM-CNR Research Centre, La Sapienza University, Rome, Italy

Carmelo Carlo-Stella, Arianna Giacomini, Silvia L. Locatelli, Cristiana Lavazza and Alessandro M. Gianni
Medical Oncology, Fondazione IRCCS Istituto Nazionale Tumori and University of Milano, Italy